Telehealth: A Multidisciplinary Approach

Editorial Advisor

JOEL J. HEIDELBAUGH

ELSEVIER

1600 John F. Kennedy Boulevard • Suite 1800 • Philadelphia, Pennsylvania, 19103-2899

http://www.theclinics.com

CLINICS COLLECTIONS
ISSN 2352-7986, ISBN-13: 978-0-323-84864-0

Editor: John Vassallo (j.vassallo@elsevier.com)

Clinics Collections (ISSN 2352-7986) is published by Elsevier Inc., 360 Park Avenue South, New York, NY 10010-1710. Business and editorial offices: 1600 John F. Kennedy Boulevard, Suite 1800, Philadelphia, PA 19103-2899. **POSTMASTER:** Send address changes to *Clinics Collections*, Elsevier Health Sciences Division, Subscription Customer Service, 3251 Riverport Lane, Maryland Heights, MO 63043. **Customer Service: Telephone: 1-800-654-2452** (U.S. and Canada); **1-314-447-8871** (outside U.S. and Canada). **Fax: 314-447-8029.** E-mail: **journalscustomerserviceusa@elsevier.com** (for print support); **journalsonlinesupport-usa@elsevier.com** (for online support).

Reprints. For copies of 100 or more of articles in this publication, please contact the Commercial Reprints Department, Elsevier Inc., 360 Park Avenue South, New York, NY 10010-1710. Tel.: 212-633-3874; Fax: 212-633-3820; E-mail: reprints@elsevier.com.

Contributors

EDITOR

JOEL J. HEIDELBAUGH, MD, FAAFP, FACG
Departments of Family Medicine and Urology, University of Michigan Medical School, Ann Arbor, Michigan, USA; Ypsilanti Health Center, Ypsilanti, Michigan, USA

AUTHORS

KIMBERLY PEDDICORD ANDERSON, PhD
Director, Department of Psychology, The Center for Eating Disorders at Sheppard Pratt, Baltimore, Maryland, USA

AMBER B. AMSPOKER, PhD
Assistant Professor, VA HSR&D Center for Innovations in Quality, Effectiveness and Safety, Michael E. DeBakey VA Medical Center, (MEDVAMC 152), Baylor College of Medicine, Houston, Texas, USA

CYNTHIA BAUTISTA, PhD, APRN, FNCS
Associate Professor, Egan School of Nursing and Health Studies, Fairfield University, Fairfield, Connecticut, USA

WILLIAM BENDER, MD, MPH
Assistant Professor of Medicine, Division of Pulmonary, Allergy, Critical Care and Sleep Medicine, Emory University School of Medicine, Atlanta, Georgia, USA

HAYWOOD L. BROWN, MD
Professor of Obstetrics and Gynecology, Associate Dean, Diversity, Morsani College of Medicine, Vice President Institutional Equity, University of South Florida, Tampa, Florida, USA

TIMOTHY G. BUCHMAN, PhD, MD, FACS, FCCP, MCCM
Professor of Surgery, Anesthesiology, and Biomedical Informatics, Emory University School of Medicine, Atlanta, Georgia, USA

JOSIP CAR, MD, PhD, DIC, MSc, FFPH, FRCP (Edin)
Associate Professor of Health Services Outcomes Research, Director, Health Services Outcomes Research Programme, Director, Centre for Population Health Sciences, Principal Investigator, Population Health & Living Laboratory, Centre for Population Health Sciences, Lee Kong Chian School of Medicine, Nanyang Technological University, Singapore, Singapore

LAURA E. CARR, MD
Fellow in Neonatology, Division of Neonatology, Department of Pediatrics, University of Arkansas for Medical Sciences, Little Rock, Arkansas, USA

NG KEE CHONG, MBBS, MMed(Paeds), FAMS (Singapore), FRCPCH (UK), eMBA
Senior Consultant, Medical Innovation & Care Transformation, Division of Medicine, KK Women's & Children's Hospital, Duke-NUS School of Medicine, Singapore, Singapore

WALTER D. CONWELL, MD, MBA
Associate Dean for Equity, Inclusion, and Diversity, Assistant Professor, Department of Clinical Science, Kaiser Permanente Bernard J. Tyson School of Medicine, Pasadena, California, USA

VICTOR CUETO, MD, MS
Division of General Internal Medicine, Department Internal Medicine, Assistant Professor, Rutgers New Jersey Medical School, Newark, New Jersey, USA

GISELLE DAY, MPH
Research Associate, VA South Central Mental Illness Research, Education and Clinical Center (a Virtual Center), VA HSR&D Center for Innovations in Quality, Effectiveness and Safety, Michael E. DeBakey VA Medical Center, (MEDVAMC 152), Houston, Texas, USA

STEPHANIE C. DAY, PhD
Assistant Professor, VA South Central Mental Illness Research, Education and Clinical Center (a Virtual Center), Baylor College of Medicine, Houston, Texas, USA

DIRK F. DE KORNE, PhD, MSc
Duke-NUS School of Medicine, Deputy Director, Medical Innovation & Care Transformation, KK Women's & Children's Hospital, Singapore, Singapore; Adjunct Assistant Professor, Erasmus School of Health Policy and Management, Erasmus University Rotterdam, Rotterdam, Netherlands; Director, Care & Welfare, SVRZ Cares in Zeeland, Middelburg, SVRZ, Middelburg, Netherlands

NATHANIEL DeNICOLA, MD, MSHP
Department of Obstetrics and Gynecology, The George Washington University, Washington, DC, USA

BRADFORD L. FELKER, MD
VA Puget Sound Health Care System, Seattle Division, Department of Psychiatry and Behavioral Sciences, University of Washington, Seattle, Washington, USA

BARRY G. FIELDS, MD, MSEd
Associate Professor of Medicine, Department of Pulmonary, Allergy, Critical Care, and Sleep Medicine, Emory University School of Medicine, Atlanta VA Health Care System, Atlanta, Georgia, USA

TERRI L. FLETCHER, PhD
Investigator, Houston VA HSR&D Center for Innovations in Quality, Effectiveness and Safety, Michael E. DeBakey VA Medical Center (MEDVAMC 152), Assistant Professor, Department of Psychiatry and Behavioral Sciences, Baylor College of Medicine, Investigator, VA South Central Mental Illness Research, Education and Clinical Center (a Virtual Center), Department of Veterans Affairs, Houston, Texas, USA

JENNIFER L. FOGEL, PhD
Division of Endocrinology, Department of Pediatrics, Children's Hospital Los Angeles, Los Angeles, California, USA

PABLO MORENO FRANCO, MD
Division of Transplant Medicine, Department of Critical Care Medicine, Mayo Clinic, Jacksonville, Florida, USA

MARINELLA DeFRE GALEA, MD
Chief, Department of Spinal Cord Injury and Disorder, Director, Amyotrophic Lateral
Sclerosis Program, Co-Director, Multiple Sclerosis Regional Center, The James J. Peters
VA Medical Center, Bronx, New York, USA; Assistant Professor, Department of Physical
Medicine and Rehabilitation, Icahn School of Medicine at Mount Sinai, Assistant
Professor, Columbia University, School of Medicine, New York, New York, USA

SASHIKUMAR GANAPATHY, MB BCh Bao, MRCPCH(UK), MSc
Adjunct Assistant Professor, Emergency Medicine, KK Women's & Children's Hospital,
Duke-NUS School of Medicine, Singapore, Singapore

PRAMOD K. GURU, MBBS, MD
Department of Critical Care Medicine, Mayo Clinic, Jacksonville, Florida, USA

KELSEY HALBERT, MSN, RN, CNL, SCRN, CNRN
Nurse Navigator, Yale New Haven Hospital, New Haven, Connecticut, USA

RICHARD W. HALL, MD
Professor, Neonatology, Division of Neonatology, Department of Pediatrics, University of
Arkansas for Medical Sciences, Little Rock, Arkansas, USA

ASHLEY HELM, MA
Research Associate, VA South Central Mental Illness Research, Education and Clinical
Center (a Virtual Center), VA HSR&D Center for Innovations in Quality, Effectiveness and
Safety, Michael E. DeBakey VA Medical Center, (MEDVAMC 152), Houston, Texas, USA

CHERYL A. HIDDLESON, MSN, RN, CENP, CCRN-E
Director, Emory eICU Center, Emory Healthcare Inc., Atlanta, Georgia, USA

WILBUR C. HITT, MD, FACOG, FACOEM
Associate Professor, Department of Obstetrics and Gynecology, Florida International
University, Miami, Florida, USA

JULIANNA HOGAN, PhD
Investigator, Houston VA HSR&D Center for Innovations in Quality, Effectiveness and
Safety, Michael E. DeBakey VA Medical Center (MEDVAMC 152), Assistant Professor,
Department of Psychiatry and Behavioral Sciences, Baylor College of Medicine,
Investigator, VA South Central Mental Illness Research, Education and Clinical Center (a
Virtual Center), Department of Veterans Affairs, Houston, Texas, USA

CALEB HSIEH, MD, MS
Pulmonary, Critical Care and Sleep Medicine, David Geffen School of Medicine at UCLA,
Los Angeles, California, USA

JULIANNA C. HSING, BA
Master of Science Candidate, Department of Epidemiology and Population Health,
Stanford School of Medicine, Stanford, California, USA

SHABANA KHAN, MD
Director of Telepsychiatry, Assistant Professor, Department of Child and Adolescent
Psychiatry, Hassenfeld Children's Hospital at NYU Langone Health, New York, New York,
USA

SIWON LEE, MD, PhD
Resident, Department of Obstetrics and Gynecology, Mount Sinai Medical Center, Miami
Beach, Florida, USA

JAN A. LINDSAY, PhD
Investigator, Houston VA HSR&D Center for Innovations in Quality, Effectiveness and Safety, Michael E. DeBakey VA Medical Center (MEDVAMC152), Associate Professor, Department of Psychiatry and Behavioral Sciences, Baylor College of Medicine, Investigator, VA South Central Mental Illness Research, Education and Clinical Center (a Virtual Center), Department of Veterans Affairs, Houston, Texas, USA

TIFFANY T. LIU
Research Intern, Center for Policy, Outcomes and Prevention, Stanford School of Medicine, Stanford, California, USA

JASMIN MA, BS
Research Assistant, Center for Policy, Outcomes and Prevention, Stanford University School of Medicine, Stanford, California, USA

CALLIE A. MARGIOTTA, BS
Arkansas Children's Research Institute, Little Rock, Arkansas, USA

LINDSEY A. MARTIN, PhD
Assistant Professor, VA HSR&D Center for Innovations in Quality, Effectiveness and Safety, Michael E. DeBakey VA Medical Center, (MEDVAMC 152), Baylor College of Medicine, Houston, Texas, USA

RUSSELL A. McCANN, PhD
Department of Psychiatry and Behavioral Sciences, University of Washington School of Medicine, Seattle, Washington; VA Puget Sound Health Care System, American Lake Division, Lakewood, Washington, USA

MEGHAN M. McGINN, PhD
VA Puget Sound Health Care System, Seattle Division, Department of Psychiatry and Behavioral Sciences, University of Washington School of Medicine, Seattle, Washington, USA

WALTER T. McNICHOLAS, MD, FERS
Department of Respiratory and Sleep Medicine, School of Medicine, University College Dublin, St. Vincent's University Hospital, St. Vincent's Hospital Group, Dublin, Ireland

BURTON N. MELIUS, MBA
Senior Manager, Consulting and Implementation, Southern California Permanente Medical Group, Pasadena, California, USA

FRANSCESCA MIQUEL-VERGES, MD
Associate Professor, Division of Neonatology, Department of Pediatrics, University of Arkansas for Medical Sciences, Little Rock, Arkansas, USA

CLARE NESMITH, MD
Assistant Professor, Division of Neonatology, Department of Pediatrics, University of Arkansas for Medical Sciences, Little Rock, Arkansas, USA

CLIONA O'DONNELL, MB BCh BAO
UCD School of Medicine, Health Sciences, Centre, University College Dublin, Belfield, Dublin, Ireland; Department of Respiratory and Sleep Medicine, St. Vincent's University Hospital, Elm Park, Dublin, Ireland

TAMARA T. PERRY, MD
Department of Pediatrics, University of Arkansas for Medical Sciences, Arkansas
Children's Research Institute, Little Rock, Arkansas, USA

SHAWN PURNELL, MD, MS
Department of Surgery, Houston Methodist Hospital, Houston, Texas, USA

UJJWAL RAMTEKKAR, MD, MBA, MPE
Associate Medical Director, Partners for Kids (ACO), Assistant Professor, Division of Child
and Adolescent Psychiatry, Nationwide Children's Hospital, Ohio State University,
Columbus, Ohio, USA

JENNIFER K. RAYMOND, MD, MCR
Division of Endocrinology, Department of Pediatrics, Children's Hospital Los Angeles,
Associate Professor of Clinical Pediatrics, Keck School of Medicine of the University of
Southern California, Los Angeles, California, USA

TALAYEH REZAYAT, DO, MPH
Pulmonary, Critical Care and Sleep Medicine, David Geffen School of Medicine at UCLA
Los Angeles, California, USA

SASHA M. ROJAS, MS
VA Puget Sound Health Care System, Seattle Division, Seattle, Washington; University of
Arkansas, Fayetteville, Arkansas, USA

MILENA S. ROUSSEV, PhD
VA Puget Sound Health Care System, Seattle Division, Seattle, Washington, USA

SILKE RYAN, MD, PhD
UCD School of Medicine, Health Sciences Centre, University College Dublin, Belfield,
Dublin, Ireland; Department of Respiratory and Sleep Medicine, St. Vincent's University
Hospital, Elm Park, Dublin, Ireland

LEE M. SANDERS, MD, MPH
Division of General Pediatrics, Department of Pediatrics, Associate Professor
of Pediatrics, Division Chief, Stanford School of Medicine, Stanford, California,
USA

DEVANG K. SANGHAVI, MBBS, MD
Department of Critical Care Medicine, Mayo Clinic, Jacksonville, Florida, USA

SHARON SCHUTTE-RODIN, MD, DABSM, FAASM, CBSM
Adjunct Professor of Medicine, University of Pennsylvania Perelman School of Medicine,
Penn Sleep Center, Philadelphia, Pennsylvania, USA

ERIKA M. SHEARER, PhD
VA Puget Sound Health Care System, Seattle, Washington; VA Puget Sound Health Care
System, American Lake Division, Lakewood, Washington, USA

LAURA ELIZABETH SPROCH, PhD
Research Coordinator, Department of Psychology, The Center for Eating Disorders at
Sheppard Pratt, Baltimore, Maryland, USA

MELINDA A. STANLEY, PhD
Professor Emeritus, Baylor College of Medicine, Houston, Texas, USA

TARA VENABLE, MD
Assistant Professor, Division of Neonatology, Department of Pediatrics, University of Arkansas for Medical Sciences, Little Rock, Arkansas, USA

C. JASON WANG, MD, PhD
Director, Center for Policy, Outcomes, and Prevention, Associate Professor of Pediatrics (General Pediatrics), Medicine (Primary Care Outcomes Research), and Health Research and Policy, Co-Chair, Mobile Health and Other New Technologies, Center for Population Health Sciences, Stanford School of Medicine, Stanford, California, USA

PAUL H. WISE, MD, MPH
Richard E. Behrman Professor in Child Health and Society, Professor, Department of Pediatrics, Stanford School of Medicine, Stanford, California, USA

MICHELLE R. ZEIDLER, MD, MS
Pulmonary, Critical Care and Sleep Medicine, David Geffen School of Medicine at UCLA, Los Angeles, California, USA

FEIBI ZHENG, MD, MBA, FACS
Assistant Professor of Surgery, Weill Cornell Medical College, Adjunct Assistant Professor of Surgery, Texas A&M, Assistant Member, Houston Methodist Research Institute, Assistant Director of Surgical Quality and Population Health, Department of Surgery, Houston Methodist Hospital, Houston, Texas, USA

BARRY ZUCKERMAN, MD
Professor and Chair Emeritus, Department of Pediatrics, Boston University School of Medicine, Boston, Massachusetts, USA

Contents

Telehealth and telemedicine services can be a solution for improving accessibility and reducing the cost of health care. Challenges remain in designing, implementing, and sustainably scaling telehealth solutions. Research is lacking on the health impacts and cost-effectiveness of telehealth; more data are needed in the evaluation of telehealth programs, adjusting for potential participant bias and extending the time frame of evaluating impact. In addition, rethinking and addressing the economic incentives and payment for telehealth services, as well as the medical-legal framework for provider competition across geographic regions (and jurisdictions), are needed for greater adoption of telehealth services.

As part of an efficient, continuously improving care delivery system, telehealth can increase patient engagement by creating new or additional ways of communicating with patients' physicians. Telehealth has the potential to increase patient and primary care provider access to specialists, provide specialist support to rural providers, assist with on-going monitoring and support for patients with chronic conditions, and reduce health care expenses by maximizing the use of specialists without the need to duplicate coverage in multiple locations. Current and future physicians will need to develop competencies that will enable them to navigate this new telehealth landscape.

Sleep telemedicine practitioners must ensure their practice complies with all applicable institutional, state, and federal regulations. Providers must be licensed in any state in which they provide care, have undergone credentialing and privileging procedures at outside facilities, and avoid real or perceived conflicts of interest while providing that care. Internet-based prescribing remains limited to certain circumstances. Whether or not a malpractice insurance policy covers telemedicine depends on the insurer, especially if interstate care is provided. All telemedicine programs must protect patient health information. Similarly, bioethical principles of autonomy, beneficence, nonmaleficence, and justice apply to both in-person and telemedicine-based care.

evidence of benefits for communication and counseling, and from remote patient monitoring of chronic conditions. However, the benefits and costs of telehealth programs are highly dependent on the technology used, the medical condition studied, and the health care context.

Telehealth has improved delivery of health care worldwide by improving access to and the quality of health care and by improving the global shortage of health professionals through collaboration and training. Although many telehealth efforts have been reported in adult health care settings, it is important to examine telehealth efforts in the pediatric setting. Children who are most commonly ill and malnourished are often those of underserved populations of the developing world. This article examines current uses of pediatric telehealth in a global setting and discusses key approaches to how telehealth may become successfully integrated and scaled in those settings.

Optimal perinatal regionalization is a proven evidence-based strategy to lower infant mortality. Telemedicine can engage community stakeholders, providers, and patients to facilitate optimal perinatal regionalization leading to lower infant mortality. Rural community caregivers and administrators can participate in forming optimal perinatal guidelines without leaving their community. The visual picture created by telemedicine facilitates better transport decisions; ensuring infants who are transferred to larger centers truly need it while supporting smaller nurseries by providing better consultation services and back transport of patients when appropriate. Telemedicine can also provide educational opportunities to community practices, leading to better evidence-based care.

Pediatric patients with uncontrolled asthma often live in underserved areas such as rural communities where few pediatric asthma specialists exist. There are significant costs associated with acute asthma exacerbations, which are increasingly prevalent in these high-risk populations. Telemedicine is a viable option when addressing barriers in access to care and cost-efficiency. Implementing telemedicine in schools and other local community settings, as well as implementing innovative technology such as smartphone applications, can reduce the burden of asthma; increase patient satisfaction; and, most importantly, improve pediatric asthma outcomes.

especially in the postpartum period for breastfeeding and lactation assistance and for postpartum depression follow-up.

Telepsychiatry is used to deliver care to children and adolescents in a variety of settings. Limited literature exists on telepsychiatry education and training, and the vast majority does not address considerations unique to practicing telepsychiatry with youth. Without relevant education, clinical experience, and exposure to technology, child and adolescent psychiatrists may be resistant to integrating telepsychiatry into their practice. Additional research is needed to assess the current state of telepsychiatry education and training in child and adolescent psychiatry fellowship programs.

There is increasing evidence that the delivery of mental health services via clinical video telehealth (CVT) is an effective means of providing services to individuals with access barriers, such as rurality. However, many providers have concerns about working with individuals at risk for suicide via this modality, and many clinical trials have excluded individuals with suicide risk factors. The present article reviews the literature, professional guidelines, and laws that pertain to the provision of mental health services via CVT with high-risk patients and provides suggestions for adapting existing best-practice recommendations for assessing and managing suicide risk to CVT delivery.

The delivery of teletherapy is an important advancement in clinical care for the treatment of eating disorders (EDs). Specifically, it seems to improve access to highly specialized ED treatment. Research on the application of videoconferencing-based psychotherapy services for EDs is minimal; however, results suggest that this treatment format leads to significant improvements in clinical symptoms and is well accepted by patients. General telemedicine guidelines and administrative and clinical recommendations specific to the treatment of ED patients have been identified. With careful planning and thoughtful application, Internet-based therapy seems to be a valuable resource for practitioners seeking to disseminate specialized ED treatments.

Intensive care unit (ICU) telemedicine is an established entity that has the ability to not only improve the effectiveness, efficiency, and safety of critical care, but to also serve as a tool to combat staffing shortages and resource-limited environments. Several areas for future innovation exist within the field, including the use of advanced practice providers, robust inclusion in medical education, and concurrent application of advanced machine learning. The globalization of critical care services will also likely be predominantly delivered by ICU telemedicine. Limitations faced by the field include technical issues, financial concerns, and organizational elements.

The health care delivery system is complex. New technologies offer new treatment options. The process of quality improvement includes system re-engineering. Telemedicine intensive care is an evolving area of delivery. Its core characteristic is the need for a merger of human and machine activity. Optimal use of quality improvement tools can lead to improved patientcentered outcomes. This article outlines how quality improvement tools can be used to facilitate the patient-centered collaboration with a focus on defining evidence-practice gaps, developing actionable metrics, analyzing the impact of proposed interventions, quantifying resources, prioritizing improvement plans, evaluating results, and diffusing best practices.

Insomnia is a significant public health concern. Cognitive behavioral therapy for insomnia (CBT-i) is considered first-line treatment. The use of telemedicine for CBT-i allows for increased access to providers for patients who are geographically remote as well as to self-directed CBT-i modalities that do not require the involvement of a therapist. Tele-CBT-i modalities include video conferencing with a CBTi therapist in an individual or group setting or use of Web or mobile applicationbased CBT-i modules with varying levels of support from a therapist. Multiple studies and meta-analyses support the efficacy of tele-CBT-i when compared with face-to-face CBT-i and placebo.

Obstructive sleep apnea (OSA) telehealth management may improve initial and chronic care access, time to diagnosis and treatment, between-visit care, e-communications and e-education, workflows, costs, and therapy outcomes. OSA telehealth options may be used to replace or supplement none, some, or all steps in the evaluation, testing, treatments, and management of OSA. All telehealth steps must adhere to OSA guidelines. OSA telehealth may be adapted for continuous positive airway pressure (CPAP) and non-CPAP treatments. E-data collection enhances uses for individual and group analytics, phenotyping, testing and treatment selections, high-risk identification and targeted support, and comparative and multispecialty therapy studies.

Stroke can cause severe disability and death in the adult population. Many stroke patients do not have access to resources required to provide a timely diagnosis and treatment. Telestroke can provide these patients the accurate diagnosis and appropriate treatment they require. Telestroke has been linked to improved functional outcomes in the treatment of acute ischemic strokes. There are several barriers to providing a telestroke service, such as licensure and liability, reimbursement, technology, and financial issues. It is important to recognize these barriers and begin to implement strategies to overcome them. Telestroke use is cost-effective by reducing stroke complications and disabilities.

Telerehabilitation refers to the virtual delivery of rehabilitation services into the patient's home. This methodology has shown to be advantageous when used to enhance or replace conventional therapy to overcome geographic, physical, and cognitive barriers. The exponential growth of technology has led to the development of new applications that enable health care providers to monitor, educate, treat, and support patients in their own environment. Best practices and well-designed Telerehabilitation studies are needed to build and sustain a strong Telerehabilitation system that is integrated in the current health care structure and is costeffective.

New telehealth platforms and interventions have proliferated over the past decade and will be further spurred by the COVID-19 pandemic. Emerging literature examines the efficacy and safety of these interventions. Early pilot studies and trials demonstrate equivalent outcomes of telehealth interventions that seek to replace routine postoperative care in low-risk patients who have undergone low-risk surgeries. Studies are underway to evaluate interventions in higher-risk populations undergoing more complex procedures. Tele-ICU platforms demonstrate promise to provide specialized, high-acuity care to underserved areas and may also be used to augment compliance with evidence-based protocols.

Preface

Articles featured within the *Clinics* series continue to provide physicians, nurse practitioners, physician assistants, and many other health care professionals across all medical disciplines with robust and current information that they immediately incorporate in their practices. For nearly 100 years, the expansive reach of the *Clinics* across all disciplines of medicine remains at the forefront of high-quality medical literature.

This collection of articles dedicated to telehealth is highly relevant to our rapidly changing and adapting practices, as we are currently in the midst of the COVID-19 pandemic. Prior to the pandemic, many practices across a multitude of disciplines had either conceived or began to embrace telehealth to augment communication with patients and meet their needs.

This collection of articles centered on telehealth draws from our vast *Clinics* database to provides multidisciplinary teams with practical clinical advice in this evolving facet of health care. The issue features articles from the *Obstetrics and Gynecology Clinics of North America, Sleep Medicine Clinics, Pediatric Clinics of North America, Critical Care Clinics, Heart Failure Clinics, Dermatologic Clinics, Physical Medicine and Rehabilitation Clinics of North America, Rheumatic Disease Clinics of North America,* and *Surgical Clinics.*

I hope that you find this issue to be informative and provocative, and the material to be groundbreaking and timely. I encourage you to share this issue with your colleagues in the hope that it will promote new perspectives, stimulate thought toward research and innovation, and guide high-quality health care for your patients.

Joel J. Heidelbaugh, MD, FAAFP, FACG
Departments of Family Medicine
and Urology
University of Michigan Medical School
Ann Arbor, MI 48103, USA

Ypsilanti Health Center
200 Arnet, Suite 200
Ypsilanti, MI 48198, USA

E-mail address:
jheidel@umich.edu

Clinics Collections 10 (2021) xvii
https://doi.org/10.1016/j.ccol.2020.12.048
2352-7986/21/© 2020 Published by Elsevier Inc.

Design, Adoption, Implementation, Scalability, and Sustainability of Telehealth Programs

C. Jason Wang, MD, PhD[a],*, Tiffany T. Liu[b,1], Josip Car, MD, PhD[c,d],
Barry Zuckerman, MD[e]

KEYWORDS

- Telehealth • Telemedicine • Design and implementation of telehealth
- Scalability and sustainability • Health care • Health technology

KEY POINTS

- Improving the design and adoption of telehealth may include customization of telehealth services using a human-centered, design thinking process, matching technology to patients' needs, and fixing technological issues such as maintenance of information technology infrastructure, data security and privacy, and interoperability of patient records.
- More robust research on telehealth outcomes that accounts for participant and cost-effectiveness is necessary for its greater adoption.
- The current medical-legal framework for health care delivery is a barrier to scaling telehealth. Policymakers must rethink and address the economic incentives and payment of telehealth services, the medical-legal issues surrounding virtual care, and the effects of increased competition across geographic areas and jurisdictions.

INTRODUCTION

As telehealth programs become prevalent, it is now more urgent and pertinent to ensure its successful integration into the existing health care systems of care. Recently, there has been an increase in consumer technology such as telecommunication tools (eg, Facetime, Skype, WebEx, GoToMeeting, Zoom), as well as a growth

This article originally appeared in *Pediatric Clinics*, Volume 67, Issue 4, August 2020.
[a] Center for Policy, Outcomes, and Prevention, Stanford University School of Medicine, 117 Encina Commons, Stanford, CA 94305, USA; [b] Center for Policy, Outcomes and Prevention, Stanford University School of Medicine, Stanford, CA, USA; [c] Department of Primary Care and Public Health, Imperial College London, London W6 8RP, UK; [d] Centre for Population Health Sciences, Nanyang Technological University, Clinical Sciences Building, 11 Mandalay Road, Singapore 308232, Singapore; [e] Department of Pediatrics, Boston University School of Medicine, 801 Harrison Ave, Boston, MA 02118, USA
[1] Present address: 117 Encina Commons, Stanford, CA 94305.
* Corresponding author. 117 Encina Commons, Stanford, CA 94305.
E-mail address: cjwang1@stanford.edu

Clinics Collections 10 (2021) 1–8
https://doi.org/10.1016/j.ccol.2020.12.001
2352-7986/21/© 2020 Elsevier Inc. All rights reserved.

of app-based online consultation platforms (eg, Babylon Health, MDLIVE, LiveHealth, Express Care Virtual). However, matching patients with appropriate technologies and experience remains a significant challenge; patients and providers face additional difficulties navigating virtual care on top of traditional health care delivery. Moreover, telehealth programs need to overcome the lack of traditional face-to-face interaction that allows dialogue to be mapped against facial features and visual cues.[1] Telehealth practitioners should carefully consider the customer experience and their business model; many industries now have both online and off-line presence, such as the retail industry (see the Zappos example in **Box 1**).[2]

In health care, understanding patients' level of interest (or lack thereof) and reasons for using telehealth technologies is only the first step in understanding the full scope and impact of current telehealth programs. Health systems should also consider many more factors when designing and evaluating telehealth care, including human-technology interaction, social factors, technology infrastructure, privacy and security, and organization of health care systems.

DESIGN AND ADOPTION

As technology advances and users continuously adapt to new forms of technology in telehealth, several challenges arise in the design and adoption of telehealth technology. One of the most fundamental aspects of designing telehealth is understanding the patient experience and customizing telehealth to fit user's needs and wants. The first step to holistically capture the patient experience is through the customization and matching of technology to patients. The design thinking process (empathize, define, ideate, prototype, and test) has been widely used as a strategy to assess the needs and wants of users and to rigorously define and test prototypes to develop interventions.[3–10] The most useful telehealth programs benefit greatly from the design thinking process as researchers engage in many iterations of user feedback and customization to tailor programs to fit patients' tastes as closely as possible. At present, this process is often not incorporated into the telemedicine systems; 1 study found that only 61% of information system projects meet customer requirement specifications,[11] and 63% of projects exceed their estimated budgets because of inadequate initial user analysis.[12] Inadequate use of the design thinking may lead to a waste of resources on creating and adopting telemedicine that users do not want or use. However, the design thinking process is often time consuming and expensive, and can be difficult to scale depending on the diversity of patients needed to give appropriate feedback in different practice settings.

One example of successful usage of design thinking in implementing telemedicine is the ongoing telehealth study by the Veterans Health Administration (VHA). The VHA Care Coordination/Home Telehealth network, established in 2003, allows health

---

Box 1

Online Shoe Shopping

One of the fastest-growing industries now is online shoe shopping. Previously, the existence of this industry seemed unimaginable because people assumed that shoe shopping necessitates trying shoes on in person. Zappos, a shoe-selling platform, transformed the customer shopping experience through an innovative new business model of allowing customers to buy multiple shoes online, trying them on at home, and returning ones that they do not want. Its focus on developing customer loyalty and retaining repeat buyers allowed the company to universalize the concept of online shoe shopping.

care providers to customize patient telehealth over multiple years through a combination of remote patient monitoring devices and analysis of ongoing user data and feedback. This comprehensive telehealth program resulted in a 20% reduction in VHA hospital admissions in 2010, and overall patient satisfaction greater than 86% throughout the study.[13] However, this successful implementation required a massive network of providers, robust funding, and years of technology customization. Such individualized customization may be too slow, expensive, and time consuming to scale up. As more telehealth programs are designed and administered, researchers will need to determine ways to select representative patient groups to test their prototypes and efficiently iterate their programs, while balancing available funding for implementation.

Another important issue to consider in telehealth adoption is the need for expansion and improvement in information technology (IT) infrastructure and data security. Rural areas can uniquely benefit from reduced transportation costs from telehealth, but there is often a lack of the broadband capacity to fully implement and scale telehealth in rural regions.[14] In general, expanding telehealth, especially in rural and small practice settings, is hindered by a limited capacity to accommodate bandwidth-heavy telehealth programs. Furthermore, telehealth requires an extensive care team: effective implementation of telehealth often requires receiving and processing data from various devices, which need to be analyzed and translated into clinical information for physicians and other health care providers. Not only are telehealth programs expensive in the installation, operations and maintenance of technological systems also require the hiring and training of key personnel to navigate telehealth technology and to continuously maintain and update IT systems to ensure compliance. Because medical data must be kept private and secure, technology for telehealth often prioritizes defense against security breaches. Telecommunications contain many nodes during storage and transmission, including the device, Wi-Fi routers, Internet service providers, carriers' cellular towers, and cloud storage farms. Each of these nodes contains hardware and software vulnerable to hacking attacks or leaks; therefore, ensuring data security during storage and transit requires stringent privacy policy and security protocols and personnel vigilance.

In addition to complying with the technical requirements, researchers must also account for how technology alters the nature of the patient-doctor relationship. Telehealth practitioners may need to determine an appropriate so-called Web-side manner to account for the loss of a traditional in-person patient-doctor connection. As virtual care becomes more common, care providers must find strategies to make the patients feel comfortable, heard, and understood; to convey empathy and compassion virtually; and to pick up body language or emotional cues from the patients through a screen.[15,16]

OUTCOMES OF TELEHEALTH: EFFECTIVENESS, COST-EFFECTIVENESS, AND PARTICIPANT BIAS

As telehealth solutions are poised to become substitutes for traditional health care services in many clinical arenas, there is a lack of conclusive evidence on the outcomes of telehealth implementation.[17] In a study by the Deloitte Center for Health Solutions, 53% of respondents who have used virtual care visits said that they did not believe the provider they met was as competent or professional as a doctor in an in-person visit. Only a third of respondents said they thought that they had received all the necessary medical information during their virtual care visit.[18] Quality indicators for telehealth care should ideally be developed with input from experts in various specialties of clinical care, quality of care, information technology, and patient representatives. Moreover, gaps in knowledge on telehealth outcomes should include the impact of telemedicine on different patient groups, and over a longer-term period. At present, many telehealth studies have evaluation periods between 6 and 12 months, which might be too short to truly assess the effectiveness of telehealth.[19]

Because of the relative novelty of telehealth, there are few robust studies on the cost-effectiveness of telehealth compared with traditional health care.[19] One study from The UK Whole System Demonstrator project revealed that, after a 12-month implementation of telehealth, there was a reduction in mortality and hospital admissions, but telemedicine was not cost-effective because it served as an add-on to traditional treatments.[20,21] This study challenges the validity of what people regard as a core benefit of telehealth: its ability to replace traditional health care at a much lower cost. Similar to other newly introduced technologies, telehealth programs must establish appropriateness criteria for use to guard against provider or patient overuse and prevent provider-driven demand or moral hazard from patients that leads to increase in health care costs.

In addition, current telehealth research must overcome research sample bias that does not involve a representative, objective pool of participants. For example, people who join telehealth studies tend to already have a positive view of telemedicine. Those who decline to participate worry about health interference, independence, and privacy,[22] all of which are salient barriers to telehealth implementation. Going forward, randomized controlled trials of telehealth in primary care settings, specialty services, and by medical conditions may be necessary to advance the understanding of telehealth.

TRAINING, SCALABILITY, SUSTAINABILITY, AND INTEGRATION
Business Model

There is limited research into a scalable business model for telehealth, and care providers struggle to develop an economically sustainable reimbursement system for telehealth. At present, most states stipulate private insurers to pay for telehealth, but states vary in their requirements of how much those parties ought to pay. For example, some states require insurers to pay for any and all telehealth services, whereas others, such as New Jersey, only require insurers to pay for telehealth programs if they cost less than comparable in-person services.[23] In addition, reimbursements by health insurance programs such as Medicare are not consistent across various types of telemedicine services, and reimbursement policies have not been standardized among various private payers. Furthermore, payers such as Medicare do not recognize the home as a reimbursable originating site of care,[24] except for remote physiologic monitoring.[25] Medicare reimbursement is mostly limited to specific institutions, nonmetropolitan areas, and places with certain current procedural terminology codes.[26]

However, in places with capitated reimbursement, such as the US Veterans Affairs, telehealth programs such as home-based chronic disease management and remote patient monitoring have flourished. Using data from 17,025 patient participants, researchers found a 19% reduction in hospital admissions and a 25% reduction in length of hospital stay through telehealth solutions.[27] It is possible that, in order to overcome barriers to scaling telehealth, new payment and reimbursement systems should be established to align incentives between patients, providers, insurance companies, and other third-parties.

Licensure and Medical-Legal Issues

Another issue hampering wide scalability of telehealth is the licensure and cross-jurisdictional regulations of medical practice. In the United States, most doctors are licensed to practice in their own states,[28] but telehealth can transcend state borders. For certain specialty services with physician shortages, patients cannot reap the benefits of telehealth until health care providers are allowed to offer services to patients outside of their home states, and, in some cases, outside of the country. Regulators should rethink ways to assess eligibility and licensure for telehealth when traditional licensing rules are obsolete in the advent of new technology. They shall also evaluate litigations and other challenges that arise from the medical-legal issues of virtually seeing patients across state borders.

Integrating with Traditional Health Care Services

The emergence of telehealth in the retail space is also worth mentioning, especially with regard to competition within the health care landscape. For example, CVS Health's launch of the MinuteCinic in 2006[29] and Walgreen's 2018 launch of digital health platform Find Care Now signal the expansion of the retail health care market and a shift away from traditional hospital health care.[30] Smaller health care providers may innovate in telehealth to compete with larger health care systems because the value of physical space and infrastructure has depreciated. The inclusion of retail telehealth providers from virtually any geographic location may result in greater competition and erosion of patient loyalty,[31] destabilizing the existing health care system. With the increase in retail telehealth comes new questions about defining ownership of patient-provided data. Many companies may become covered entities under the Health Insurance Portability and Accountability Act (HIPAA), because they now see patients through telemedicine. The lack of clarity regarding the conditions under which personal data become protected health information and the potential legal obligations under existing policies such as HIPAA can impede scalability and sustainability of these platforms if left unaddressed.

Furthermore, integration of telehealth into traditional health care may require challenging adjustments in the current delivery of care. New interorganizational approaches and changes to current health care systems need to be developed because the feasibility and adoption of telehealth services depend on their integration into current organizational practices and workflows,[32] as well as their compatibility with vastly diverse patient populations, physician preferences, and hospital settings.[33,34] One framework to consider is the eHealth-enhanced chronic care model. In this model, physicians involve nurses, pharmacists, or dietitians in coaching the patient through telehealth in between physical hospital visits.[35] This approach combining telehealth with in-person health care can complicate health care delivery, because they require new systems and curriculum for training and management that do not currently exist. Specifically, the lack of proper training and education for medical staff and lack of management support in telehealth impedes implementation of services that incorporate telemedicine into the current health care delivery system.[15,34,36,37] Thus, optimizing care for patients that includes telehealth without detracting from the existing benefits of in-person hospital visits will become an important consideration in the successful scaling of telehealth.

Another barrier to integrating telehealth is the interoperability of patient data; namely, the ability to access, use, and change data across various platforms.[38] The lack of interoperability standards for patient records thereby is an important issue to consider in the integration of telemedicine into health care.[39,40] As people use more diversified telehealth resources instead of 1 central health provider's services, communication and standardization of data across different platforms, service providers, and payer organizations are necessary to protect the integrity of patient data. In a similar vein, the universality of technology invokes the issue of reliability and accuracy, especially for important medical or health information. For example, anyone can make a health app or educational resource that qualifies as telemedicine, but there is currently no system in place to ensure that experts regularly check and verify medically important information. These emergent concerns will define the responsibility and liability of stakeholders, including but not limited to patient users, doctors and nurses, insurance companies, hospitals, and the government regulators.

SUMMARY

Telehealth is a growing health care service with various barriers to successful widespread implementation. To adopt new technologies such as telemedicine, stakeholders often expect strong evidence of potential benefits, which requires longitudinal, comprehensive research. Lack of definitive data on the medical benefits, cost-effectiveness, and cost benefits of telemedicine has been both an economic and social challenge to adoption of telehealth. Improving technological issues such as technology customization and expansion of broadband infrastructure, as well as the reevaluation of the legal processes for handling malpractice claims, privacy and security issues, and data breaches, may be necessary for full adoption of telehealth.

DISCLOSURE

The authors have nothing to disclose.

REFERENCES

1. Rothwell E, Ellington L, Planalp S, Crouch B. Exploring challenges to telehealth communication by specialists in poison information. Qual Health Res 2012; 22(1):67–75.
2. Goldstein S. How Tony Hsieh Transformed Zappos With These 5 Core Values. Inc Mag 2017.
3. Roberts JP, Fisher TR, Trowbridge MJ, Bent C. A design thinking framework for healthcare management and innovation. Healthc (Amst) 2016;4(1):11–4.
4. Eckman M, Gorski I, Mehta K. Leveraging design thinking to build sustainable mobile health systems. J Med Eng Technol 2016;40(7–8):422–30.
5. Beaird G, Geist M, Lewis EJ. Design thinking: Opportunities for application in nursing education. Nurse Educ Today 2018;64:115–8.
6. Velu AV, van Beukering MD, Schaafsma FG, et al. Barriers and facilitators for the use of a medical mobile app to prevent work-related risks in pregnancy: a qualitative analysis. JMIR Res Protoc 2017;6(8):e163.
7. Gorski I, Bram JT, Sutermaster S, Eckman M, Mehta K. Value propositions of mHealth projects. J Med Eng Technol 2016;40(7–8):400–21.
8. Basir M, Ahamed S, Iqbal), Jones C, et al. The preemie prep for parents (p3) mobile app - a new approach to educating expectant parents who are at risk for preterm delivery. Pediatrics 2018;141(1 MeetingAbstract):17.
9. Knight-Agarwal C, Davis DL, Williams L, Davey R, Cox R, Clarke A. Development and pilot testing of the eating4two mobile phone app to monitor gestational weight gain. JMIR mHealth uHealth 2015;3(2):e44.
10. Ledford CJW, Canzona MR, Cafferty LA, Hodge JA. Mobile application as a prenatal education and engagement tool: A randomized controlled pilot. Patient Educ Couns 2016;99(4):578–82.

11. Williams D, Williams D, Kennedy M. Towards a model of decision-making for systems requirements engineering process management. Available at: http://citeseerx.ist. psu.edu/viewdoc/summary?doi=10.1.1.106.5868. Accessed September 23, 2019.

12. Wallach D, Scholz SC. User-centered design: why and how to put users first in software development. In: Maedche A, Botzenhardt A, Neer L, editors. Software usability in small and medium sized enterprises in Germany: an empirical study. Germany: Springer; 2012. p. 11–38. https://doi.org/10.1007/978-3-642-31371-4_2.

13. Broderick A, Codirector MBA. Case studies in telehealth adoption: the Veterans Health Administration: taking home telehealth services to scale nationally. The Commonwealth Fund 2013;4(1657).

14. Schadelbauer R. Anticipating economic returns of rural telehealth. 2017. Available at: www.ntca.org. Accessed February 10, 2020.

15. van Galen LS, Wang CJ, Nanayakkara PWB, Paranjape K, Kramer MHH, Car J. Telehealth requires expansion of physicians' communication competencies training. Med Teach 2019;41(6):714–5.

16. Heath S. Patients interested in telehealth tech, but improvements are key. Patient Engagement Hit. 2018. Available at: https://patientengagementhit.com/news/ patients-interested-in-telehealth-tech-but-improvements-are-key.   Accessed February 10, 2020.

17. Currell R, Urquhart C, Wainwright P, Lewis R. Telemedicine versus face to face patient care: effects on professional practice and health care outcomes. Cochrane Database Syst Rev 2000;(2):CD002098.

18. Abrams K, Korba C. Consumers are on board with virtual health options: Can the health care system deliver? Deloitte Insights. 2018. Available at: https://www2. deloitte.com/content/dam/insights/us/articles/4631_Virtual-consumer-survey/DI_ Virtual-consumer-survey.pdf. Accessed February 10, 2020.

19. Wootton R. Twenty years of telemedicine in chronic disease management–an evidence synthesis. J Telemed Telecare 2012;18(4):211–20.

20. Dinesen B, Nonnecke B, Lindeman D, et al. Personalized telehealth in the future: A global research agenda. J Med Internet Res 2016;18(3). https://doi.org/10. 2196/jmir.5257.

21. Car J, Huckvale K, Hermens H. Telehealth for long term conditions: Latest evidence doesn't warrant full scale roll-out but more careful exploration. BMJ 2012;344(7865). https://doi.org/10.1136/bmj.e4201.

22. Sanders C, Rogers A, Bowen R, et al. Exploring barriers to participation and adoption of telehealth and telecare within the Whole System Demonstrator trial: A qualitative study. BMC Health Serv Res 2012;12(1). https://doi.org/10.1186/ 1472-6963-12-220.

23. Fanburg JD, Walzman JJ. Telehealth and the law: the challenge of reimbursement. Medical Economics 2018;95(20). Available at: https://www. medicaleconomics.com/article/telehealth-and-law-challenge-reimbursement. Accessed February 10, 2020.

24. Org M, Lazur B, Bennett A, King V. Milbank Memorial Fund • Www the Evolving policy Landscape of telehealth services delivered in the home and other Nonclinical settings issue Brief. 2019. Available at: www.milbank.org.

25. Centers for Medicare & Medicaid Services. Document 2019-24086. Office of the Federal Register 2019. Available at: https://www.federalregister.gov/documents/ 2019/11/15/2019-24086/medicare-program-cy-2020-revisions-to-payment-policies-under-the-physician-fee-schedule-and-other.   Accessed   February   10, 2020.

26. Institute of Medicine. Challenges in telehealth. The Role of Telehealth in an Evolving Health Care Environment: Workshop Summary. Washington, DC: The National Academies Press; 2012. p. 17–30.
27. Bartolini E, McNeill N. Getting to value: eleven chronic disease technologies to watch. 2012. Available at: www.nehi.net.
28. Balestra M. Telehealth and legal implications for nurse practitioners. The Journal for Nurse Practitioners 2017;14(1):33–9.
29. Dalen JE. Retail clinics: a shift from episodic acute care to partners in coordinated care. Am J Med 2016;129(2):134–6.
30. Graham J. Walgreens introduces new digital marketplace featuring 17 leading health care providers. Walgreens; 2018. Available at: https://news.walgreens.com/press-releases/general-news/walgreens-introduces-new-digital-marketplace-featuring-17-leading-health-care-providers.htm. Accessed February 10, 2020.
31. Smith A. How telemedicine technology is changing the competitive landscape. Chiron Health. 2016. Available at: https://chironhealth.com/blog/how-telemedicine-technology-is-changing-the-competitive-landscape/2019. Accessed February 10, 2020.
32. King G, Richards H, Godden D. Adoption of telemedicine in Scottish remote and rural general practices: a qualitative study. J Telemed Telecare 2007;13(8):382–6.
33. Vuononvirta T, Timonen M, Keinänen-Kiukaanniemi S, et al. The compatibility of telehealth with health-care delivery. J Telemed Telecare 2011;17(4):190–4.
34. Al-Qirim N. Championing telemedicine adoption and utilization in healthcare organizations in New Zealand. Int J Med Inform 2007;76(1):42–54.
35. Cueto V, Wang C, Sanders L. Impact of a mobile application-based health coaching and behavior change program on participant engagement and weight status of overweight & obese children: a retrospective cohort study. JMIR mHealth uHealth 2019;7(11):e14458.
36. Lewis ER, Thomas CA, Wilson ML, Mbarika VWA. Telemedicine in acute-phase injury management: A review of practice and advancements. Telemed J E Health 2012;18(6):434–45.
37. Stronge AJ, Rogers WA, Fisk AD. Human factors considerations in implementing telemedicine systems to accommodate older adults. J Telemed Telecare 2007;13(1):1–3.
38. What is Interoperability in Healthcare? Healthcare Information and Management Systems Society. Available at: https://www.himss.org/what-interoperability. Accessed February 10, 2020.
39. Porter ME, Teisberg EO. Redefining health care: creating value-based competition on results. Boston: Harvard Business Review Press; 2006.
40. Ackerman MJ, Filart R, Burgess LP, Lee I, Poropatich RK. Developing next-generation telehealth tools and technologies: patients, systems, and data perspectives. Telemed J E Health 2010;16(1):93–5. https://doi.org/10.1089/tmj.2009.0153.

Impact of Telehealth on Health Economics

Burton N. Melius, MBA[a],*, Walter D. Conwell, MD, MBA[b]

KEYWORDS

• Telehealth • Patient engagement • Health economics • Care delivery

KEY POINTS

- As part of an efficient, continuously improving care delivery system, telehealth can increase patient engagement by creating new or additional ways of communicating with patients' physicians.
- Telehealth has the potential to increase patient and primary care provider access to specialists, provide specialist support to rural providers, assist with on-going monitoring and support for patients with chronic conditions, and reduce health care expenses by maximizing the use of specialists without the need to duplicate coverage in multiple locations.
- Current and future physicians will need to develop competencies that will enable them to navigate this new telehealth landscape.

With the recent outbreak of the COVID-19 pandemic, health care organizations were forced to change the way they delivery care quickly. The pandemic caused many previously existing barriers to fall quickly in the need to be able to provide care safely and effectively, while at the same time preserving scare resources for patients in need. The expansion of telehealth services was a solution that could be implemented and/or expanded quickly and that met both of those criteria.

There has been a desire by health care organizations to shift the delivery of health care from higher cost settings to lower cost settings (eg, from the main operating room to ambulatory surgery centers) and to bring care from the hospital to community settings so it is closer to home for patients. Telemedicine is a vehicle that allows care delivery to stay closer to home, whether it is in a rural clinic far from a major metropolitan area or a smaller community hospital that may not have a specialist on site. Telemedicine allows rural clinics or community hospitals to connect with specialists anywhere in the world and receive consultative support and even care oversight by the specialist or a team of specialists.[1,2]

This article originally appeared in *Sleep Medicine Clinics*, Volume 15, Issue 3, September 2020.
[a] Southern California Permanente Medical Group, East Walnut Street, Pasadena, CA 91188, USA; [b] Department of Clinical Science, Kaiser Permanente Bernard J. Tyson School of Medicine, 98 South Los Robles Avenue, Pasadena, CA 91101, USA
* Corresponding author.
E-mail address: Burton.N.Melius@kp.org

Clinics Collections 10 (2021) 9–18
https://doi.org/10.1016/j.ccol.2020.12.002
2352-7986/21/© 2020 Elsevier Inc. All rights reserved.

Moving toward an effective, efficient, and continuously improving health system is an important goal for the US health care system, allowing it to contain costs while providing safe care with high-quality outcomes.[1] In 2018, health care spending in the United States reached $3.6 trillion or $11,172 per person. This figure equates to 17.7% of the gross domestic product[3] (for comparison, in 2017, the United Kingdom spent $3,858, Japan spent $4,169, Canada spent $4755, and France spent $4380; the United States was at $10,246 in 2017 based on data from The World Bank from 2019). Even with this high rate of health care spending per capita, according to a recent data release by the Centers for Disease Control and Prevention, the United States ranked 55th in the world for maternal mortality, which is a sentinel public health indicator.[4]

As part of an efficient, continuously improving care delivery system, telehealth can increase patient engagement by creating new or additional ways of communicating with patients' physicians. In the landmark report by the Institute of Medicine (IOM) titled *Crossing the Quality Chasm: A New health System for the 21st Century*, patient-centeredness was listed as 1 of the 6 aims for health care improvement. Patient-centeredness was defined as "respectful of and responsive to individual patient preferences, needs, and values and ensuring that patient values guide all clinical decisions."[5] In 2012 the IOM followed up with *Best Care at Lower Cost: The Path to Continuously Learning Health Care in America*. In this report, they listed 7 characteristics of an effective, efficient, and continuously improving health system of which one is "engaged, empowered patients."[5] Increased patient engagement is associated with better health outcomes, a better care experience, and lower health care costs.

Families indicate that patients want their providers to take a holistic, rather than a disease-based, approach to their care. They want clinicians to coordinate their care and communicate effectively across care settings. They want tools to help them manage their health conditions. Patients see efforts to engage them in their care as a path toward shared decision making and getting help from their clinicians in better understanding their health conditions. Of the patients surveyed who reported having 1 or more chronic conditions, almost all agreed that their care should be well coordinated, but only half reported that their care actually was coordinated. The question for many health care executives now is how to build a patient-centered health care system and deliver high-quality care in ways that are beneficial for both their patients and their bottom lines.[5]

This article explores areas where telehealth can provide value in the care delivery system, how to assess the value of telemedicine, ways of completing an economic analysis, and the role of telemedicine in medical education.

WHAT VALUE CAN TELEHEALTH PROVIDE

Telehealth has the potential to increase patient and primary care provider access to specialists, provide specialist support to rural providers, assist with on-going monitoring and support for patients with chronic conditions, and reduce health care expenses by maximizing the use of specialists without the need to duplicate coverage in multiple locations. Telemedicine has already been implemented for patients who live remotely, have limited access to specialists, or may have chronic conditions that require regular monitoring. Examples include monitoring care for patients with heart conditions or diabetes through the transmissions of echocardiograms for faster expert diagnosis and the frequent monitoring of patients with diabetes or heart failure via telephone or videoconference. In dermatology and ophthalmology, videoconferencing and image transmission allow long-distance consultations with experts for faster diagnosis and treatment while also avoiding travel costs for patients and families.[2]

Telehealth opens the door to many streams of communication among patients and clinicians and creates opportunities for patients to become engaged in their health care planning. New telehealth capabilities also improve patient engagement. Structured help lines, telemonitoring of physiologic data such as weight and blood pressure, and telecoaching in order to provide patients with structured after-care contact with clinicians can improve patients' decision making, confidence, and satisfaction. Recognizing the transformative potential of patient-engaged care, new methods of organizing and paying for health care tie reimbursement to performance based on measures of patient satisfaction and engagement.[5]

ASSESSING THE ECONOMIC IMPACT OF TELEHEALTH

To understand the true value of telehealth for an organization, it is necessary to understand the value telehealth will bring. This understanding requires some type of economic evaluation where the costs and consequences of telemedicine can be identified, measured, and compared with any alternatives. In the case of telemedicine, the alternatives normally include the conventional system of delivering health care and telemedicine. A comparison would allow a decision to be made on which option represents the best use of organizational resources.[6] This decision is essential because there are typically limited resources that are unable to meet all the needs without driving an organization into debt, so choices must be made as to how limited resources will be allocated.[6] Understanding and applying economic methods in health research is vital to promote the efficiency and sustainability of health care, one of the core goals that telehealth aims to achieve.[7]

As mentioned earlier, economic evaluations provide information about whether health care technologies represent an efficient use of resources by comparing the costs and benefits of one health care technology with another. Because health care budgets are limited, resources should be allocated to technologies where the ratio of incremental costs to incremental benefits lies within a given cost-effectiveness threshold. This ratio (or threshold) represents the society's willingness to pay for an additional unit of health.[8] Given the innovative nature of telehealth interventions and the dynamic nature of technology, conducting an economic analysis in this area should involve the incorporation of societal values and the preferences of users, something that is possible with cost-benefit analysis.[7]

As part of the assessment of the economic value of telemedicine, it is necessary to estimate the economic benefits to a program. To do this, it is helpful to look at it from the client or patient's perspective, the physician or health care provider's perspective, and the perspective of any other stakeholders. From the patient's perspective, there is (1) increased access to health care, (2) faster and potentially more accurate diagnosis and treatment, (3) reduced waiting time, (4) increased medication adherence, (5) an increased ability for self-care, (6) avoided travel expenditures, and (7) decreased risk of job loss or time away from work. The first 4 of these benefits have the additional potential benefit of reduced morbidity and possible avoided mortality.[2,7]

Looking at the benefits from the physician or provider's perspective, there might be (1) avoided office visits, (2) increased medication adherence, (3) easier and increased knowledge transfer among practitioners, (4) increased accuracy and faster diagnosis, (5) increased patient satisfaction, and (6) clinical confirmation (second opinion). These benefits may be a mixed bag for physicians; the patients can access them faster through telehealth but the physicians may lose revenue because of avoided office visits.[2,6]

Other stakeholders may include the hospital, the insurer, pharmaceutical companies, and the employer. As an example, the hospital may see reduced length of stay, avoided readmissions, avoided emergency room visits, and even avoided hospitalizations. These things need to be accounted for in the economic analysis. From the hospital perspective, these may not necessarily be positive things because they may drive down revenue, although they may be offset by increased quality outcomes driven by telehealth consults with distant specialists that ultimately have a positive impact on the reputation and brand of the hospital. Although the reduced hospital stays or admissions may decrease revenue in the short term, the increased recognition of high-quality outcomes could increase revenue in the long term through additional contracts with other insurers. The benefits to other stakeholders are fewer, but, for employers, it may mean less time off needed for workers so there is less of a loss of productivity. There is the possibility of increased or easier access to health care for a special population; for example, prisoners.[2] It is important to consider all stakeholders and ensure an adequate understanding of the benefits of telemedicine from their perspectives.

There are 2 additional points to consider when conducting an economic evaluation. In terms of telemedicine, the technology is changing rapidly. In a 2013 article in the *MIT News* on predicting the progress of technology, research showed that Moore's Law and Wright's Law best predict how technology improves. Moore's Law states that the number of components on a computer chip double every 18 months. Wright's Law states that the rate of improvement increases exponentially over time.[9] The implication of these 2 laws is evident in telemedicine because any lessons and conclusions derived from economic evaluations of telemedicine programs may lose validity in a short period of time because of the rapid and continuous decline in equipment prices caused by continuously improving and changing technology.[2]

The second point to consider when conducting a cost analysis is whether the costs and consequences of interventions and their alternatives can be adapted from one context to another.[1] Although this is not the primary consideration, there is value in considering this, particularly in a larger organization where there may be multiple projects in subsequent years. Being able to generalize results against other analyses allows comparison with other organizations and across settings internally to an organization.[1] Rigorous benefit-cost analyses of telemedicine programs could provide credible and comparative evidence of their economic viability and thus lead to the adoption and/or expansion of the most successful programs. As part of the analysis, it would be important to show that telehealth strategies can help slow the growth of health care spending without compromising access, effectiveness, and safety.[2] Tailoring analysis methods appropriately to the intervention and context is vital to produce findings that can be generalized outside of the research environment.[7]

TYPES OF ECONOMIC EVALUATION

The type of analysis to be used often depends on the business question to be answered. In the case of telemedicine, the question may be whether it is less expensive to insert telemedicine into an existing care pathway, replace an existing process, or introduce a completely new service. If investing in telemedicine costs more and is more effective, the decision maker would need information on how much more beneficial it is for the costs involved.[1] If specific outcome measures show equal or better patient outcomes than usual care, then the next step is to assess the differences in costs using standard costing techniques. However, lower cost is not always the best path of action. In addition, clinical outcomes may be better with a combination of traditional approach and telemedicine, even if that leads to a higher cost. There may be additional components of the economic evaluation that are challenging to place a value on but are important considerations. For example, better quality outcomes may lead to increased market share, potential good will with the community, and peer recognition as a leader in high-quality health care delivery. On the reverse side, this type of recognition may lead to what is known as adverse selection, where sicker patients, or patients with more challenging chronic conditions and complex situations, may choose to use services. These positive and challenging situations need to be accounted for in any economic analysis.

To complicate things further, there are several categories of costs that need to be accounted for. Fixed costs account for things like equipment/technology, office space, and depreciation. Variable costs cover maintenance and repairs, telecommunication costs, administrative support, supplies, training, and wages for staff and technicians. There may even be additional costs such as marketing or travel.[2] From a cost perspective, telehealth interventions have been shown to reduce mortality and hospitalizations for patients with chronic heart disease.[5] Each type of analysis has strengths and weaknesses when it comes to accounting for costs and intangibles such as good will and adverse selection.

Three of the most common economic evaluation methods are cost analysis, cost-effectiveness analysis, and benefit-cost analysis. What follows is a short description of each.[2,6,7]

Cost Analysis

This type of evaluation is the most basic, assessing the costs associated with the service, any potential cost savings, plus any changes in revenue. This type of analysis is typically a comparison of multiple options that cost out different variations of how to deliver the service. The assumption is that the options will all have similar results. This type of evaluation typically does not include an analysis of the options. It may include some aspect of the cost of the outcome; for example, one option may have a longer length of stay in an inpatient setting than another. However, it typically does not include an analysis of the quality of one outcome compared with another.

Cost-Effectiveness Analysis

Cost-effectiveness analysis (CEA) is a more inclusive evaluation in that it considers both costs and outcomes. This type of analysis evaluates both the costs and outcomes of the program and expresses the results as a cost per unit of outcome. Although a CEA evaluation is more comprehensive in that it includes outcomes, it does have a drawback in that it is only able to evaluate a single outcome.

Benefit-Cost Analysis

This is the most comprehensive of the 3 types of cost analysis. The benefit-cost analysis allows the evaluation of options with multiple outcomes. It takes the benefits of the option and quantifies them by placing a monetary value that then can be combined with the costs. This approach allows a more equal comparison with other options to determine whether a program is economically justified and better than alternative uses of the same resources. In addition, the costs and benefits are discounted to account for the present value of the future costs and benefits, which allows for comparison across options that have different periods of time. It allows for the comparison of one option that may start this year with other options that start in different years. The dollars in future years will have been inflated by a specific percentage to account for average inflation, but then discounted back to current value to allow an "apples-with-apples" comparison of options.

Cost-Utility Analysis

The cost-utility analysis is the most comprehensive of the economic evaluation models and is considered the gold standard because it captures the value of the gains in health-related quality of life. Although it is the most comprehensive, it may also be challenging to use because telehealth interventions are frequently intended to provide greater efficiency, convenience, and access for patients and it may be difficult or unrealistic to anticipate a measurable improvement in health-related quality of life. However, it may be reasonable to anticipate that the gains in convenience and access lead to gains in overall quality of life.[7]

It may be valuable to discuss several factors to keep in mind in the evaluation of telehealth programs. First, suitable outcome indicators and measures must be identified, and reliable and valid instruments to measure the socioeconomic benefit of telehealth must be developed and consistently applied. Second, relevant frameworks may need to be developed to capture monetary and nonmonetary measures in addition to any unintended consequences. Third, telehealth programs should be implemented and evaluated in a culturally aware and culturally sensitive manner. In addition, evaluations should include examination of the social, organizational, and policy aspects of telehealth.[10]

It is key to note here that consistency in measures that assess the effectiveness of a treatment modality has important implications in decision making. There are analyses where telemedicine services may be used to replace the tradition face-to-face encounters between patients and health care physicians and providers. In these cases, it may be adequate to consider disease-specific measures to estimate the effectiveness of one modality (face to face) rather than another (telemedicine). The downside to this approach is that the outcomes measures may not be generalizable if the disease-specific measures are different. With that caveat, if specific outcome measures show equal or better patient outcomes than usual care, then the next step is to assess the differences in costs using standard costing techniques.[1]

In most real-life situations, a telehealth solution is rarely a complete substitute for a face-to-face encounter; there is typically some combination of face to face and telemedicine, which requires a thorough understanding of each of the options analyzed in addition to understanding the current care pathway. Understanding the cost and benefits of an analysis is only the beginning of the decision-making process. In projecting whether a telehealth program will be a success or failure, there are additional factors that are beneficial to keep in mind: the reliability of equipment and software plus the level of technical support; political, economic, and/or budgetary issues; whether there is a perceived need for telehealth services; aptitude and ability to train the workforce and turnover levels; level of cooperation between in organizations with multiple entities or that are part of networks.[11]

VALUE OF TELEHEALTH TO THE HEALTH CARE SYSTEM

Telehealth can provide value to the health care system in a variety of ways; however, the cost-effectiveness of telemedicine may depend on many factors, including the service that is being evaluated; whether it is the physician, hospital, or patient's perspective; the type of analysis completed; how the outcomes are quantified; how fast the technology is accepted; and the overall usage or uptake rate of the service.[1,8] In addition, the stakeholders bearing the costs may differ from those experiencing the benefits, which in most cases are patients and employers. It is important to be clear about the viewpoint chosen (provider, patient, society) for the analysis and how this affects the results.[1]

In addition to cost-effectiveness, the success of a program is also something to be considered. Success in telehealth can be taken to reflect the extent to which it makes a "sustained, worthwhile contribution to the operation of health services and the maintenance or improvement of health status."[12] The development of the information superhighway; fiber optic and broadband networks, combined with new methods to digitally compress information; and even the advent of consumer wearables and robotics with audio and visual capabilities all make it possible to provide consultations, real-time interpretation of images, and management of chronic conditions in a way that was not possible just a few years ago.[13]

Telehealth also has the ability to engage patients in their own care and this move toward engaging patients in their own care is not simply the right thing to do, it is quickly becoming the norm amid growing evidence that patient-engaged care is associated with better health outcomes, better care experience for patients, and lower health care costs. Patient-centeredness, the idea that care should be designed around patients' needs, preferences, and circumstances, is a central tenet of health care delivery. Engaged, powerful patients are central to achieving better outcomes at a better value.[5] However, telemedicine evaluations should ensure that the technology is safe and generates as much benefit as conventional means before any decision about implementation is made.[11]

Current and future physicians will need to develop competencies that will enable them to navigate this new telehealth landscape. Efforts within medical education to develop and enhance physician telehealth competency are discussed next.

VALUE OF TELEHEALTH IN MEDICAL EDUCATION

Before the COVID-19 pandemic, the American Medical Association (AMA) and other professional and regulatory bodies recognized that future physicians would need to develop competencies that would enable them to navigate a telehealth landscape. These entities encouraged medical schools across the country to accelerate the work of developing and integrating telehealth into medical school curricula. The rate of integration had remained slow but steady. According to data from the Academy of American Medical Colleges (AAMC), during the 2013 to 2014 academic year only 44% of medical schools reported having incorporated telehealth into their clerkship curricula and 27% into their preclerkship curricula (**Fig. 1**). These numbers had increased to 68% and 44% respectively as of the 2017 to 2018 academic year. The observation that medical schools had found more opportunities to include telehealth into clerkship courses is notable and likely reflects the increasing integration of telehealth into routine clinical practice. The breadth of experiences for clerkship students is also notable and ranged from unplanned exposure to telehealth during patient care to more robust exposure during structured telehealth electives. The rate of incorporation of telehealth education into preclerkship courses had lagged behind that of clerkship courses, though many schools had identified opportunities for growth. Based on 1 survey, 71% of sampled schools have incorporated didactic learning about telehealth, 53% offered real patient telehealth experiences for preclerkship students, 59% had incorporated standardized patient encounters, and 29% had incorporated telehealth exposure into student scholarly projects.[14] Barriers to integration of telehealth in medical school curricula were numerous and reflected barriers to health care integration such as concerns regarding reimbursement, electronic medical

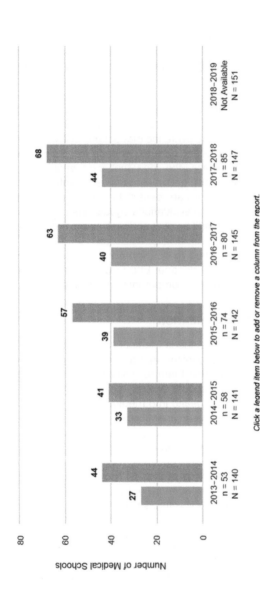

Fig. 1. Number of medical schools including telemedicine in required and elective courses. Survey item: check the topics listed that are included in the curriculum as part of a required course and/or an elective course. Note: data for telemedicine were not collected in 2018 to 2019. *n* indicates the total number of medical schools that included the topic in either a required or an elective course in the given academic year. *N* indicates the total number of medical schools that participated in the survey for the given academic year. (Source: LCME Annual Medical School Questionnaire Part II, 2013-2014 through 2018-2019. Courtesy of the American Association of Medical Colleges, Washington DC; with permission.)

record system capabilities and integration, privacy issues, licensure requirements, and patient satisfaction concerns.[15] At the start of 2020, it was thought that these intransigent issues would continue to create barriers for years to come, but then the COVID-19 pandemic occurred.

The COVID-19 pandemic has been a catalyst for the rapid integration of telehealth into health care delivery systems and medical education. The AAMC and individual schools of medicine are working to develop telehealth-related competency sets and reliable professional activity frameworks. Once developed, these tools will allow medical schools to define telehealth-related learning objectives and ultimately develop more robust learning activities that align with the new telehealth landscape. Some of these activities will occur in virtual patient care settings where much of primary care and subspecialty care is now occurring. For example, within the Kaiser Permanente system, more than 90% of primary care visits and greater than 50% of some subspecialty visits have been converted to virtual visits in response to the pandemic. The distinctive value-based Kaiser Permanente model has allowed for this transition in a rapid, agile, and seamless manner. As the new Kaiser Permanente Bernard J. Tyson School of Medicine prepares to welcome its first class of students, who will begin clinical experiences within their first year, we are working to understand how we can adapt and capitalize on the virtual care transformation to deliver a unique and innovative learner experience. Other medical schools are similarly evaluating their systems to identify new telehealth learning opportunities.

Although the current pandemic has created an unprecedented opportunity to show the value of telehealth to medical education, there are important questions that need to be answered. How will medical students develop the vital clinical and emotional skills needed for future face-to-face clinical interactions? How will student development be assessed toward the telehealth competencies? Are there unforeseen equity, inclusion, and diversity-related implications for learners and patients secondary to the rapid integration of telemedicine into medical education? There are no simple answers to these questions, but the community of medical educators, led by the AAMC, have created spaces for discussion, to share best practices, and to collaborate on medical education research to address these questions.[16] Outcomes related to this collaborative work will help to determine the long-term landscape of telehealth medical education. Regardless of the exact details of that landscape, there is little doubt that medical education will be forever changed by the COVID-19 pandemic.

In response to the COVID-19 pandemic, health care organizations have accelerated their adoption of telehealth, and medical education is adapting to ensure that the next generation of physicians have the skills needed to thrive in this new telehealth environment. These trends may allow the US health care system to contain costs while continuing to provide high-quality care and more equitable health care outcomes.

REFERENCES

1. Bergmo TS. Can economic evaluation in telemedicine be trusted? A systematic review of the literature. Cost Eff Resour Alloc 2009;7(1):1–10.

2. Dávalos ME, French MT, Burdick AE, et al. Economic evaluation of telemedicine: review of the literature and research guidelines for Benefit–Cost analysis. Telemed J E Health 2009;15(10):933–48.

3. CMS historical health care expenditures. 2019. Available at: https://www.cms.gov/Research-Statistics-Data-and-Systems/Statistics-Trends-and-Reports/National HealthExpendData/NationalHealthAccountsHistorical. Accessed May 28, 2020.

4. Belluz J. We finally have a new U.S. maternal mortality estimate. It's still terrible. 2020. Available at: https://www.vox.com/2020/1/30/21113782/pregnancy-deaths-us-maternal-mortality-rate. Accessed May 28, 2020.
5. Cosgrove DM, Fisher M, Gabow P; et al. Ten strategies to lower costs, improve quality, and engage patients: the view from leading health system CEOs. Health Aff 2013;32(2):321–7. Available at: https://search.proquest.com/docview/1347785405.
6. McIntosh E, Cairns J. A framework for the economic evaluation of telemedicine. J Telemed Telecare 1997;3(3):132–9.
7. Snoswell C, Smith AC, Scuffham PA, et al. Economic evaluation strategies in tele-health: obtaining a more holistic valuation of telehealth interventions. J Telemed Telecare 2017;23(9):792–6.
8. Mistry H. Systematic review of studies of the cost effectiveness of telemedicine and telecare. Changes in the economic evidence over twenty years. J Telemed Telecare 2012;18:1–6.
9. Chandler D. Massachusetts institute of technology; how to predict the progress of technology. 2013. Available at: http://news.mit.edu/2013/how-to-predict-the-progress-of-technology-0306. Accessed May 30, 2020.
10. Jennett PA, Scott RE, Hall LA, et al. Policy implications associated with the socio-economic and health system impact of telehealth: a case study from Canada. Telemed J E Health 2004;10(1):77–83.
11. Bergmo TS. Economic evaluation in telemedicine – still room for improvement. J Telemed Telecare 2010;16(5):229–31.
12. Hailey D, Crowe B. A profile of success and failure in telehealth – evidence and opinion from the successes and failures in telehealth conferences. J Telemed Telecare 2003;9(2_suppl):22–4.
13. Pelletier-Fleury N, Lanoé J, Philippe C, et al. Economic studies and 'technical' evaluation of telemedicine: the case of telemonitored polysomnography. Health Policy 1999;49(3):179–94.
14. Waseh S, Dicker A. Telemedicine training in undergraduate medical education: mixed methods review. JMIR Med Educ 2019;5(1):e12515.
15. US telemedicine industry benchmark survey. 2017. Available at: https://www.healthlawinformer.com/wp-content/uploads/2017/05/2017- telemed-us-industry-survey.pdf.
16. Resource hub, 2020 Coronavirus (COVID-19) resource hub. 2020. Available at: https://www.aamc.org/coronavirus-covid-19-resource-hub#medicaleducation. Accessed May 13, 2020.

Regulatory, Legal, and Ethical Considerations of Telemedicine

Barry G. Fields, MD, MSEd*

KEYWORDS

- Telemedicine • Interstate licensure compact • Informed consent • Stark law
- Ryan Haight act • Protected health information

KEY POINTS

- Telemedicine practitioners should follow applicable practice regulations at the facility, state, and federal levels.
- Streamlined multistate medical licensing now exists through the Interstate Medical Licensure Compact.
- Practitioners should collaborate with their malpractice insurers to ensure appropriate coverage.
- The same ethical, conflict of interest, and personal health information protection obligations exist for practicing telemedicine as practicing in-person medicine.

INTRODUCTION

Telemedicine has been regulated almost as long as it has existed. Five states had adopted legislation by 1992, a number that grew to 15 states within 3 years. A quarter of a century later, all 50 states now have laws pertaining to telemedicine.[1] Federal statutes and any facility-based regulations are superimposed on that state-based legislation, resulting in a tangle of rules than can frustrate even the most committed sleep telemedicine practitioner.

The purpose of this article is not to stymie the field with lists of regulations, laws, and ethical dilemmas. On the contrary, it is meant to guide telemedicine practitioners and other stakeholders (heath system administrators, practice managers, and so forth) through the broad brushstrokes of these topics while identifying useful resources for more in-depth study (**Box 1**). Even if this article does not provide answers to every applicable question, it should aid these individuals in learning which questions to ask.

Much of the article can be summarized in 3 words: know your state. Or, more precisely, know your state's rules (distant site) and the rules pertaining to the states in

This article originally appeared in Sleep Medicine Clinics, Volume 15, Issue 3, September 2020. Department of Pulmonary, Allergy, Critical Care, and Sleep Medicine, Emory University School of Medicine, Atlanta VA Health Care System, Atlanta, GA, USA
* Atlanta VA Sleep Medicine Center, 250 North Arcadia Avenue, Decatur, GA 30030.
E-mail address: barry.fields@emory.edu

> **Box 1**
> **Major legal and regulatory considerations**
>
> - Informed consent
> - Licensing
> - Clinical privileges and credentials
> - Internet prescribing
> - Conflicts of interest
> - Malpractice insurance
> - Protected health information

which your patients reside (originating sites). States have instituted different regulations regarding practices before, during, and after clinic encounters. For instance, some states require patients to complete a written informed consent form before telemedicine visits can begin. Others require an in-person visit be performed before engaging in telemedicine-based follow-up. Learning these details about the states in which care is provided is essential; disobeying telemedicine regulations can have professional and legal consequence for both providers and their workplaces, as the following case study illustrates.

A CASE STUDY: HAGESETH V. SUPERIOR COURT

In 2005, a California resident attempted to purchase fluoxetine online for his ongoing moderate depression. The Web site operators, based outside the United States, forwarded his request and associated questionnaires to Colorado psychiatrist Dr Christian Hageseth. Dr Hageseth neither conducted a face-to-face evaluation of the patient nor was licensed to practice medicine in California. After reviewing the questionnaire information, Dr Hageseth issued an online prescription for the medication. A Mississippi pharmacy filled the prescription and sent it to the patient. Several weeks later, the patient completed suicide. Postmortem bloodwork revealed detectable fluoxetine levels. The San Mateo County District Attorney charged Dr Hageseth with practicing medicine in California without a license. He challenged the charges, claiming that the court lacked jurisdiction because his prescribing behavior took place outside of California. However, the California Court of Appeals ruled against this challenge and Dr Hageseth pled guilty. He was sentenced to 9 months in prison.[2]

Although *Hageseth v. Superior Court* involves a particular form of telemedicine (Internet-based prescribing), it raises many questions that are applicable to other forms of telemedicine as well:

1. Should a patient provide informed consent before beginning telemedicine-based treatment, absolving the prescriber of all or most potential harms that could arise?
2. Can a provider licensed in one state treat a patient located in another state?
3. Are providers allowed to order medication over the Internet (controlled substance or not) for patients they have never evaluated beyond questionnaires?
4. Must providers have the same privileges at a health care facility–based originating site as they would if physically providing care there?
5. What conflict of interest regulations apply?
6. Does medical malpractice insurance cover telemedicine?
7. What personal health information (PHI) regulations should be considered?

Each of these topics is reviewed here, followed by a discussion of ethical standards as they pertain to sleep telemedicine, such as: what are the ethical duties of prescribers who have never physically met, or even interacted, with their patients?

INFORMED CONSENT

Informed consent requirements vary by state; there is no federal policy. Some states require a written acknowledgment form completed and signed by the patient, whereas other states have no such requirements. As noted in the Ethics section later, informed consent is an important part of telemedicine initiation whether documentation to that effect is required or not. The Federation of State Medical Boards (FSMB) suggests the following elements be included in informed consent:[3]

- Documentation of the patient, provider, and credentials
- Type of telemedicine being used (face to face, online prescribing, and so forth)
- Recognition that the practitioner may decide whether managing a particular condition is appropriate via telemedicine
- Security measures taken to protect PHI, and potential privacy risks
- Clause holding providers harmless for information loss caused by technical failure
- Requirement for patient consent to forward PHI to a third party

Of course, these are only suggestions for states and their providers. Individual telemedicine practitioners may wish to develop their own informed consent forms in conjunction with legal counsel not only to enhance patient disclosure processes but also to reduce potential legal exposure should negative outcomes arise. *Hageseth v. Superior Court* reveals a potential vulnerability when no such documentation of risk acknowledgment exists. Among other deficiencies, Dr Hageseth had no record of patient consent to his method of care.

LICENSING

In general, practitioners must be licensed in the states in which their originating site patients reside. Licensing requirements vary significantly by state; knowing both originating state and distant state rules before implementing a telemedicine program is essential. Detailed information is available through the National Telehealth Policy Resource Center, a component of the Center for Connected Health Policy (CCHP): https://www.cchpca.org/about/projects/national-telehealth-policy-resource-center.

The CCHP notes that 9 states issue special licenses or certificates allowing out-of-state licensed practitioners to practice telemedicine with patients in their states: Alabama, Louisiana, Maine, Minnesota, New Mexico, Ohio, Oregon, Tennessee, and Texas. State-specific rules apply regarding what constitutes telemedicine, and whether these practitioners are then prohibited from opening brick-and-mortar practices in the state.[2]

Federal legislation easing interstate licensing restrictions has slowly materialized with the advent of the Interstate Medical Licensure Compact (IMLC), developed by FSMB. Twenty-nine states, the District of Columbia, and Guam are now part of the IMLC, with more states joining annually. Although a license obtained through the IMLC costs physicians more than licenses obtained conventionally (standard state licensing fee plus FSMB fee), significant time and effort is saved because a single online application may be used to apply for licensure in multiple states. There are specific physician qualifications to participate, including maintaining unrestricted licensure in the state of principle licensure, remaining board certified in the specialty of practice, and having no history of disciplinary actions against the license. The FSMB outlines additional qualifications on their Web site: www.fsmb.org. Consulting the IMLC Web site in the context of our case study shows that Dr Hageseth would still be prohibited from treating California patients through telemedicine unless he obtained a California medical license through traditional methods; although Colorado is part of the IMLC, California is not.

Like many other specialties, sleep medicine is becoming more focused on a team-based model of care.[4] Therefore, licensing concerns are not only limited to physicians and advanced care providers (ACPs; physician assistants and nurse practitioners) but also to nurses and polysomnogram (PSG) technicians. Nurses must hold licenses in both the state in which they reside and the state in which the patient is located. Similar to the IMLC, a nursing licensure compact now exists among 25 states. Interstate PSG technician licensing is more variable; individual state policy should be consulted. For instance, some medical boards (eg, Idaho, Tennessee, New York, and California) have specific technician licensing requirements.[5] In addition, nurses and technicians must consider scope of practice when conducting telemedicine visits. Like ACPs, their allowable scope can differ among states. In sum, sleep nurses and technicians should ensure that they are both (1) licensed in the state where the patient is located (if applicable for technicians) and (2) practicing within the scope of practice regulations in that state. In another nuance, nurses may only take orders from physicians or ACPs licensed in the patient's state; orders from providers unlicensed in that state are invalid.[6]

CLINICAL PRIVILEGES AND CREDENTIALS

Like traditional care providers, telemedicine providers must obtain treatment privileges and be credentialed at any health care facility in which they practice. This requirement can lead to substantial administrative burden on both the provider and the facility. However, facilitated processes do exist for federally defined Critical Access Hospitals. Congress created this designation in 1997 in response to many rural hospitals closing in the late 1980s and early 1990s. Therefore, part of the federal government's goal is to stabilize the number of practitioners available to provide care within them; telemedicine-based care is a vital part of this strategy. In 2011, Centers for Medicare and Medicaid Services (CMS) decreased the burden on both distant-site providers and Critical Access Hospitals (originating sites) by allowing providers' distant-site credentials to be accepted at originating sites. This credentialing by proxy option is available to hospitals meeting specific criteria:[7]

- Written agreement between originating and distant site
- Distant site is a Medicare-participating hospital or telemedicine entity
- Telemedicine provider is privileged at distant-site hospital, with those privileges provided to originating site
- Telemedicine provider holds a license in originating site's state
- Originating site hospital reviews provider's performance and provides this information to distant-site hospital
- Originating site hospital informs distant-site hospital of all adverse events and complaints related to the telemedicine provider

Therefore, sleep providers wishing to conduct telemedicine visits to a Critical Access Hospital need not repeat the credentialing process at that facility as long as they have completed it at a distant site. If that Critical Access Hospital is located in a state in which the provider is licensed, the process (from a legal and regulatory standpoint) is even more straightforward.

INTERNET PRESCRIBING

As telemedicine has grown, so have concerns about practitioners' prescribing controlled substances for patients whom they have never physically seen or examined. States vary in their Internet-based prescribing regulations, especially when the prescriber resides out of state. Any policies from both the medical and pharmacy boards should be reviewed before implementing a telemedicine program in any state in which the care occurs.

Like several areas discussed, federal law overlays state policy. The Ryan Haight On-line Pharmacy Consumer Protection Act of 2008 regulates this area. The act, designed to prevent illegal distribution and dispensing of controlled substances via the Internet, added new provisions to the already-established Controlled Substances Act. Its overall message is that no controlled substance "may be delivered, distributed, or dispensed by means of the Internet without a valid prescription."[8] A key part of the "valid prescription" definition is that the prescriber, or a covering prescriber, must perform at least 1 in-person medical evaluation of the patient.[8]

Although the act recognizes the practice of telemedicine as an exception to this rule, it stops short of delineating a special registration pathway that would allow telemedicine practitioners to prescribe through the Internet without in-person evaluation. The act states: "The Attorney General may issue to a practitioner a special registration to engage in the practice of telemedicine."[8] Although this special registration process was never enacted, changes are afoot. Substance Use-Disorder Prevention that Promotes Opiate Recover and Treatment (SUPPORT) for Patients and Communities Act of 2018 set a 10/24/19 deadline for the Attorney General to activate that provision.

As of this writing, there is no finalized, public guidance in response to that deadline. However, it is anticipated that telemedicine practitioners will soon learn of a specific registration process that will allow them to comply with Drug Enforcement Agency (DEA) regulations and the Ryan Haight Act while still performing telemedicine without in-person examination requirements.

CONFLICTS OF INTEREST

Sleep telemedicine providers must adhere to the same federal standards regarding real or perceived conflicts of interest as they would as in-person sleep medicine providers. These situations include providing or accepting goods or services simply to encourage referrals (anti-kickback laws). For instance, if a distant-site provider purchases telemedicine equipment for a Critical Access Hospital with hopes of establishing it as an originating site, that action could be viewed as a form of inducement. If such behavior results in remuneration to the offender under a federal health care program, it is an Anti-Kickback Statute–associated felony punishable by steep fines and/or imprisonment.[5]

Another potential conflict of interest occurs when telemedicine providers leverage their programs to increase business traffic to their own business ventures. The federal self-referral law, or Stark Law, applies to every practitioner whether care is provided through telemedicine or in-person methods. For instance, the Stark Law prohibits providers from billing Medicare if selling patients durable medical equipment from a company in which they have a financial stake. Sleep testing is outside of the Stark Law and, therefore, a sleep provider ordering testing in a self-owned sleep laboratory is permissible as long as the laboratory is not performed in a hospital (and, even then, it may be allowed in some situations). Stark Law does not apply if nonfederal reimbursement is sought for goods and services.

In addition to federal rules addressing conflicts of interest, many states possess their own legislation regarding kickbacks, self-referrals, and the like. Sleep telemedicine providers should familiarize themselves with applicable laws at all originating sites; it is these rules against which their conduct will be judged if seeking federally sourced reimbursement.

MALPRACTICE INSURANCE

This topic, more than any other, is most heavily dependent on a practitioner's specific situation. Before implementing any telemedicine program, liability exposure should be mitigated. There are 2 primary questions to consider. Does the malpractice policy cover (1) telemedicine and (2) care provided outside of the states in which the clinician currently practices? Telemedicine-related claim coverage should be stipulated explicitly in the policy documents. Similarly, policies must indicate the jurisdictions in which claims are covered; practitioners may find that although *intrastate* telemedicine may be within their policy's coverage, *interstate* telemedicine is not. These malpractice insurance considerations extend beyond practitioners (physicians, ACPs) to other sleep medicine teammates as well, such as nurses.[6]

PROTECTED HEALTH INFORMATION

Providers' approach to PHI during telemedicine should be the same as it is for in-person visits. Health Insurance Portability and Accountability Act (HIPAA) requirements must be followed in addition to any state, local, or institutional/organizational standards. Software used should be patched with the latest security updates, and the operating system used should be up to date. Notably, PHI is not limited to medical reports. Patients' email addresses, phone numbers, street addresses, and so forth are all in this category and must all be protected. State privacy laws vary in their stringency depending on the technology used; the National Telehealth Policy Resource Center provides more state-specific information: https://www.cchpca.org/about/projects/national-telehealth-policy-resource-center.

Any communication and data storage systems should be encrypted and password protected, with telemedicine practitioners educated on best practices to protect PHI. Inactivity timeout functionality is recommended. Only authorized users should have access to telemedicine systems, with unauthorized access attempts recorded and reviewable.[9] Collaboration with data security experts/computer technicians is generally recommended. Audio and video recording is discouraged given patient consent considerations and susceptibility to hacking.[6]

Sleep telemedicine is unique in its significant reliance on store-and-forward telemedicine technology in patient assessment and decision making. Protected access to previous sleep testing is often required, with any data from that testing transferred directly into the secure patient records. Providers must use positive airway pressure (PAP) data collection platforms offering cybersecurity protection of patient data on their Web site. These sites are restricted either to a practice group or an individual provider (eg, Airview and EncoreAnywhere).

ETHICS

Like any emerging technology, telemedicine-related hardware and software come with no ethical dilemmas in themselves. It is how this technology is used that can create ethical conundrums. The American Medical Association (AMA) outlines ethical obligations between a patient and provider along a continuum reflecting the type of telemedicine used (levels of accountability).[10] At 1 end of this continuum are Web sites providing only indirect interaction between a patient and provider. Although the medical professional is responsible for the general accuracy of content presented, there is no direct responsibility and little accountability for how readers will use that information. Web sites guiding patients through the steps of insomnia treatment are good examples. Further along the continuum are non–real-time platforms for patients' sleep study data, so-called asynchronous or store-and-forward telemedicine. In this scenario, the distant-site provider is responsible for making an accurate diagnosis that will guide the patient's care. However, it could be another provider who makes treatment decisions based on those findings. Both the interpreting and treating providers share responsibility for keeping with in-person standards (confidentiality, adequate training to perform the task, and so forth).[10]

When telemedicine and treatment initiation are provided by the same person (as in *Hageseth v. Superior Court*), more ethical dilemmas arise. The following ethical discussion focuses on provider-patient interactions at the most interactive end of the telemedicine spectrum: real-time, synchronous, clinical video telehealth (CVT). Four widely accepted principles of medical ethics should be respected in developing and sustaining any sleep CVT program:[11]

1. Autonomy: patients' right to make decisions about their medical care
2. Beneficence: a provider's duty to benefit the patient in all situations
3. Nonmaleficence: a provider's duty to harm neither the patient nor society during the care of that patient
4. Justice: a provider's duty to ensure fairness in medical decisions, implying equal distribution of scarce resources and new treatments, and upholding applicable laws and legislation

Autonomy

If a sleep medicine patient's autonomy in decision making is to be supported, the patient needs as much information as possible about both the care recommended and the manner in which it is provided (ie, telemedicine vs in-person care). Respecting this principle begins when the patient is first referred to the sleep clinic. If both telemedicine and in-person care options exist, and the condition is likely equally well managed through both modalities, then the patient should be made aware of both options. It should not be assumed that a patient would prefer a telemedicine encounter to an in-person evaluation, even if the individual lives far from a sleep center or experiences disability. Conversely, it should not be assumed that a local patient free from disability would be best served by in-person care. In either case, patients should receive information about both treatment formats at the time of scheduling without an opt-in or opt-out bias guiding the discussion. Once both options are fully presented, patients can then make a more informed decision about how they wish to receive their care.

This decision-making process incorporates several assumptions. First, because it is typically scheduling staff who initiate communication with patients, it behooves practitioners and practice managers to ensure these individuals are themselves informed enough about telemedicine to educate patients effectively. Supporting patients' autonomy is heavily dependent on accurate information sharing at this point of initial contact; withholding information either voluntarily or unwittingly undermines these efforts. Second, the decision-making process described assumes that practitioners are just as able to treat one patient through telemedicine as any other. This situation is not always the case. As described in relation to licensing, practitioners may not have the licensing and credentials to treat a patient if the visit originates from another state;

legal considerations sometimes preclude patient choice. Third, telemedicine can be difficult to explain over the phone even for the most experienced scheduling personnel and savviest of patients. Nuances, including audio quality, telemedicine presenter interaction, and loss of physical practitioner-patient touch, may not be fully appreciated until the patient arrives for the first telemedicine visit. Autonomy must then be supported if a patient wishes to reverse an earlier decision and pursue in-person care; it should be made explicit to the patient that initiating telemedicine does not preclude future in-person visits.

Respecting patients' autonomy goes beyond choices in health care setting. Sleep telemedicine practitioners must ensure patient privacy to the same extent they would during in-person visits. It should not be assumed that information gleaned from patient encounters (verbal information, sleep testing results, PAP data) may be shared with any other entity unless specified by the patient. Other individuals in the room with the patient at the originating site should be identified, and providers should ask patients explicitly if they will allow others to remain in the room throughout the interview no matter what material is discussed. Similarly, providers at the distant site should identify anyone else in the room with them, including trainees, nurses, or administrative staff. A patient's autonomy is eroded if anyone, on either side of the interaction, has access to the PHI without the patient's knowledge and permission.

Beneficence

Once patients choose to participate in a telemedicine-based treatment pathway, providers and associated personnel must uphold the highest standards of care during their sleep medicine journeys. Part of that obligation comes through education. It is not feasible to assume that clinicians can transition seamlessly from in-person patient care to telemedicine-based care without training, both didactic and experiential. Although multiple specialties have recognized this need and committed themselves to formalizing telemedicine education (dermatology, emergency medicine, neurology), sleep medicine has lagged behind. Recent research shows that most physicians without telemedicine experience are uncomfortable evaluating new patients (75%) and making diagnosis and treatment decisions through telemedicine (95%).[11] However, studies with providers having more telemedicine experience reveal more positive attitudes toward the modality. Providers think that telemedicine's impact on patient-provider interactions is neutral to, or even more positive than, in-person visits.[12,13]

Beyond an initial visit, sleep telemedicine providers should use patient satisfaction and quality improvement monitoring to ensure the principle of beneficence remains upheld. In 2015, the American Academy of Sleep Medicine (AASM) introduced a series of quality measures for adult obstructive sleep apnea (OSA),[14] pediatric OSA,[15] narcolepsy,[16] restless legs syndrome (RLS),[17] and insomnia.[18] Although designed to be measured and tracked in more traditional, in-person environments, every quality measure may also be adapted for the telemedicine clinic. For instance, the same RLS symptom severity questionnaires used in an in-person clinic may also be used for telemedicine; questionnaires can be located at an originating clinic for center-to-center (C2C) telemedicine or emailed to a patient for center-to-home (C2H) telemedicine. The responses can then be transmitted to the distant site using encrypted systems with the patient's permission. In the OSA realm, most PAP machines have wireless data download capability. Treatment adherence and effectiveness can be reviewed via the Internet with a patient using screen-share technology. Therefore, by subtle adaptations to in-person clinic practice, telemedicine in no way precludes practitioners from ensuring beneficence for their patients while meeting AASM quality measure goals.

Nonmaleficence

Although telemedicine has been used to decrease travel burden on patients, the modality can also have unintended negative effects. The principle of nonmaleficence addresses this issue. Fear can be a significant issue among patients and families even if they initially agree to partake in the technology. As alluded to earlier, telemedicine-naive patients may relish the prospect of staying home or close to home for their sleep medicine care. However, considering the full implications of the visit as it draws nearer can be unsettling. Unfamiliar technology coupled with an unknown medical provider far away can prove stressful, even overwhelming.[11] Providers and other staff members should remain sensitive to these concerns and how they evolve over time. Patients may be calmed to learn that telemedicine is simply a tool to provide standard medical care, staff will be available to assist with the technology (especially for C2C visits), and patients may choose to switch to in-person care at any time. These techniques can decrease the unintended burden on patients often already encumbered by other issues and concerns.

In addition to these important but well-intentioned challenges to the principle of nonmaleficence, more malignant threats exist. Telemedicine-associated equipment can be expensive. Therefore, practitioners must use it for many patients to recuperate the cost and obtain a profit. A conflict of interest can then arise when patients who might otherwise have been offered in-person care are scheduled for telemedicine-based care, regardless of their wishes (diminishing their autonomy), medical complexity, and providers' experience with the technology. As one bioethicist wrote, "At that moment the technological imperative transforms the healing profession into a healthcare enterprise and our patients become a means to an end."[11] Nevertheless, the same reimbursement restrictions that have slowed sleep telemedicine's growth have also curbed the potential for its misuse. Because practitioners receive little to no additional reimbursement for telemedicine encounters compared with in-person visits, there is less motivation to choose one modality rather than the other (especially once telemedicine technology costs have been recovered). It is yet to be seen how changes in health care reimbursement as a whole may affect how nonmaleficence is maintained.

Justice

Ideally, every patient should have the same access to telemedicine for part or all of their sleep medicine care. However, the same provider shortages that plague the specialty also apply to telemedicine. The AASM estimates there are only about 7500 board-certified sleep specialists to serve more than 350 million Americans. Therefore, there is 1 sleep specialist for about every 43,000 Americans, with most sleep providers concentrated in states such as New York, Florida, Texas, and California.[4] There are current efforts to widen the training pipeline, but real shortages in terms of provider numbers and geography will persist. It is this area where telemedicine has greatest potential to improve treatment equity and justice.

However, there are significant challenges to consider. Socioeconomically disadvantaged Americans face the same limited access to telemedicine care as they would in-person care. Fiscally responsible telemedicine programs rely on adequate reimbursement to sustain them, typically from public payors, private payors, and out-of-pocket from patients. Uninsured or underinsured Americans often lack each of these sources, perpetuating telemedicine inaccessibility. Another factor affecting justice in telemedicine dissemination is geography. Although one benefit of telemedicine is overcoming geographic challenges, rural patients accessing C2C telemedicine often travel long distances to do so. Difficulties accessing reliable transportation, missed work hours, and variable weather conditions are all potential burdens. Although C2H telemedicine can ameliorate some of these issues, it relies on patients possessing feasible equipment (smartphone, tablet, computer) to make the connection. Furthermore, some payors who cover C2C visits do not reimburse for C2H visits. For instance, as of early 2020, Medicare only covered C2H for specific purposes, which do not include sleep medicine. Long term plans to sustain temporary, Covid-19 related coverage benefits for C2H telemedicine are yet to be determined.

Telemedicine program developers must consider each of these factors in designing programs enhancing justice and access equity among all patients served. The US Department of Veterans' Affairs (VA) system has made progress in this regard. Supported by the VA MISSION Act, computer tablets with webcams can be sent to veterans for variable amounts of time. With those devices, any veteran may choose to participate in C2H using the VA-issued hardware. Use outcomes are being tracked, but preliminary data show significant impact among veterans throughout the nation.[19]

SUMMARY

Navigating the regulatory system underlying sleep telemedicine in 2020 requires preparation, commitment, and attention to detail; however, so does navigating the same system for in-person care. Telemedicine is unique in some ways. Prescribers may need to consider multiple states' regulations, and work through nuances such as multistate licensing and credentialing. In other ways, telemedicine is simply another way to practice medicine. Conflict of interest (real or perceived) should be avoided, PHI should be protected, and the highest of ethical standards should be upheld. With that recognition of more similarity than dissimilarity will come improved processes to streamline interstate licensing and credentialing requirements, while loosening online prescribing rules that currently inhibit telemedicine-based care. That progress at federal and state levels will then lead sleep telemedicine to more completely fulfill the promise it has held for more than 2 decades.

DISCLOSURE

The author has nothing to disclose.

REFERENCES

1. Waller M, Stotler C. Telemedicine: a primer. Curr Allergy Asthma Rep 2018; 18(10):54.
2. Becker CD, Dandy K, Gaujean M, et al. Legal perspectives on telemedicine part 1: legal and regulatory issues. Perm J 2019;23:18–293.
3. Federation of State Medical Boards. Model policy for the appropriate use of telemedicine technologies in the practice of medicine 2014. Available at: https://www.fsmb.org/siteassets/advocacy/policies/fsmb_telemedicine_policy.pdf. Accessed January 30, 2019.
4. Watson NF, Rosen IM, Chervin RD, Board of Directors of the American Academy of Sleep Medicine. The past is prologue: the future of sleep medicine. J Clin Sleep Med 2017;13(1):127–35.
5. Venkateshiah SB, Hoque R, Collop N. Legal aspects of sleep medicine in the 21st century. Chest 2018;154(3):691–8.
6. Brous E. Legal considerations in telehealth and telemedicine. Am J Nurs 2016; 116(9):64–7.

7. Center for connected health policy. Available at: https://www.cchpca.org/telehealth-policy/credentialing-and-privileging. Accessed January 30, 2020.
8. Stupak B. H.R.6353 - Ryan Haight online pharmacy consumer protection Act of 2008. 2008. Available at: https://www.congress.gov/bill/110th-congress/house-bill/6353/text. Accessed January 30, 2020.
9. Singh J, Badr MS, Diebert W, et al. American Academy of Sleep Medicine (AASM) position paper for the use of telemedicine for the diagnosis and treatment of sleep disorders. J Clin Sleep Med 2015;11(10):1187–98.
10. Chaet D, Clearfield R, Sabin JE, et al, Council on Ethical and Judicial Affairs American Medical Association. Ethical practice in telehealth and telemedicine. J Gen Intern Med 2017;32(10):1136–40.
11. Fleming DA, Edison KE, Pak H. Telehealth ethics. Telemed J E Health 2009;15(8):797–803.
12. Kobb R, Hoffman N, Lodge R, et al. Enhancing elder chronic care through technology and care coordination: report from a pilot. Telemed J E Health 2003;9(2):189–95.
13. Marcin JP, Ellis J, Mawis R, et al. Using telemedicine to provide pediatric subspecialty care to children with special health care needs in an underserved rural community. Pediatrics 2004;113(1 Pt 1):1–6.
14. Aurora RN, Collop NA, Jacobowitz O, et al. Quality measures for the care of adult patients with obstructive sleep apnea. J Clin Sleep Med 2015;11(3):357–83.
15. Kothare SV, Rosen CL, Lloyd RM, et al. Quality measures for the care of pediatric patients with obstructive sleep apnea. J Clin Sleep Med 2015;11(3):385–404.
16. Krahn LE, Hershner S, Loeding LD, et al. Quality measures for the care of patients with narcolepsy. J Clin Sleep Med 2015;11(3):335.
17. Trotti LM, Goldstein CA, Harrod CG, et al. Quality measures for the care of adult patients with restless legs syndrome. J Clin Sleep Med 2015;11(3):293–310.
18. Edinger JD, Buysse DJ, Deriy L, et al. Quality measures for the care of patients with insomnia. J Clin Sleep Med 2015;11(3):311–34.
19. Zulman DM, Chang ET, Wong A, et al. Effects of intensive primary care on high-need patient experiences: survey findings from a veterans affairs randomized quality improvement trial. J Gen Intern Med 2019;34(Suppl 1):75–81.

The Role of Text Messaging and Telehealth Messaging Apps

Sashikumar Ganapathy, MB BCh Bao, MRCPCH(UK), MSc[a,b],
Dirk F. de Korne, PhD, MSc[b,c,d,e],
Ng Kee Chong, MBBS, MMed(Paeds), FRCPCH, AMS(Singapore)[a,b],
Josip Car, MD, PhD[f,*]

KEYWORDS

- Text-based messaging • Applications • Telehealth • Legal issues • Technology

KEY POINTS

- The rapid advancement of technology experienced worldwide in the recent past continues to leave a significant effect wherever the technology is applied.
- Currently, various telecommunication tools, such as the Internet, email, and videoconferencing, are used in the health care context to exchange information among doctors and patients regarding different health problems, ranging from acute to chronic conditions, such as minor injuries, febrile conditions, weight management, smoking cessation, medication adherence, depression, anxiety, and stress.
- One particular telecommunication tool that is gaining wider popularity is the use of text messaging, whose use comes with low costs, quick delivery, increased safety, and lower intrusiveness compared with telephone calls.

INTRODUCTION

The rapid advancement of technology experienced worldwide in the recent past continues to leave a significant effect wherever the technology is applied. Currently, various telecommunication tools, such as the Internet, email, and videoconferencing, are used in the health care context to exchange information among doctors and

This article originally appeared in Pediatric Clinics, Volume 67, Issue 4, August 2020.
[a] KK Women's & Children's Hospital, 100, Bukit Timah Road 229899 Singapore; [b] Duke-NUS School of Medicine, Singapore, Singapore; [c] Medical Innovation & Care Transformation, KK Women's & Children's Hospital, Singapore, Singapore; [d] Erasmus School of Health Policy and Management, Erasmus University Rotterdam, Rotterdam, Netherlands; [e] Care & Welfare, SVRZ Cares in Zeeland, Middelburg, SVRZ, Koudekerkseweg 143, Middelburg 4335 SM, Netherlands; [f] Centre for Population Health Sciences, Lee Kong Chian School of Medicine, Nanyang Technological University, Singapore, Clinical Sciences Building, 11 Mandalay Road, Singapore 308232, Singapore
* Corresponding author.
E-mail address: josip.car@ntu.edu.sg
Twitter: @dirkdekorne (D.F.K.); @ejosipcar (J.C.)

Clinics Collections 10 (2021) 31–39
https://doi.org/10.1016/j.ccol.2020.12.004
2352-7986/21/© 2020 Elsevier Inc. All rights reserved.

patients regarding different health problems, ranging from acute to chronic conditions, such as minor injuries, febrile conditions, weight management, smoking cessation, medication adherence, depression, anxiety, and stress.[1] Indeed, "(t)he rapid expansion of mobile health (mHealth) programs through text messaging provides an opportunity to improve health knowledge, behaviors, and clinical outcomes, particularly among hard-to-reach populations."[2] Rathbone and Prescott[3] state that "Studies have found that 31% of mobile phone owners use them to access health information; 19% have also installed a mobile app that relates to a current medical condition or to manage their health and well-being." Another study showed that "over 56% of healthcare settings use mHealth to aid clinical practice."[4] One particular telecommunication tool that is, gaining wider popularity is the use of text messaging, whose use comes with low costs, quick delivery, increased safety, and lower intrusiveness compared with telephone calls.[5]

TEXT MESSAGING IN TELEHEALTH

Currently, text messaging is being used in telemedicine and telehealth where patients and doctors use their different electronic gadgets, such as personal computers, tablets, or mobile phones, to communicate through text-based messaging transmitted as short message services (SMS) over networks of mobile operators or the Internet. This is where mobile and computer applications, such as WhatsApp, WeChat, FaceTime, Messenger, Line, and Viber, among others, come into use. This article examines the role of these and other text messaging apps in telehealth, with an overview on whether these apps meet HIPAA and other considerations.

As is the case with any other set-up, people will use the most efficient, convenient, and cost-effective platform available. The use of text messaging services and apps comes in with what most of their users desire, particularly concerning the cost in terms of money and time, and convenience, the latter arising from the ability of mobile devices to have several communications tools/apps in a single mobile device.[1] Because of their low cost and reliance, text messaging apps are widely used to share information used for various purposes, including administrative, health disease management, education, telepathology, health and behavior change, diagnoses and management, triage, home monitoring, or screening.[6] According to Kamel and colleagues,[7] telemedicine services implemented in urology, where patients perform video visits, have saved patients of Los Angeles VA Hospital considerable costs in the money and time they spent per visit. Used this way, WhatsApp, for instance, has been able to eliminate geographic constraints that are common concerning physical visits to health service providers. The use of WhatsApp and generally other telehealth apps encourage not only seeking initial clinical but also ongoing expert clinical care among health care professionals.[8] Hence, one of the roles of text messaging and messaging apps in telehealth is reducing the cost while improving the convenience of sharing information.

Text messaging and messaging apps also play a key role in strengthening health care systems. Besides enhancing the accessibility of health care services, text messaging and messaging apps can open up access to health care services for patients in remote areas. As health care services get closer to the people, more patients are likely to benefit from emergency referrals, whereas other groups of people, such as community workers, midwives, especially those in remote areas, are able to receive the support that is otherwise limited or absent.[2,9] The use of text messaging and messaging apps also makes it easier for community health workers to collect data remotely.[2]

The host of services and capacities of mobile devices will also benefit users in various ways, such as to support various health interventions, among them health promotion and disease prevention, treatment compliance, health information systems and point-of-care support, data collection and disease surveillance, and emergency medical response.[2] For instance, the messaging services and apps enhance the delivery of information related to health practices and prevention of diseases, thereby promoting healthy behaviors. Besides, patients and providers benefit from common uses of text messaging services and apps, including setting and/or passing reminders for appointments, monitoring dermatologic lesions, remote screening and diagnosis, creation of patient self-reports, storages and forwarding of results, skin self-examination and burns, health behavior reminders concerning the use sunscreen, and monitoring compliance for prevention and treatment.[2,3,6,10] Health professionals, such as doctors and community health workers, also benefit from clinical support that telemedicine is able to offer concerning functions, such as access to real-time data, and creating clinic and hospital records on the outbreak of diseases through monitoring of patient attendances. Concerning this role, some of the text-messaging initiatives that are in use include Text4baby, TXT4Tots, SmokeFreeTXT, QuitNowTXT, Health Alerts On-the-Go, Text Alert Toolkit, and SmokeFree Moms.[2]

Evidence exists on the acceptance, usage, and effectiveness of text messaging programs in telehealth. Studies on the use of SMS reminders show that the use of text messaging help improves patient-medical compliance, and that text messages make a better choice for users based on ease of use, low costs of use, and rapid and automated delivery of messages.[11] According to research by the US Department of Health and Human Services, descriptive studies have provided insights into not only patient preferences for text messaging concerning the receipt of health information and reminders but also retention in health interventions after enrollment,[2] hence the reason text messaging can safely be made a regular practice.

APPLICATIONS IN ADULT CARE

For telehealth in the general (adult) population, messaging apps have been used to stimulate compliance and self-management in patients with chronic issues. Automatic text reminders for ambulatory visits are common, but also reminders for tests and vaccinations.[12,13] Maugalian and colleagues[14] reviewed the use of text messaging in oncology, and described examples of successful text messaging interventions, including addressing behavioral change, attendance to screening and follow-up appointments, adherence to treatment, and assessment of symptoms and quality of life.

Huo and colleagues[15] show how a text message intervention resulted in better glycemic control in patients with diabetes mellitus and coronary heart disease. Having the text messages sent by the patient's family or friends showed an increased effect on health-related lifestyle issues[16,17] and mental health.[18–20] Comparable examples are known from smoking cessation,[21,22] addiction,[23,24] and patients on hemodialysis.[25]

SEXINFO, an innovation developed by the US Agency for Healthcare Research and Quality Health Care Innovations Exchange with the intention of creating awareness about the high rates of spread of gonorrhea in San Francisco, proved effective in the use, sharing, and satisfaction with messages, and a high number of inquiries and referrals.[26] One great aspect of the SEXINFO innovation is that it capitalized on the inseparability concerning access and use of mobile technology to reach the target audience. In Australia, the use of text message interventions to teach youths about sexually transmitted infections showed greater use compared with emails; "the use of text messages related to sexual health suggests that text messaging offers promise for reaching teens about health information, referrals, and testing reminders."[2]

In New York, text messaging interventions used for delivery of immunization reminders among English- and Spanish-speaking expectant women and parents of adolescents showed an improved rate of vaccinations and that the parents of adolescents were uniformly satisfied based on simplicity, brevity, and personalization.[27,28] The same positive result of the interventions showed that pregnant women were interested in the programs concerning encouragement to take vaccines and talk to clinicians during pregnancy.[27] The same can apply for other categories of people given the ever-increasing use of mobile technology across the globe, including patients with human immunodeficiency virus/AIDS for whom evidence shows that reminders are helpful in adherence to medications and hence suppression of viral load.[29]

APPLICATIONS IN PEDIATRIC CARE

As in health care in general, the use of text messaging has also been applied in pediatric care only recently. One of the first studies on text messaging was done in Denmark and indicated that SMS reminders reduced nonattendance at the pediatric outpatient clinic.[30]

In 2012, a systematic review studied the evidence using text messaging as a tool to deliver healthy lifestyle behavior intervention programs in pediatric and adolescent populations.[31] They found 37 relevant articles and concluded the high potential of text messaging–delivered health care behavior interventions that work as a reminder system for chronic disease management in these populations.

In 2013, a Harvard qualitative study using focus groups concluded that "text messaging is a promising medium for supporting and encouraging pediatric obesity-related behavior changes."[32] Similarly, a Johns Hopkins survey indicated that "caregivers of children would be interested in communicating with healthcare providers following an ED visit."[33] In a trauma resilience and recovery program, mental health symptoms postinjury were tracked via a 30-day text messaging program and screening for post-traumatic stress disorder via a questionnaire was completed via telephone screens.[34] Standardized text messages improved the 30-day follow-up for American College of Surgeons National Surgical Quality Improvement Program scores.[35] In pediatric tonsillectomy patients, text messaging was used to improve communication and overall experience.[36] In pediatric asthma, real-time capture of peak flow rate meter readings was done with SMS.[37]

In diabetes care, Stephens and colleagues[38] show how behavioral intervention technologies and artificial intelligence could help in pediatric obesity and prediabetes treatment support. Moreover, encouragement for influenza vaccines was successfully given by text messaging in a pediatric population.[39–41]

The role of text messaging for disease monitoring was also studied in childhood nephrotic syndrome.[42] Text messages soliciting home urine protein results, symptoms, and medication adherence were sent to a caregiver who responded by texting. The system reliably captured number of disease relapses and time-to-remission compared with data collected by conventional visits.

Text messaging may also play an important role in obtaining and using patient-reported outcomes. Mellor and colleagues[43] show that text messaging permits valid assessment of the Pediatric International Knee Documentation Committee and Pediatric Functional Activity Brief Scale scores in adolescents.[43] They conclude that "questionnaire delivery by automated text messaging allows asynchronous response and may increase compliance and reduce the labor cost of collecting PRO's [patient-reported outcomes]."

In a study in patients after neonatal intensive care unit discharge, Flores-Fenlon and colleagues[44] concluded that smartphones and text messaging were associated with higher parent quality-of-life scores and enrollment in early intervention.[44]

USE OF CROSS-PLATFORM MESSAGING APPLICATIONS

Such apps as WhatsApp, WeChat, and Line are ubiquitous cross-platform messaging and voice-over Internet protocol/Internet protocol freeware services.

Currently, WhatsApp Messenger is one of the most widely used mobile apps in telehealth; however, various sources have indicated that this application and likes have serious limitations with regard to privacy and data security. Many attribute the widespread use of WhatsApp Messenger to its extensive capabilities, such as to share high-quality photographs, videos, and voice messages, and to make voice and video calls, videos on top of text-based messages. In addition, WhatsApp Messenger uses an Internet connection that can use a mobile data plan or Wi-Fi, which makes it more affordable than the conventional SMS modality. With quality, reliability, and low cost, WhatsApp Messenger has become one of the most preferred messaging apps among patients and health professionals because the information shared (images and videos) is of sufficient detail as would be needed to make adequate diagnosis and initial treatment, leading to better efficacy compared with other modalities that can serve the same purpose.[6] The WhatsApp Group feature that is part of WhatsApp Messenger is also an excellent platform for text blasting/bulk messaging because it allows sharing information to 256 people at once, or by the use of the app's Broadcast Lists where information can be repeatedly shared to preselected and saved list of recipients, eliminating the need to select the recipients each time.[7] In this case, for instance, a health professional can create a group and add relevant members, after which the professional will instantly share a piece of educational or related information to all members, which is faster than having to share the information to each recipient individually.

Results of research examining the usefulness of WhatsApp in clinical decision-making and patient care showed that the mobile app is a "low-cost and fast technology with the potential of facilitating clinical communications, enhancing learning, and improving patient care while preserving their privacy."[7] When used on patients battling with smoking relapse, WhatsApp provides enhanced discussion and social support, which proved effective in helping the patients reduce relapse to rates of 2 and 6 months as the authors continue to narrate. Additionally, when used among emergency surgery teams in a London hospital, WhatsApp was attributed to a flattened hierarchy that allowed all participants (students, residents, and experienced consultants) to actively and freely contribute to the discussions. These authors also found WhatsApp to be a better platform for case discourses, increasing awareness on patient-related information, improving the efficiency of the handover process, and reducing the duration of ancient morning handover processes among orthopedic residents. These are just a few examples of the situations where the use of WhatsApp in health care has proved beneficial. Various bodies, however, suggest taking serious steps to ensure compliance with data protection laws when introducing text messaging services. To safeguard data privacy and confidentiality, mobile messaging should only take place through a secure health care messaging application, and in Europe the National Health Service has provided detailed instructions for its practice.

In Asia WeChat and Line are the WhatsApp equivalent. In China, WeChat is used to expand human immunodeficiency virus testing by reaching key parts of the population, among them nonheterosexuals who rarely do testing.[45] However, there are considerable security concerns. The population whom the said study targeted were apprehensive about using the platform and participating in the intervention for fear that the information shared through the app would reach their families, which would then have exposed their sexual orientation.

LEGAL IMPLICATIONS

Despite the increasing use and promising potential benefits, the use of text messaging and messaging apps in telemedicine is limited by whether they are compliant with US HIPAA regulations, Europe's General Data Protection Regulation, and Singapore's Personal Data Protection Act, among other bodies. For instance, HIPAA is particular about sharing of protected health information as a text message.[7] HIPAA's security rule includes specific security standards for the disclosure and storage of electronic health information and requires safeguarding of PHI [protected health information]. This means that before a messaging app is used, its security standards must meet some threshold. Besides, texting is shown to have a unique set of risks that without management compromise the privacy and security of the shared information. For example, this could happen if the mobile devices are lost or recycled.[46]

In a study reported in 2014, pediatric hospitalists were surveyed on their use of text messaging. Forty-six percent of the 97 respondents worried privacy laws can be violated by sending/receiving text messages, and 30% reported having protected health information in text messages.[47] However, only 11% reported their institution offered encryption software for text messaging.

In pediatric dermatology, text messaging and cell phone cameras have facilitated curbside consultations and a recent survey indicated that they increase access and promote collegiality; but they are also usually not compensated, consume considerable time, risk liability exposure for providers, and potentially compromise confidentiality.[48]

The information a patient discloses to a physician is confidential and should be treated as such.[40] Hence, before any of these apps are put into wide telemedical use, a thorough evaluation is needed to ensure consistency and compliance with ethical practices. Notably, HIPAA does not bar the use of any mode of communication, including texting, but care should be taken to enhance the safety and privacy of information shared.[8,46] Such apps as WhatsApp Messenger are deploying end-to-end encryption that enhances the safety of information shared, which can make them among the HIPAA-compliant messaging apps. Generally, HIPAA recommends using messaging apps under secure encrypted networks with access and audit controls.[49]

This paper has discussed the role of text messaging and messaging applications including technical and legal issues. The reviews of current examples of text messaging in adult and pediatric practice show uptake has been increasing substantially in the past 3 years, especially to stimulate adherence and self-management in patients with chronic diseases. In pediatric care text messaging has been used for behavior intervention and outcomes tracking. Although applications are promising, especially efficiencies and selected, the potential of nonsynchronic messaging in the formal delivery of care is still in the neonatal phase compared with its grown-up existence in day-to-day modern life.

REFERENCES

1. Shah O, Matlaga B. Emerging technologies in renal stone management, an issue of urologic clinics, EBook. Elsevier Health Sciences; 2019.
2. US Department of Health and Human Services. Health resources and services administration. Using health text messages to improve consumer health

knowledge, behaviors, and outcomes: an environmental scan. Rockville (MD): US Department of Health and Human Services; 2014.
3. Rathbone AL, Prescott J. The use of mobile apps and SMS messaging as physical and mental health interventions: systematic review. J Med Internet Res 2017; 19(8):e295.
4. Franko OI, Tirrell TF. Smartphone app use among medical providers in ACGME training programs. J Med Syst 2012;36(5):3135–9.
5. Kannisto KA, Koivunen MH, Välimäki MA. Use of mobile phone text message reminders in health care services: a narrative literature review. J Med Internet Res 2014;16(10):e222.
6. Morris C, Scott RE, Mars M. Instant messaging in dermatology: a literature review. Stud Health Technol Inform 2018;254:70–6.
7. Kamel Boulos M, Giustini D, Wheeler S. Instagram and WhatsApp in health and healthcare: an overview. Future Internet 2016;8(3):37.
8. Mars M, Scott RE. WhatsApp in clinical practice: a literature. The promise of new technologies in an age of new health challenges. Stud Health Technol Inform 2016;231:82–90.
9. Giordano V, Koch H, Godoy-Santos A, et al. WhatsApp messenger as an adjunctive tool for telemedicine: an overview. Interact J Med Res 2017;6(2):e11.
10. Schilling L, Bennett G, Bull S, et al. Text messaging in healthcare research toolkit. Center for Research in Implementation Science and Prevention (CRISP), University of Colorado School of Medicine; 2013.
11. Schwebel FJ, Larimer ME. Using text message reminders in health care services: a narrative literature review. Internet Interv 2018;13:82–104.
12. Esteban-Vasallo M, Domínguez-Berjón M, García-Riolobos C, et al. Effect of mobile phone text messaging for improving the uptake of influenza vaccination in patients with rare diseases. Vaccine 2019;37(36):5257–64.
13. Lee HY, Lee MH, Sharratt M, et al. Development of a mobile health intervention to promote Papanicolaou tests and human papillomavirus vaccination in an underserved immigrant population: a culturally targeted and individually tailored text messaging approach. JMIR Mhealth Uhealth 2019;7(6):e13256.
14. Mougalian SS, Gross CP, Hall EK. Text messaging in oncology: A review of the landscape. JCO clinical cancer informatics 2018;2:1–9.
15. Huo X, Spatz ES, Ding Q, et al. Design and rationale of the Cardiovascular Health and Text Messaging (CHAT) Study and the CHAT-Diabetes Mellitus (CHAT-DM) Study: two randomised controlled trials of text messaging to improve secondary prevention for coronary heart disease and diabetes. BMJ 2017;7(12):e018302.
16. Haider R, Hyun K, Cheung NW, et al. Effect of lifestyle focused text messaging on risk factor modification in patients with diabetes and coronary heart disease: a sub-analysis of the TEXT ME study. Diabetes Res Clin Pract 2019;153:184–90.
17. Mayberry LS, Bergner EM, Harper KJ, et al. Text messaging to engage friends/family in diabetes self-management support: acceptability and potential to address disparities. J Am Med Inform Assoc 2019;26(10):1099–108.
18. Stevens GJ, Hammond TE, Brownhill S, et al. SMS SOS: a randomized controlled trial to reduce self-harm and suicide attempts using SMS text messaging. BMC Psychiatry 2019;19(1):117.
19. Thomas K, Bendtsen M. Mental health promotion among university students using text messaging: protocol for a randomized controlled trial of a mobile phone–based intervention. JMIR Res Protoc 2019;8(8):e12396.
20. Xu DR, Xiao S, He H, et al. Lay health supporters aided by mobile text messaging to improve adherence, symptoms, and functioning among people with

schizophrenia in a resource-poor community in rural China (LEAN): A randomized controlled trial. PLoS Med 2019;16(4):e1002785.

21. Cartujano-Barrera F, Arana-Chicas E, Ramírez-Mantilla M, et al. "Every day I think about your messages": assessing text messaging engagement among Latino smokers in a mobile cessation program. Patient Prefer Adherence 2019;13:1213.

22. Nolan MB, Warner MA, Jacobs MA, et al. Feasibility of a perioperative text messaging smoking cessation program for surgical patients. Anesth Analg 2019;129(3):e73–6.

23. Bendtsen M. Text messaging interventions for reducing alcohol consumption among harmful and hazardous drinkers: protocol for a systematic review and meta-analysis. JMIR Res Protoc 2019;8(4):e12898.

24. Mastroleo NR, Celio MA, Barnett NP, et al. Feasibility and acceptability of a motivational intervention combined with text messaging for alcohol and sex risk reduction with emergency department patients: a pilot trial. Addict Res Theory 2019;27(2):85–94.

25. Stevenson J, Campbell KL, Brown M, et al. Targeted, structured text messaging to improve dietary and lifestyle behaviours for people on maintenance haemodialysis (KIDNEYTEXT): study protocol for a randomised controlled trial. BMJ Open 2019;9(5):e023545.

26. Levine D, McCright J, Dobkin L, et al. SEXINFO: a sexual health text messaging service for San Francisco youth. Am J Public Health 2008;98(3):393–5.

27. Kharbanda EO, Vargas CY, Castaño PM, et al. Exploring pregnant women's views on influenza vaccination and educational text messages. Prev Med 2011; 52(1):75–7.

28. Stockwell MS, Kharbanda EO, Martinez RA, et al. Text4Health: impact of text message reminder–recalls for pediatric and adolescent immunizations. Am J Public Health 2012;102(2):e15–21.

29. Lauffenburger JC, Choudhry NK. Text messaging and patient engagement in an increasingly mobile world. Circulation 2016;133(6):555–6.

30. Kruse L, Hansen L, Olesen C. Non-attendance at a pediatric outpatient clinic. SMS text messaging improves attendance. Ugeskr Laeger 2009;171(17):1372–5.

31. Militello LK, Kelly SA, Melnyk BM. Systematic review of text-messaging interventions to promote healthy behaviors in pediatric and adolescent populations: implications for clinical practice and research. Worldviews Evidence-Based Nurs 2012;9(2):66–77.

32. Sharifi M, Dryden EM, Horan CM, et al. Leveraging text messaging and mobile technology to support pediatric obesity-related behavior change: a qualitative study using parent focus groups and interviews. J Med Internet Res 2013; 15(12):e272.

33. Dudas RA, Pumilia JN, Crocetti M. Pediatric caregiver attitudes and technologic readiness toward electronic follow-up communication in an urban community emergency department. Telemed J E Health 2013;19(6):493–6.

34. Ridings LE, Anton MT, Winkelmann J, et al. Trauma resilience and recovery program: addressing mental health in pediatric trauma centers. J Pediatr Psychol 2019;44(9):1046–56.

35. Taylor SL, Meyer JM, Munoz-Abraham AS, et al. Standardized text messages improve 30-day patient follow-up for ACS pediatric NSQIP cases. Pediatr Surg Int 2019;35(4):523–7.

36. Newton L, Sulman C. Use of text messaging to improve patient experience and communication with pediatric tonsillectomy patients. Int J Pediatr Otorhinolaryngol 2018;113:213–7.

37. Gahleitner F, Legg J, Holland E, et al. The validity and acceptability of a text-based monitoring system for pediatric asthma studies. Pediatr pulmonology 2016;51(1):5–12.
38. Stephens TN, Joerin A, Rauws M, et al. Feasibility of pediatric obesity and prediabetes treatment support through Tess, the AI behavioral coaching chatbot. Translational behavioral medicine 2019;9(3):440–7.
39. Hofstetter AM, Vargas CY, Camargo S, et al. Impacting delayed pediatric influenza vaccination: a randomized controlled trial of text message reminders. Am J Prev Med 2015;48(4):392–401.
40. Sloand E, VanGraafeiland B, Holm A, et al. Text message quality improvement project for influenza vaccine in a low-resource largely Latino pediatric population. J Healthc Qual 2019;41(6):362–8.
41. Stockwell MS, Kharbanda EO, Martinez RA, et al. Effect of a text messaging intervention on influenza vaccination in an urban, low-income pediatric and adolescent population: a randomized controlled trial. JAMA 2012;307(16):1702–8.
42. Wang C-s, Troost JP, Greenbaum LA, et al. Text messaging for disease monitoring in childhood nephrotic syndrome. Kidney Int Rep 2019;4(8):1066–74.
43. Mellor X, Buczek MJ, Adams AJ, et al. Collection of common knee patient-reported outcome instruments by automated mobile phone text messaging in pediatric sports medicine. J Pediatr Orthop 2020;40(2):e91–5.
44. Flores-Fenlon N, Song AY, Yeh A, et al. Smartphones and text messaging are associated with higher parent quality of life scores and enrollment in early intervention after NICU discharge. Clin Pediatr 2019;58(8):903–11.
45. Zhao Y, Zhu X, Pérez AE, et al. MHealth approach to promote oral HIV self-testing among men who have sex with men in China: a qualitative description. BMC Public Health 2018;18(1):1146.
46. Storck L. Policy statement: texting in health care. On Line J Nurs Inform 2017;21(1).
47. Kuhlmann S, Ahlers-Schmidt CR, Steinberger E. TXT@ WORK: pediatric hospitalists and text messaging. Telemed J E Health 2014;20(7):647–52.
48. Khorsand K, Sidbury R. The shadow clinic: emails, "curbsides," and "quick peeks" in pediatric dermatology. Pediatr Dermatol 2019;36(5):607–10.
49. Drolet BC, Marwaha JS, Hyatt B, et al. Electronic communication of protected health information: privacy, security, and HIPAA compliance. J Hand Surg 2017;42(6):411–6.

Personalized Implementation of Video Telehealth

Jan A. Lindsay, PhD[a,b,c,]*, Stephanie C. Day, PhD[a,c],
Amber B. Amspoker, PhD[b,c], Terri L. Fletcher, PhD[a,b,c],
Julianna Hogan, PhD[a,b,c], Giselle Day, MPH[a,b], Ashley Helm, MA[a,b],
Melinda A. Stanley, PhD[c], Lindsey A. Martin, PhD[b,c]

KEYWORDS

- Telemedicine • Veterans • Mental health • Implementation
- Health services research • Delivery of health care

KEY POINTS

- Implementing video telehealth to home (VTH) within large medical systems relies heavily on a flexible implementation strategy that involves external and internal facilitation.
- Providing mental health treatment via VTH allows patients and providers to overcome many barriers to treatment and provides patients greater choice about when and where they receive their care.
- Implementing a sustainable VTH program should start small by identifying dedicated clinical champions and celebrating early successes.
- Measuring multiple variables to evaluate the breadth and depth of VTH delivery and the implementation strategy can increase impact.

This article originally appeared in *Psychiatric Clinics*, Volume 42, Issue 4, December 2019.
The authors report no financial conflicts of interest.
This work was supported by a grant from the VA Office of Rural Health, Salt Lake City Resource Center and partly supported by the use of facilities and resources of the Houston VA HSR&D Center for Innovations in Quality, Effectiveness and Safety (CIN13-413) and the VA South Central Mental Illness Research, Education and Clinical Center. The opinions expressed are those of the authors and not necessarily those of the Department of Veterans Affairs, the US government, or Baylor College of Medicine.
[a] VA South Central Mental Illness Research, Education and Clinical Center (a virtual center);
[b] Houston VA HSR&D Center for Innovations in Quality, Effectiveness and Safety, Michael E. DeBakey VA Medical Center (MEDVAMC152), 2002 Holcombe Boulevard, Houston, TX 77030, USA; [c] Department of Psychiatry and Behavioral Sciences, Baylor College of Medicine, One Baylor Plaza, Houston, TX 77030, USA
* Corresponding author. Houston VA HSR&D Center for Innovations in Quality, Effectiveness and Safety, Michael E. DeBakey Veterans Affairs Medical Center, (MEDVAMC 152), 2002 Holcombe Blvd., Houston, TX 77030.
E-mail address: Jan.Lindsay2@va.gov

Clinics Collections 10 (2021) 41–52
https://doi.org/10.1016/j.ccol.2020.12.005
2352-7986/21/Published by Elsevier Inc.

INTRODUCTION

Notable logistical, financial, and stigma-related barriers to engaging in and being retained in mental health (MH) care exist. Those who seek MH care often have difficulty accessing specialty or evidence-based treatment and may not receive an adequate dose to address their MH issues.[1,2] Telehealth programs for MH care, specifically, clinical videoconferencing, have not reached their potential in increasing access to care, largely due to system complexities in implementation,[3–5] including technical difficulties for support staff and challenges of integration into clinical workflow.[6] Although patient satisfaction with telehealth programs is high, provider adoption is slow. For example, providers have concerns over the impact of video technology on the provider-patient relationship, logistical (eg, scheduling) issues, and complexities associated with the technology.[6–9] Implementation approaches with concrete steps and guidance are needed to fully leverage telehealth technology for widespread use.

Initially, MH telehealth in the Veterans Health Administration (VHA) was conducted clinic-to-clinic, allowing providers at a large facility to remotely deliver care to patients in another clinic location. However, this approach did not fully address logistical, financial, and transportation barriers, given the patients still had to travel to the community clinic. Video telehealth to home (VTH) is another form of telehealth that enables patients to connect with MH provider directly from home or another convenient, private location of their choice (**Fig. 1**). VTH can increase access to care and retention in MH treatment and is as effective as in-person care.[10]

Developing telehealth programs within a hospital or clinic system has often involved creating silos (ie, providers within a medical center who deliver care only via telehealth) or telehealth centers (ie, providers in a remote/distant location who use telehealth delivery to address gaps or personnel shortages). These models allow providers to become extremely proficient in telehealth delivery of care and overcome provider shortage concerns in underserved areas by allowing providers in one geographic region to provide care to patients in another. However, silo and telehealth center models eliminate the possibility of meeting with patients in person when necessary or when preferred by patients because providers often are in geographically distant locations and/or do not have access to traditional office space.

Integrated models of VTH maximize patient choice by offering the option to meet with providers either in person or virtually, as preferred. When many providers across a clinic or health care system are trained to deliver care via VTH as one aspect of their clinical role, patients and providers can collaboratively determine the mode of delivery (eg, all in-person, all VTH, a combination of in-person and VTH) that is most convenient and clinically appropriate. For example, a patient with transportation or childcare

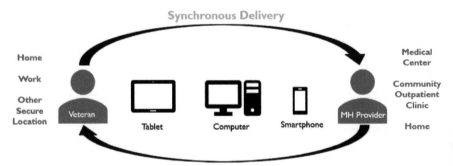

Fig. 1. VA video connect technology.

barriers can request a VTH appointment instead of canceling. Similarly, a provider can ask a patient who is decompensating to come in person to the next appointment.

Despite notable benefits of VTH for patient care and clinical practice and high levels of patient satisfaction,[11–14] VTH utilization in the VHA has not expanded as quickly as expected or desired, demonstrating a need for effective and replicable implementation approaches that increase uptake of VTH among providers and clinics. This article describes a clinical demonstration project for which the authors developed a specific implementation approach, Personalized *I*mplementation for *V*ideo *T*elehealth (PIVOT), to increase adoption of VTH across a large, urban VA Medical Center (VAMC). Development of PIVOT for implementation of VTH was anchored in Implementation Facilitation,[15] a strategy responsive to contextual factors that promotes the uptake of innovations in health care settings through activities, including stakeholder engagement, innovation messaging, and technical support, among others.[15–18] The adaptive nature of this approach allows responsiveness to technological and contextual changes, both nationally and locally, that affect VTH implementation.

The authors first provide historical context about the use of VTH in the VHA Health Care System. Thereafter, they describe the development and application of PIVOT, a strategy that allowed them to maximize patient choice and incorporate VTH into general practice, compared with a silo or telehealth center approach. They review how the use of PIVOT helps to engage health-system leadership and key stakeholders and identify Internal Facilitators and Clinical Champions to promote change. The authors describe their implementation process and strategies used to meet implementation goals, with a special focus on formative and summative outcomes that demonstrate how PIVOT led to overall satisfaction and sustained growth of VTH at this VAMC. They also offer recommendations for implementing a VTH program using the PIVOT strategy.

VIDEO TELEHEALTH TO HOME IN THE VA: HISTORICAL OVERVIEW

Several developments over the past 5 years within the VHA expanded the reach of telehealth and significantly changed the VTH technology platform (**Table 1**).

PERSONALIZED IMPLEMENTATION OF VIDEO TELEHEALTH

The PIVOT approach (**Fig. 2**) developed as the authors sought to fully integrate VTH into existing MH clinics over 5 years (FY14 through FY18) at the Houston VAMC. The Houston project was the next iteration that built on a smaller-scale implementation effort in Jackson, MS, which used a similar approach but focused solely on the delivery of evidence-based psychotherapies to increase access to rural patients.[19] The Houston VAMC serves approximately 130,000 Veterans at its main campus and network of 11 community clinics. To maximize patient choice, VTH was incorporated into general practice across multiple MH clinics (rather than training specific providers to deliver only VTH) as one option for care delivery, improving continuity of care and increasing the likelihood that VTH would be sustained and integrated into routine clinical care.

Evolving technological innovations and VHA priorities necessitated a nimble implementation approach to allow real-time communication about technology and policy changes to MH leadership and providers at the Houston VAMC. The PIVOT approach can be adapted to address different health-system contexts and specific innovations. It uses expert External Facilitators (licensed clinicians with expertise in implementation science and telehealth technology); Internal Facilitators (individuals with knowledge of the hospital system and existing relationships with providers who are empowered to

Table 1
Historical developments of video telehealth to home within the VHA system

Year	Developments in VA	Details
2013	Approval to provide MH via VTH	Cumbersome for patients and providers (software-based, required usernames & passwords to connect)
2017	Expansion of telehealth	Support for telehealth services across state lines (no official policy) Focus on Veterans in remote or rural areas
2017	National introduction of VA Video Connect platform	More user friendly (web-based program, eliminates usernames and passwords); allows delivery of MH care via personal computer, tablet or smartphone, with VHA providing device if necessary Mandate that >5% Veterans will receive some care through telehealth to home or mobile device in FY18
2018	Expansion of telehealth services into the home and other non-VA settings	Official policy approving anywhere-to-anywhere delivery All telehealth services within VHA under umbrella of federal supremacy Mandate that 100% of MH providers be trained in VTH by end of FY20

be local VTH point of contact); and Clinical Champions (providers located in satellite community or specialty MH clinics who inform colleagues and patients about VTH) to increase uptake of VTH throughout a medical system. External Facilitators simultaneously gather and coalesce information while training, supporting, and empowering on-site Internal Facilitators to implement and sustain VTH. The External Facilitators' credentials and expertise maximize their credibility as the authors engage key stakeholders in implementing VTH.

The first step of PIVOT is an initial meeting with External Facilitators, health-system leadership, and key stakeholders (eg, information technology, MH leadership, site telehealth lead) to discuss nationally established, system-wide implementation goals; present evidence for VTH; and consult about where to initiate implementation efforts. External Facilitators then identify on-site Internal Facilitators, often community or specialty clinic supervisors, with knowledge of the local system, influence, and existing relationships with providers. The focus on long-term sustainability necessitates training Internal Facilitators in VTH delivery and empowering each to become a local VTH expert, with support from External Facilitators. External Facilitators also help Internal Facilitators identify Clinical Champion providers across clinics and disciplines (eg, psychiatry, psychology, social work, masters-level counselors) to maximize uptake. Ideally, one Clinical Champion is identified in each satellite community or specialty MH (ie, posttraumatic stress disorder [PTSD], General MH, Women's Health, Substance Dependence Treatment, Primary Care MH Integration) clinic where VTH implementation will occur. External Facilitators train Clinical Champions in VTH delivery, then mentor and empower Internal Facilitators to provide support and guidance to ensure consistent, positive VTH messaging. External Facilitators continue to provide Internal Facilitators with support, resources (ie, note templates, emergency guidance), and troubleshooting to help them create and sustain a VTH program.

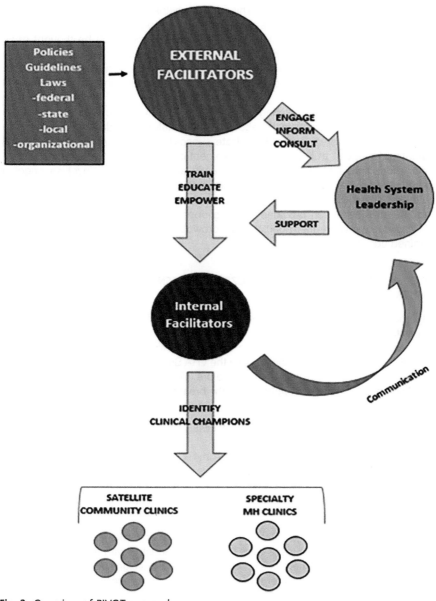

Fig. 2. Overview of PIVOT approach.

Throughout the implementation process, External Facilitators review and compile multilevel (federal, state, local, organizational) best practices, ethical guidelines, laws, and mandates concerning VTH delivery, technology, and compensation. During early stages of implementation, External Facilitators are responsible for communicating the latest developments in VTH policy to site leadership and Internal Facilitators. In preparation for sustainability, Internal Facilitators are encouraged to take an active role in expanding and sustaining the innovation, with guidance from External Facilitators on how to access information directly and to communicate with site leadership about relevant changes. This process helps External Facilitators shift responsibilities to Internal Facilitators and allows greater communication between Internal Facilitators and leadership. The transition to sustainment can be thought of as titrating external efforts down and placing a greater emphasis on engagement at the local level. During the sustainment phase, the role of External Facilitators transforms to a consultative role, with responsibility for active problem-solving shifting to Internal Facilitators.

The initial focus on empowering early adopter clinical champions, who identified themselves as being enthusiastic about the VTH-delivery modality, enabled us to quickly enter the system and demonstrate success, before VHA instituted national mandates. However, truly integrated implementation of VTH, or any innovation, requires more than engagement of a few early adopters. PIVOT involves ongoing communication with MH providers, clinic leadership, site leadership, and national telehealth to clarify expectations and shift the system's perceptions about VTH. The authors' iterative approach provided ongoing opportunities to assess the benefits of VTH and communicate them back to MH providers, thus increasing motivation and sustained adoption.

OUTCOME EVALUATION OF PERSONALIZED IMPLEMENTATION FOR VIDEO TELEHEALTH

Outcome evaluation of VTH implementation included both quantitative and qualitative data collection. To test the impact of this implementation approach, the authors compared rates of VTH use in Houston VAMC and affiliated community clinics to national VHA data, which were collected via the VHA Support Service Center Capital Assets Databases. They chose to examine the prevalence of 5 outcomes at the Houston VAMC and national levels to capture both the breadth and depth of a sustainable telehealth clinic:

1. Linear change in number of patients receiving MH services via VTH from FY13 to FY18,
2. Linear change in number of VTH visits from FY13 to FY18,
3. Number of MH providers delivering services via VTH in FY18,
4. Number of unique specialty-care MH clinics offering VTH services in FY18, and
5. Number of community clinics active in delivering VTH at any point from FY14 to FY18.

As nationwide data were positively skewed (all Shapiro-Wilks $Ps < 0.0001$), five 1-sample median (Sign) tests were used to compare Houston with the median nationwide value on each outcome. Sites identified by VHA as designated telemental health hubs (n = 11) were excluded from analyses because they received temporary dedicated funding for staff to deliver telehealth, as part of a larger national initiative. **Table 2** presents demographic data for patients who received VTH in Houston between FY14 and FY18.

Change in the number of unique patients receiving VTH and the number of VTH visits for the Houston VAMC and nationwide from FY14 to FY18 are presented in **Figs. 3** and **4**. Houston showed a significantly greater increase in the number of unique Veterans receiving VTH (linear slope = 59.71) and the number of VTH encounters (linear slope = 248.91) than other VAMCs (median slopes of 9.51 and 38.11, respectively), Sign Test M = -58.5 and -55.5, respectively, both $Ps < 0.0001$. In fact, the increase in the number of patients receiving VTH and VTH visits was 6.3 and 6.5 times (respectively) greater for Houston relative to median national improvement.

Table 2 Demographic data for the patients who received VTH in Houston between FY14 and FY18 (N = 619)	
	N (%)
Male	405 (65.43%)
Age (y)	
20–29	83 (13.41%)
30–39	229 (37.00%)
40–49	128 (20.68%)
50–59	101 (16.32%)
60–69	51 (8.24%)
70–79	24 (3.88%)
80–89	3 (0.48%)
Urban Residence	491 (79.32%)
OEF/OIF/OND[a]	
Yes	212 (34.25%)
No/Unknown	407 (65.75%)

[a] Veterans returning from the recent conflicts in Iraq and Afghanistan.

Furthermore, Houston had 47 MH providers who provided VTH in FY18, which was significantly greater (3.92 times greater) than the national median (ie, 12 providers), Sign Test M = −58.5, $P<0.0001$. Depth of VTH integration was evidenced by a significantly greater number of unique specialty MH clinics offering VTH in Houston in FY18 (n = 7) and a greater number of community clinics active in delivering VTH at any point from FY14 to FY18 (n = 7), numbers that were significantly greater (3.5 and 7 times greater, respectively) than the national median of 2 and 1 (respectively), Sign Test M = −61 and −55.5, respectively, both $Ps < 0.0001$.

To inform ongoing implementation efforts, the authors gathered qualitative feedback from VTH providers about their experiences with this modality. Providers noted how VTH enabled patients to receive care for low-incidence MH issues (ie, obsessive-compulsive disorder), more effectively treated certain disorders (ie, ability to see home environment of patients with hoarding; patients with agoraphobia do not need to resolve anxiety to receive care), and reach patients who would otherwise not engage in care due to issues or conditions that make coming to a VAMC or community clinic

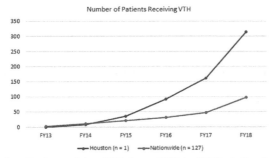

Fig. 3. Number of patients receiving VTH from FY13 to FY18 at the Houston VAMC and Nationwide.

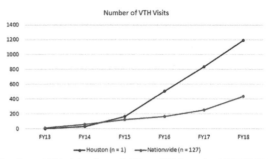

Fig. 4. Number of unique VTH visits from FY13 to FY18 at the MEDVAMC and Nationwide.

difficult (ie, PTSD, military sexual trauma, and chronic pain or physical disability). Providers also highlighted logistical and clinical concerns (eg, handling emergency situations over video, whether providing care into the home was "enabling" avoidant behavior) that the authors were able to preemptively address with newly trained VTH providers. One notable contextual change that providers described as affecting implementation efforts was Hurricane Harvey. See sidebar for additional information describing conditions in Houston during part of this project. The authors believe that these conditions contributed, in part, to their successful outcome by illustrating the usefulness of VTH, especially in times of crisis/natural disaster.

The authors conducted qualitative interviews with a representative, diverse sample of Veterans (n = 30) who had at least 3 MH visits via VTH to evaluate Veteran satisfaction with VTH. Veterans reported liking the convenience of VTH, as well as the comfort and privacy of receiving MH care at home. Most patients (83.3%) reported at least one barrier to engaging in MH treatment, with anxiety about leaving home being the most commonly identified barrier to accessing in-person care at a VAMC or affiliated clinic (67%). Distance/travel time (63%), taking time off work (50%), lack of comfort at VA (43%), and physical limitations (37%) were reported as other notable barriers.

RECOMMENDATIONS FOR IMPLEMENTING A VIDEO TELEHEALTH TO HOME PROGRAM

During the demonstration project, the authors identified several recommendations for implementing VTH. **Table 3** presents an overview and expansion of PIVOT recommendations to illustrate how this personalized implementation strategy might be effectively adapted for use outside VHA medical centers.

Engage Leadership Early and Often

When implementing VTH, either in a VA or non-VA setting, engaging leadership early in the implementation process is essential. For example, in the authors' demonstration project, engaging the telehealth coordinator at the local site, the clinic supervisor where implementation is taking place, and the lead of MH services at the facility promoted uptake. Leadership buy-in is critical to highlighting the importance of VTH implementation to providers at the facility, including the investment of resources to support implementation and the identification of incentives to promote adoption (eg, provider-level: flexible work schedule, telework options; clinic-level: conserves valuable resources such as space). Regularly communicating implementation progress and outcome metrics (see last point below) helps to foster ongoing leadership engagement.

Table 3
Application of Personalized Implementation for Video Telehealth

Recommendation	Considerations & Adaptations
Engage leadership early and often	• Obtain leadership buy-in and investment of resources • Establish ongoing communication to inform leadership on implementation progress/changes • Provide periodic feedback on outcome metrics from available data sources • Identify incentives to motivate provider adoption of VTH
Make facilitation key	• External facilitators provide expertise in innovation, engage leadership, and track policy changes • Local site internal facilitators need (1) protected time to support implementation and (2) training in facilitation and the clinical innovation
Start small to optimize success	• Engage stakeholders at every level of the organization • Collaboratively set realistic implementation goals • Early adopter providers and/or clinics to pilot the implementation plan • Identify motivating aspects/elements to boost provider and leadership adoption (eg, patient success stories; reduced no-shows)
Ensure flexibility	• Each site has unique barriers/facilitators • Adapt the implementation strategy to meet site needs • Capitalize on opportunities to illustrate the value of the innovation to ambivalent stakeholders
Assess multiple outcomes	• Identify outcome metrics of value to stakeholders • Identify persons responsible for outcome assessment • Additional outcome metrics are needed beyond those in national directives/policies • Revisit outcomes and how to measure/assess sustainability

Make Facilitation Key

External facilitation is key for developing successful, sustainable VTH programs again with likely relevance to both VA and non-VA systems. Based on the authors' experiences, national mandates or training requirements are insufficient to increase innovation uptake and create real practice change, particularly for complex technology-based innovations such as VTH. Using a facilitation approach such as PIVOT allows personalized assessment of the local medical system and a thorough understanding of the barriers and facilitators to implementing the innovation as well as offering external motivation, feedback about progress, and practical assistance to increase adoption. Several resources are available to support the use of external facilitation. The Agency for Healthcare Research and Quality (www.ahrq.gov), the North American Primary Care Research Group (International Conference on Practice Facilitation, www.napcrg.org), and the VA's Quality Enhancement Research Initiative (www. queri.research.va.gov) provide guidance in gaining facilitation skills to implement and sustain clinical innovations.

Start Small to Optimize Success

By starting with a "grassroots" facilitation approach, the authors were able to identify a few highly motivated providers and offer personalized "concierge" facilitation to maximize provider engagement and success. Their ability to help move providers from not only becoming trained in VTH to actively delivering care via VTH further enhanced their credibility with and buy-in from key stakeholders (eg, medical center leadership, Internal Facilitators, other potential VTH providers). Starting small also enabled them to control the message and reduce misinformation about the technology, directly addressing concerns and disseminating updates as they became available. A "grassroots" approach can help identify early adopters and clinics within a health system where the implementation plan can be piloted and adapted to the local context.

Ensure Flexibility

Technology-based innovations, including VTH, are complicated and constantly changing. VTH involves an interrelated web of logistical, technological, and ethical considerations. In addition to advances in technology, regulations at both the national and state levels are also growing and adapting, as MH providers consider applications of novel innovations and the ethics of their safety and effectiveness. For example, medical centers must ensure their computers and internet can maintain a stable connection while adhering to national guidelines for encryption/confidentiality and documenting providers' VTH training. Each site, clinic, and provider, regardless of health system and/or clinical setting, must be assessed for readiness to change, existing infrastructure or ability to develop infrastructure, and the negotiation between national, state, and site-specific guidelines. The External Facilitators use an Implementation Checklist developed specifically for VTH that can be adapted to unique contexts, but others may choose to create their own.

Assess Multiple Outcomes to Demonstrate Impact

Frameworks for assessing the spread of new interventions have historically focused on the number of patients reached and the total number of visits. These outcomes, however, are insufficient to demonstrate fully the impact of an innovation or implementation effort. High numbers of patients or visits could reflect simply a small number of highly productive providers rather than broad success in integrating VTH care delivery throughout a clinic or site. Tracking other outcomes, including number of providers trained *and* delivering care via VTH, number of affiliated community or specialty MH clinics offering VTH, and disciplines of providers (ie, psychiatry, psychology, social work) more accurately reflects the breadth and depth of implementation. Evaluation of implementation approaches and efforts also should include qualitative data collected in both formative (ie, evaluating the project while ongoing) and summative (ie, evaluation that occurs at or toward the end of the project) phases. These kinds of data are complementary and enrich our understanding of system-level change and how to bring best practices to our patients. Assessing outcomes during implementation and feeding this information back to key stakeholders increases motivation and momentum for practice change and enables sites to respond to challenges in real time.

SUMMARY

The PIVOT approach to implementing VTH supports patient-centered health care by integrating VTH into existing clinics and offering patients the choice to see their providers in person and/or via VTH; the evaluation data indicate a marked increase in the number of patients seen via VTH and overall satisfaction with this mode of MH care delivery. Veteran feedback highlights how VTH offers convenience and meets Veterans where they are; Veteran satisfaction with VTH-delivered MH care has important implications for retaining Veterans within the VA system.

Personalizing implementation enables greater responsiveness to provider needs and can address issues/concerns in real time to prevent the spread of misinformation about telehealth delivery (eg, that VTH is not as effective as providing care in person in the clinic setting). The evaluation data show that taking this personalized approach that is flexible to the contextual issues the providers face in their individual clinic settings can have a marked increase in the overall number of providers using VTH compared with national average.

Although the authors used PIVOT to implement VTH at one VAMC, the success of their clinical demonstration project indicates viability of this approach for larger-scale dissemination of VTH both within and outside VHA. As health care rapidly shifts toward more technology-enabled care via mobile apps to help patients track their health status, patient portals to communicate with health care providers, and asynchronous web-based care, PIVOT shows promise as a flexible implementation strategy that can be adapted for any technology-based MH care innovation. In addition, PIVOT's approach of fully integrating VTH within existing clinics meets the demand for more patient-centered and patient-driven care in public health and community settings, allowing patients to receive MH care when and where they desire to best meet their access needs.

Within large health care systems such as the VHA, there is increasing emphasis on leveraging telehealth to expand access to MH treatment and offer patients more choice in how and where they receive their care. PIVOT is responsive to these priorities by creating sustainable VTH programs that modernize care delivery from medical facilities and their affiliated community outpatient clinics, growing the number of providers capable of delivering MH care via VTH to increase access to care and provide patients more choice in how their care is delivered. Essential elements of PIVOT include encouraging leadership involvement from day one, relying on facilitation to overcome challenges, letting the program grow naturally, and being flexible, and looking at the "big picture" regarding outcomes can help implementation efforts succeed where they have, perhaps, failed before. The PIVOT approach can also be adapted to implement other technology-based innovations to expand access to MH treatment.

Side Bar

In August of 2017, Houston experienced a natural disaster, Hurricane Harvey, that caused widespread devastation (eg, catastrophic flooding, power outages, property damage). Thousands of individuals stayed in emergency shelters after being displaced from their homes and were without transportation (ie, personal cars were flooded, public transportation was limited). Providers relayed stories of Veterans with PTSD who were sleeping in makeshift shelters and reporting feeling distressed by the sound of search and rescue helicopters flying overhead. VTH offered a mechanism for providers and patients to connect and maintain continuity of MH treatment during this crisis. VTH delivery benefited both Veteran patients and providers who were unable to travel to the VAMC or were residing in a shelter or in an area temporarily inundated by flooding. Although Hurricane Harvey was impossible to anticipate, it offered unique motivation for previously reluctant providers to use VTH delivery to connect with their patients during the crisis and beyond.

REFERENCES

1. Olfson M, Marcus SC. National trends in outpatient psychotherapy. Am J Psychiatry 2010;167(12):1456–63.

2. Mojtabai R, Olfson M. National trends in psychotherapy by office-based psychiatrists. Arch Gen Psychiatry 2008;65:962–70.
3. Shigekawa E, Fix M, Corbett G, et al. The current state of telehealth evidence: a rapid review. Health Aff (Millwood) 2018;37(12):1975–82.
4. Kane CK, Gillis K. The use of telemedicine by physicians: Still the exception rather than the rule. Health Aff (Millwood) 2018;37(12):1923–9.
5. Ellimoottil C, An L, Moyer M, et al. Challenges and opportunities faced by large health systems implementing telehealth. Health Aff (Millwood) 2018;37(12): 1955–9.
6. Kruse CS, Krowski N, Rodriguez B, et al. Telehealth and patient satisfaction: a systematic review and narrative analysis. BMJ Open 2017;7(8):e016242.
7. Brooks E, Turvey C, Augusterfer EF. Provider barriers to telemental health: obstacles overcome, obstacles remaining. Telemed J E Health 2013;19:433–7.
8. Rees CS, Stone S. Therapeutic alliance in face-to-face versus videoconferenced psychotherapy. Prof Psychol Res Pract 2005;36:649.
9. Jameson JP, Farmer MS, Head KJ, et al. VA community mental health service providers' utilization of and attitudes toward telemental health care: the gatekeeper's perspective. J Rural Health 2011;27:425–32.
10. Fletcher TL, Hogan JB, Keegan F, et al. Recent advances in delivering mental health treatment via video to home. Curr Psychiatry Rep 2018;20(8):56.
11. Luxton DD, Pruitt LD, O'Brien K, et al. An evaluation of the feasibility and safety of a home-based telemental health treatment for posttraumatic stress in the U. S Military Telemed. J E Health 2015;21(11):1–7.
12. Campbell R, O'Gorman J, Cernovsky ZZ. Reactions of psychiatric patients to telepsychiatry. Ment Illn 2015;7(2):54–5.
13. Choi NG, Wilson NL, Sirrianni L, et al. Acceptance of home-based telehealth problem-solving therapy for depressed, low-income homebound older adults: qualitative interviews with the participants and aging-service case managers. Gerontologist 2013;54(4):704–13.
14. Gros DF, Lancaster CL, Lopez CM, et al. Treatment satisfaction of home-based telehealth versus in-person delivery of prolonged exposure for combat-related PTSD in veterans. J Telemed Telecare 2016;24(1):1–5.
15. Ritchie MJ, Dollar KM, Miller CJ, et al. Using implementation facilitation to improve care in the Veterans Health Administration (Version 2). Veterans Health Administration, Quality Enhancement Research Initiative (QUERI) for team-based behavioral health. 2017. Available at: https://www.queri.research.va.gov/ tools/implementation/Facilitation-Manual.pdf. Accessed February 15, 2019.
16. Baskerville NB, Liddy C, Hogg W. Systematic review and meta-analysis of practice facilitation within primary care settings. Ann Fam Med 2012;10:63–74.
17. Kirchner JE, Ritchie MJ, Pitcock JA, et al. Outcomes of a partnered facilitation strategy to implement primary care-mental health. J Gen Intern Med 2014; 29(Suppl 4):904–12.
18. Ritchie MJ, Parker LE, Kirchner JE. Using implementation facilitation to foster clinical practice quality and adherence to evidence in challenged settings: a qualitative study. BMC Health Serv Res 2017;17:294.
19. Lindsay JA, Hudson S, Martin L, et al. Implementing video to home to increase access to evidence-based psychotherapy for rural veterans. J Technol Behav Sci 2017;2(3–4):140–8.

The Impact of Telehealth on the Organization of the Health System and Integrated Care

Cliona O'Donnell, MB BCh BAO[a,b], Silke Ryan, MD, PhD[a,b], Walter T. McNicholas, MD, FERS[c,*]

KEYWORDS

- Telemedicine • Integrated care • Sleep medicine • Organization of the health system

KEY POINTS

- Prevalence of sleep-disordered breathing is growing and will need enhanced access to services and specialist input for a subset of patients.
- Telemedicine has potential to facilitate a move toward an integrated model of care, involving professionals from different disciplines and different organizations working together in a team-oriented way toward a shared goal of delivering all of a person's care requirements.
- A hub-and-spoke model of integrated care is likely to be the optimal organization of the health system with regard to sleep medicine.
- Telehealth has applications in all stages of the diagnosis, treatment, and follow-up of obstructive sleep apnea.
- Issues around consumer health technology and nonphysician sleep providers will need to be carefully evaluated in the development of a Telehealth system to promote integrated care.

INTRODUCTION

Sleep medicine is a rapidly developing field that is well-suited to initiatives such as Telehealth to provide safe, effective clinical care to an expanding group of patients. The optimal organization of the health system with regard to sleep medicine deserves special attention for a number of reasons: (1) the very high and growing prevalence of sleep disorders results in long waiting lists and a lack of specialist availability in many jurisdictions; (2) it has already integrated health technology to a greater degree

This article originally appeared in Sleep Medicine Clinics, Volume 15, Issue 3, September 2020.
[a] UCD School of Medicine, Health Sciences Centre, University College Dublin, Belfield, Dublin 4, Ireland; [b] Department of Respiratory and Sleep Medicine, St. Vincent's University Hospital, Elm Park, Dublin 4, Ireland; [c] Department of Respiratory and Sleep Medicine, School of Medicine, University College Dublin, St. Vincent's University Hospital, St. Vincent's Hospital Group, Elm Park, Dublin 4, Ireland
* Corresponding author.
E-mail address: walter.mcnicholas@ucd.ie

than other fields, with potential to continue doing so; and (3) it involves a large burden of chronic disease that requires efficient diagnosis, commencement of treatment, and continuing follow-up. Thus, an integrated care approach involving multidisciplinary teams with input from both specialist and generalist sectors, centered around providing personalized care to the individual patient, is an appropriate and achievable goal in sleep medicine, especially with the use of health technologies and telehealth to aid integration.

Sleep-disordered breathing, of which obstructive sleep apnea (OSA) is the most prevalent disorder, accounts for a large proportion of the sleep medicine patient cohort. OSA remains underdiagnosed and undertreated, and patients with OSA are at increased risk of hypertension, stroke, heart failure, diabetes, car accidents, and depression.[1] Sleep disorders affect an estimated 35% to 40% of the adult population in the United States, with a high cost burden, increased utilization of health care resources, and excess morbidity and mortality.[2] The HypnoLaus study published in 2015 involving 2168 subjects drawn from a Swiss general population and studied by home polysomnography (PSG) reported a very high prevalence for an apnea-hypopnea index (AHI) of 15 or more events per hour in 49.7% of men and 23.4% of women.[3] An AHI in the upper quartile of greater than 20.8 was independently associated with hypertension, diabetes, metabolic syndrome, and depression. The association of AHI with comorbidity is complicated by the finding that AHI rises with age,[4] whereas the association among OSA, hypertension, and cardiovascular disease is stronger in younger subjects, as is the relationship between OSA and relative mortality.[5] Furthermore, the AHI has also been shown to be poorly related to the classic symptoms of OSA, especially sleepiness.[6]

The preceding considerations illustrate the scale of the problem in the clinical assessment and management of patients with sleep-disordered breathing where personalized care is increasingly recognized as necessary to select the optimal treatment for the individual patient.[7] This review looks at the optimal organization of the health system to deliver the preceding goals, and how Telemedicine can facilitate the achievement of fully integrated care. It also will identify sleep-disordered breathing and other sleep disorders as specific examples of the potential for Telemedicine to improve integrated care.

OPTIMAL ORGANIZATION OF THE HEALTH SYSTEM TO PROMOTE INTEGRATED CARE IN SLEEP MEDICINE

The World Health Organization (WHO) defines integrated care as follows: Integrated Care is a concept bringing together inputs, delivery, management, and organization of services related to diagnosis, treatment, care, rehabilitation, and health promotion. Integration is a means to improve the services in relation to access, quality, user satisfaction, and efficiency. It involves professionals from different disciplines and different organizations working together in a team-oriented way toward a shared goal of delivering all of a person's care requirements.[8] Resources are shared, continuity of care is upheld, and the delivery process is integrated in the ideal system.[8]

Several driving forces are identified by WHO as pushing the development of integrated care among all health systems. These include demand-side factors, such as demographic change with an aging population, epidemiologic transitions, rising expectations, and patients' rights. Supply-side factors include the development of medical technologies and telemedicine, improving information systems, and economic pressures.[9]

Most of these factors are directly applicable to the field of sleep medicine. Sleep medicine is traditionally organized around specialist sleep centers that are referred patients whom they then diagnose and treat in-house, and communicate the outcomes back to the primary care referrer. Delivery of sleep services throughout Europe is limited by increasing prevalence associated with increasing age and increasing obesity, rising awareness of sleep disorders and the availability of consumer sleep technology, and improvement in available diagnostic services and information systems. The field of sleep medicine needs to evolve to meet these pressures, and movement toward a fully integrated system represents an optimal approach to the organization of health services in this context. Such integrated care involves collaboration among respiratory sleep specialists, neurologists, psychiatrists, otolaryngologists, dentists, and generalists at a medical level, and also integrating with physiologists, nurse practitioners, and industry providers to provide a cohesive, person-centered service. Such collaboration is likely to be greatly facilitated by tailored telehealth systems.

The move toward person-centered care should also be considered in the organization of the health system. This requirement includes improved communication, respectful and compassionate care of the individual, engaging patients in managing their own care, and integration of care.[10] Many health systems are currently fragmented, with poor communication of patient information between different health care providers. New ehealth technologies can support and link disjointed services across the continuum of care, such as improved electronic patient portals and the use of e-mail communication between patients and health care providers. The Health for All policy frameworks for the WHO European Region also addresses integration of services, with an emphasis on better access to family and community-oriented primary health care, supported by a flexible and responsive hospital system.[11]

As sleep also becomes more widely recognized as a pillar of health on a par with diet and exercise, more input will be required from generalists and improved referral pathways and communication with specialist services will be required. One qualitative study from 2012 found that sleep disorders are still underrecognized and not prioritized by generalists. They also found that communication between specialists and generalists in their jurisdiction was poor and led to a lack of interdisciplinary support for generalists in caring for patients with a sleep-disorder, as well as a lack of credibility for the sleep disorders specialty.[12] A recent study comparing the management of OSA by primary care physicians and specialist sleep physicians found no difference in the primary outcome of daytime sleepiness between groups after 6 months, nor in the secondary outcomes including quality of life measures, OSA symptoms, treatment adherence, and patient satisfaction. However, both diagnosis and treatment intervention in the 2 groups involved input from specialist nurses and training given to primary care physicians and nurses. They also had access to specialist support, which was availed of in a small number of cases. Furthermore, patients in this trial were deemed to be high risk for OSA based on screening, meaning that patients of uncertain diagnosis were not included in the study. This approach provides an example of a "hub-and-spoke"–type model in which access to specialist input is readily available, assisted by Telemedicine, and integrated with services provided by nurses with specialty training and industry. However, adequate resourcing and training are necessary to achieve the outcomes reported in this study.

The hub-and-spoke model ideally represents a network consisting of an anchor establishment offering a full array of services, complemented by secondary establishments that offer more limited service arrays (**Fig. 1**). Patients who need more intensive services can be re-routed to the hub for treatment.[13] The model is highly scalable and very efficient, and is well-suited to integration of care with the assistance of health technologies.

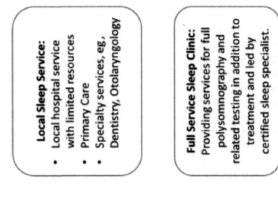

Local Sleep Service:
- Local hospital service with limited resources
- Primary Care
- Specialty services, eg, Dentistry, Otolaryngology

Full Service Sleep Clinic:
Providing services for full polysomnography and related testing in addition to treatment and led by certified sleep specialist.

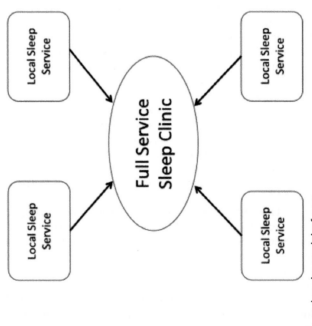

Fig. 1. Hub-and-spoke model of care.

Another research initiative toward integrated care is SMART DOCS (Sustainable Methods, Algorithms, and Research Tools for Delivering Optimal Care Study).[14] This study uses a novel patient-centered outcomes and coordinated care management approach as a new outpatient care delivery model for patients with sleep disorders. The study uses novel technologies to integrate sleep medicine care among the well-informed patient, specialist, and referring clinician. The comprehensive procedures involved include a standardized screening/intake process involving a combination of previously validated screening tools in an online questionnaire, the use of home-based diagnostic technologies and treatment adherence monitoring, actigraphy and ambulatory blood pressure monitoring, and the co-management of patients with primary care together with enhanced patient-provider data, in addition to information sharing and education.[14] These integrated procedures are greatly facilitated by telemedicine.

Thus, as seen in examples from Australia and the United States, the optimal organization of the health system with regard to sleep medicine will undoubtedly require the integration of Telemedicine to provide the most efficient, patient-centered, high-value care.

ROLE OF TELEHEALTH IN THE OPTIMAL ORGANIZATION OF HEALTH SYSTEMS

The European Commission has defined eHealth, or digital health, as follows: *The use of Information and Communication Technologies in health products, services and processes, combined with organizational change in health care systems and new skills, in order to improve health of citizens, efficiency and productivity in health care delivery, and the economic and social value of health.*[15] This definition clearly implies a key role for telehealth in the integrated organization of health care systems.

The American Telemedicine Association defines telemedicine as the use of medical information exchanged from one site to another via electronic communications to improve a patient's clinical health status,[16] and can be more broadly defined as the use of information and communications technology applications to provide health and long-term care services over a distance. In an ideal scenario, Telehealth should meet an urgent need for patient care provided at the prime point of need, favoring services in the home or in the community when possible. It offers the opportunity to deliver convenient, patient-centered, accessible care that overcomes many of the barriers present in traditional health care delivery systems, and should not simply be used as an adjunct to standard clinical care.[17] For the preceding reasons, telehealth care is a priority for Europe, as part of the "Digital Agenda for Europe," also for the UK National Health Service (NHS) as outlined in the "NHS Information Strategy," and for major health care providers in the United States such as the Department of Veterans Affairs.[18] However, most telehealth applications currently available remain segregated and require linking into more comprehensive eHealth strategies.[8]

The economic impact of telemedicine is complex to evaluate because there are different economic, social, and political factors at play. Most research studies have concluded that telemedicine systems are likely cost-effective but require better evidence.[18,19] A meta-analysis from 2008 reported that home monitoring was cost-effective in 21 of 23 studies,[20] but a report by Wootton[21] indicated a publication bias in telehealth studies looking at chronic disease management, with positive effects reported in 108 of 110 articles. Many telemedicine programs are still evolving from pilot-programs to full scale-up at regional and national levels. There is currently a lack of full assessment and evaluation of these programs, which will be essential in planning future telemedicine initiatives, as illustrated in one review of 17 telemedicine programs in Europe.[22] The development of these programs should be closely followed by those setting up sleep medicine telemedicine initiatives, as issues remain, such as confidentiality, data protection and ownership, financing, and quality of services.

The American Academy of Sleep Medicine (AASM) released a position paper on telemedicine in 2016,[2] recognizing the potential benefits and laying out conditions to promote optimal integration into clinical practice. Among other requirements, those applicable to the organization and integration of clinical care include the following:

- Telemedicine should adhere to standards of clinical care that mirror those of live office visits and include all aspects of diagnosis and treatment decisions as would be expected in a traditional encounter.
- Clinical judgment should be used to determine the scope and extent of telemedicine applications in the diagnosis of specific sleep disorders and patients.
- Live telemedicine visits should be recognized in a manner competitive or comparable with in-person visits.
- Roles, expectations, and responsibilities of providers should be defined, including both those at originating sites and distant sites.
- The care model should be a coordinated attempt to improve the value of health care delivery to the patient by sleep specialists, primary care providers, and other members of the health care team.

In 2016, the AASM also launched a telemedicine initiative called SleepTM,[23] a telemedicine platform designed specifically for the sleep field by AASM. It is primarily based around a secure video platform, but includes an interactive sleep diary and sleep log, sleep questionnaires, and the option for patients to import sleep data directly from wearable consumer sleep-monitoring devices. The aim of the program is to allow all patients access to a board-certified sleep practitioner, which has been shown in the past to be associated with better treatment adherence.[23] Follow-up will also be facilitated with the SleepTM program, and given multiple studies have shown that consistent input is necessary to maintain continuous positive airway pressure (CPAP) adherence in OSA and thus treatment benefit, this is an extremely important facet of the program.

OBSTRUCTIVE SLEEP APNEA

Several studies have looked at the feasibility or cost-effectiveness of telemedicine in the management of OSA, with some contradictory results.[24] One Spanish study found that telemedicine did not result in improved CPAP compliance and resulted in lower patient satisfaction, but it was cheaper.[25] The Tele-OSA study found that telemessaging alone and with tele-education improved CPAP compliance to what could be a clinically significant amount. The study in South Australia previously mentioned compared primary care and specialist input and found no difference in CPAP compliance between the 2 groups, but significant resources were available for both groups in terms of training provided to medical staff and patients.[26]

DIAGNOSIS

A health system that incorporates telemedicine to diagnose and treat a larger number of patients must be able to rely on accurate diagnostics as a fundamental part of management. In-laboratory PSG remains the gold standard for the diagnosis of sleep-disordered breathing, although home-based respiratory polygraphy is becoming more common and more widely available.[27] In-laboratory PSG is resource-intensive, limited by the availability of qualified staff, and expensive. A study in 2014 showed no significant difference between a 3-night home sleep study and PSG for patients without a high pretest probability of OSA.[28] It has previously been recommended that home sleep apnea testing not be used where there is ambiguity around the pretest probability or confounding comorbidities.[29,30] Masa and colleagues[29] reported that respiratory polygraphy is comparable to PSG for the diagnosis and therapeutic decision making for patients with a medium to high probability of OSA. However, data are frequently missing from home studies, which negatively affects their efficacy.[31]

Telemonitored PSG is a concept designed to overcome the disadvantages of home recordings, allowing dedicated technicians to verify the quality of the PSG recoding remotely in real time from a telemonitoring control panel. The protocols used to date have differed significantly and the evidence is therefore very weak.[31] However, a number of promising systems are attempting to overcome the problem of frequently missing data from conventional home studies.[27] As a screening tool, there are promising data looking at using nighttime pulse-oximetry telemedicine in patients at high risk for OSA.[31,32]

TREATMENT INITIATION

The treatment of OSA provides a challenge to ensure that patients can avail of specialist input when required. Mild OSA is often underrecognized in clinical practice and represents a management challenge as many different treatment options may be considered. The MERGE trial[33] involving 233 patients with mild OSA reported that quality of life significantly improved after 3 months in patients randomized to CPAP therapy compared with those randomized to supportive therapy. Notably, wireless monitoring was used to regularly review CPAP efficacy and adherence and may have helped to improve adherence.

These are patients who may not qualify for many of the studies evaluating home sleep apnea diagnosis but who may benefit from a trial of CPAP therapy. Conversely, their symptoms may not be attributable to their OSA, and inappropriate CPAP therapy may be avoided by referral to a specialist via telemedicine. A hub-and-spoke model may benefit this scenario whereby management decisions can be guided by sleep specialists and implemented by the local center. This was seen in the South Australian Primary Care study in which all patients in the Primary Care group commenced CPAP in contrast to only a proportion of patients in the Specialist group.[26] Also, mandibular advancement devices may be appropriate as an alternative to CPAP in certain subsets of patients with OSA.[34]

Phenotyping of OSA may improve the diagnosis of clinically significant OSA beyond the relatively imprecise measures of AHI and Epworth Sleepiness Scale and may benefit personalized diagnosis.[35] Gagnadoux and coworkers[36] identified 5 clusters, based on gender, presence of insomnia and comorbidities, depressive symptoms, and daytime sleepiness. CPAP use of more than 4 hours per night differed among the 5 clusters. This could provide additional prognostic information alerting the provider to those who may be at greater risk for nonadherence.[37]

Within the moderate-severe OSA group, there is established interest in the use of screening questionnaires, home sleep monitoring, and ambulatory management.[31] An initiative set up by the Veterans Health Administration used video teleconferencing, home sleep testing, modem-enabled positive airway pressure units, and automatically adjusting positive airway pressure machines to set up a fully functional telemedicine-enabled sleep Medicine service that provides care to a large, geographically disperse group of veterans. In a prospective study, they compared this telemedicine service to standard in-person care and found no difference in automatic positive airway pressure adherence after 3 months and equal patient satisfaction between groups.[38]

FOLLOW-UP

CPAP is an effective treatment for OSA but benefits are heavily dependent on patient adherence,[37] and therapeutic benefits increase with higher number of hours per night on therapy. However, compliance with CPAP is long-recognized as relatively poor in many studies and nightly compliance of more than 4 hours per night for 70% of days per week has been shown to vary between 30% and 60%.[8] Early adherence to CPAP usually predicts long-term adherence.[39] Compliance with CPAP is an area in which telemedicine is well-suited to optimization, with real-time wireless monitoring of CPAP use already available in many jurisdictions.[31] Patient's education, motivation, and active feedback can all have an impact on CPAP compliance. Conventional education and follow-up programs are expensive and require active health staff involvement. Telemedicine should be useful in the area of CPAP adherence, although some studies have been equivocal on the benefit of certain programs.[27] CPAP adherence can be objectively and remotely measured in real time. Given that remote monitoring of health status is one of the objectives of telemedicine, wireless CPAP compliance monitoring is well-suited to an integrated care system.

A large recent randomized clinical trial looked at different approaches to using telemedicine to improve adherence. The study had 4 arms, looking at a tele-education program consisting of a Web-based OSA education, a CPAP telemonitoring program with automated feedback messaging, a combination of the 2, and usual care alone. Interestingly, this study found that the automated feedback messaging improved CPAP compliance significantly, whereas the education program was not as beneficial. Sustained input from the tele-messaging service required limited provider input.[40] A similar outcome was found by a Cochrane review of educational, supportive, and behavioral interventions to improve CPAP adherence: Education alone improved adherence by only 35 minutes.[41] Furthermore, another study in Japan showed that long-term adherence rates to CPAP were improved with an intensive telemedicine follow-up program.[42] The HOPES study showed that in patients with sleep-disordered breathing after a stroke, a group in whom adherence is very challenging, a telemedicine intervention improved adherence rates in the short term at 3 months.[43] Overall, a consistent finding from studies of adherence is that sustained support and input from prescriber/clinician/nurse practitioner improves adherence and thereby improves outcomes.

Psychological measures of behavioral change constructs have been increasingly recognized as consistent predictors of CPAP adherence and as such, behavioral interventions have been most successful in optimizing adherence. However, these have not translated into routine care, primarily due to feasibility and cost issues.[44] Cognitive behavioral therapy (CBT) has been shown to be effective in small studies in improving adherence to more than 4 hours per night, and motivational enhancement therapy has also been shown to improve acceptance of but not adherence to CPAP up to a year. A Cochrane review found that behavioral therapy produces an improvement in nightly use of 1.5 hours, with a lack of cost-benefit data.[41] Given that CBT has been shown to be effective as a telemedicine-based intervention for insomnia and other sleep disorders,[45] and the resource-intensive nature of CBT for CPAP adherence, telemedicine is a potential option to enhance delivery of such programs.

OTHER SLEEP DISORDERS

Sleep disorders other than sleep-disordered breathing are also frequently underdiagnosed, underresourced, and undertreated. Conditions such as insomnia and narcolepsy have a major impact on health, with effects on psychological and cognitive functioning and decreased quality of life. There is often a poor understanding of sleep disorders such as insomnia among primary care physicians and generalists.[46] Telehealth has been used for CBT with positive results in insomnia,[47,48] agoraphobia,[49] and posttraumatic stress disorder.[50] With regard to insomnia, Web-based programs have been shown to improve sleep quality, daytime fatigue, and overall severity of insomnia. A study of Web-based versus telehealth-based CBT found that both modalities provided clear benefit in the treatment of insomnia.[48] An integrated care hub-and-spoke model using telemedicine to access specialist advice and diagnostics from a hub, with subsequent easy referral to telemedicine-based CBT could streamline currently underresourced services for common but poorly understood sleep disorders, such as insomnia.

Patients with narcolepsy often remain undiagnosed for long periods after onset of symptoms and the condition is poorly understood by many general physicians. As understanding evolves of this disease, the need for access to specialist centers increases and telemedicine based on a hub-and-spoke model of care may facilitate such access. One study showed that patients ultimately diagnosed with narcolepsy were significantly more likely to have received a diagnosis in the category of mental disorders, nervous system disorders, and congenital anomalies before their diagnosis by a sleep specialist.[51] Narcolepsy was most often diagnosed by neurologists, with internists and general practitioners diagnosing narcolepsy much less frequently. .

CONSUMER HEALTH TECHNOLOGY

As interest in sleep as a pillar of health along with diet and exercise grows, consumer sleep technology utilization continues to increase. Sleep apps remain among the most popular apps downloaded for mobile devices. Patients sharing patient-generated health data with their sleep clinician is becoming more and more common. An understanding by the sleep specialist of the accuracy and utility of these technologies is expected from the patient. However, minimal validation data exist regarding the ability of consumer sleep technologies to perform the functions that they purport to. These devices are not subject to US Food and Drug Administration oversight and therefore cannot be relied on to make clinical decisions; however, it is likely that as these devices become increasingly sophisticated, some may undergo validation and ultimately have a role in clinical care, and therefore it is important to acknowledge them as adjuncts that may help with communication with patients, goal setting, and increasing active participation.[52]

Nonetheless, investment in consumer health technology dropped from a boom of US$1.3 billion in 2014 to $300 million in 2016, possibly reflecting a reality check in terms of what can be reliably achieved by consumer health technology without rigorous validation. A further concern is the ownership of the data generated by consumer wearables.[53] Currently these data are not owned by the generating patient, but often sold to third parties.

NONPHYSICIAN SLEEP PROVIDERS

In Australia, the sleep industry is unregulated and does not have a framework to govern or review emerging pathways in the community. Potential for conflict of interest has been noted within some pathways that offer both diagnostic and treatment services.[54] Community pharmacies have developed pathways that could provide access to sleep services to a large cohort of patients; however, given that they remain unregulated, there are difficulties with this approach. Many within the pharmacy community expressed concern over appropriate practices by some sleep providers, especially

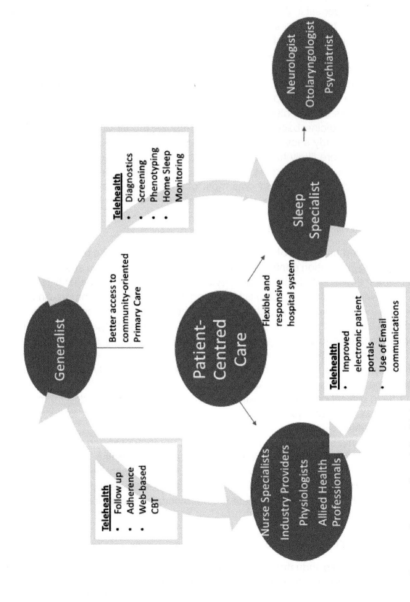

Fig. 2. Integrated care and targets for telehealth intervention.

given that many services provide both diagnostics and access to long-term, potentially expensive treatment.[55] At a basic level, there must be concern that an industry provider that provides a diagnostic sleep service and also markets CPAP devices is more likely to recommend CPAP therapy even though alternative treatment modalities may be equally appropriate. Telehealth could be used to integrate these services offered with both primary care and sleep specialist care, allowing for a greater degree of objectivity in diagnosis and management.

DISCUSSION AND SUMMARY

Sleep medicine is ideally placed to be a forerunner in truly integrated care given the availability of reliable health technology and monitoring equipment, the chronic nature of the problem, and the burgeoning prevalence and need for improved services in most jurisdictions. It crosses several specialties, and referral to the most suitable specialist service for the individual patient is important. Telemedicine can provide the links between sleep specialists, primary care, industry, and the multidisciplinary team (**Fig. 2**); however, telemedicine is a broad term describing an ever-growing field. Although there are programs and initiatives in place, it is vitally important to continue to objectively evaluate these programs to ensure safe, high-quality care is being delivered to the individual patient. Further research is required to identify the most efficient and productive methods of providing care to large numbers of people.

DISCLOSURE

The authors have nothing to disclose.

REFERENCES

1. Hilbert J, Yaggi HK. Patient-centered care in obstructive sleep apnea: a vision for the future. Sleep Med Rev 2018;37:138–47.
2. Singh J, Badr MS, Diebert W, et al. American Academy of Sleep Medicine (AASM) position paper for the use of telemedicine for the diagnosis and treatment of sleep disorders. J Clin Sleep Med 2015;11(10):1187–98.
3. Heinzer R, Vat S, Marques-Vidal P, et al. Prevalence of sleep-disordered breathing in the general population: the HypnoLaus study. Lancet Respir Med 2015; 3(4):310–8.
4. Senaratna CV, Perret J, Lodge C, et al. Prevalence of obstructive sleep apnea in the general population: a systematic review. Sleep Med Rev 2017;34:70–81.
5. Lavie P, Lavie L, Herer P. All-cause mortality in males with sleep apnoea syndrome: declining mortality rates with age. Eur Respir J 2005;25(3):514–20.
6. Deegan PC, McNicholas WT. Predictive value of clinical features for the obstructive sleep apnoea syndrome. Eur Respir J 1996;9(1):117–24.
7. Martinez-Garcia MA, Campos-Rodriguez F, Barbé F, et al. Precision medicine in obstructive sleep apnoea. Lancet Respir Med 2019;7(5):456–64.
8. Stroetmann KA, Kubitschke L, Robinson S, et al, How can telehealth help in the provision of integrated care? WHO Policy Brief, p. 39.
9. Gröne O, Garcia-Barbero M. WHO European Office for Integrated Health Care Services. Integrated care: a position paper of the WHO European Office for Integrated Health Care Services. Int J Integr Care 2001;1:e21.
10. Santana MJ, Manalili K, Jolley RJ, et al. How to practice person-centred care: a conceptual framework. Health Expect 2018;21(2):429–40.

11. World Health Organization, editor. Health21: the health for all policy framework for the WHO European Region. Copenhagen (Denmark): World Health Organization, Regional Office for Europe; 1999.

12. Hayes SM, Murray S, Castriotta RJ, et al. (Mis) perceptions and interactions of sleep specialists and generalists: obstacles to referrals to sleep specialists and the multidisciplinary team management of sleep disorders. J Clin Sleep Med 2012;8(6):633–42.

13. Elrod JK, Fortenberry JL. The hub-and-spoke organization design: an avenue for serving patients well. BMC Health Serv Res 2017;17(Suppl 1). https://doi.org/10.1186/s12913-017-2341-x.

14. Kushida CA, Nichols DA, Holmes TH, et al. Smart DOCS: a new patient-centered outcomes and coordinated-care management approach for the future practice of sleep medicine. Sleep 2015;38(2):315–26.

15. Newsroom, eHealth Action Plan 2012-2020: Innovative healthcare for the 21st century, Shaping Europe's digital future - European Commission. Available at: https://ec.europa.eu/digital-single-market/en/news/ehealth-action-plan-2012-2020-innovative-healthcare-21st-century. Accessed February 24, 2020.

16. Voran D. Telemedicine and beyond. Mo Med 2015;112(2):129–35.

17. Dinesen B, Nonnecke B, Lindeman D, et al. Personalized telehealth in the future: a global research agenda. J Med Internet Res 2016;18(3). https://doi.org/10.2196/jmir.5257.

18. McLean S, Sheikh A, Cresswell K, et al. The impact of telehealthcare on the quality and safety of care: a systematic overview. PLoS One 2013;8(8).

19. de la Torre-Díez I, López-Coronado M, Vaca C, et al. Cost-utility and cost-effectiveness studies of telemedicine, electronic, and mobile health systems in the literature: a systematic review. Telemed J E Health 2015;21(2):81–5.

20. Sv R, Mp G. A systematic review of the key indicators for assessing telehomecare cost-effectiveness. Telemed J E Health 2008;14(9):896–904.

21. Wootton R. Twenty years of telemedicine in chronic disease management – an evidence synthesis. J Telemed Telecare 2012;18(4):211–20.

22. Baltaxe E, Czypionka T, Kraus M, et al. Digital health transformation of integrated care in Europe: overarching analysis of 17 integrated care programs. J Med Internet Res 2019;21(9):e14956.

23. Watson NF. Expanding patient access to quality sleep health care through telemedicine. J Clin Sleep Med 2016;12(2):155–6.

24. Lugo VM, Garmendia O, Suarez-Giron M, et al. Comprehensive management of obstructive sleep apnea by telemedicine: clinical improvement and cost-effectiveness of a Virtual Sleep Unit. A randomized controlled trial. PLoS One 2019;14(10). https://doi.org/10.1371/journal.pone.0224069.

25. Turino C, Batlle J, Woehrle H, et al. Management of continuous positive airway pressure treatment compliance using telemonitoring in obstructive sleep apnoea. Eur Respir J 2017;49(2). https://doi.org/10.1183/13993003.01128-2016.

26. Chai-Coetzer CL, Antic NA, Rowland LS, et al. Primary care vs specialist sleep center management of obstructive sleep apnea and daytime sleepiness and quality of life: a randomized trial. JAMA 2013;309(10):997–1004.

27. Bruyneel M. Telemedicine in the diagnosis and treatment of sleep apnoea. Eur Respir Rev 2019;28(151). https://doi.org/10.1183/16000617.0093-2018.

28. Guerrero A, Embid C, Isetta V, et al. Management of sleep apnea without high pretest probability or with comorbidities by three nights of portable sleep monitoring. Sleep 2014;37(8):1363–73.

29. Masa JF, Corral J, Pereira R, et al. Therapeutic decision-making for sleep apnea and hypopnea syndrome using home respiratory polygraphy: a large multicentric study. Am J Respir Crit Care Med 2011;184(8):964–71.
30. Masa JF, Corral J, Sanchez de Cos J. Effectiveness of three sleep apnea management alternatives. Available at: https://www.ncbi.nlm.nih.gov/pmc/articles/PMC3825429/. Accessed: February 19, 2020.
31. Verbraecken J. Telemedicine applications in sleep disordered breathing: thinking out of the box. Sleep Med Clin 2016;11(4):445–59.
32. Chai-Coetzer CL, Antic N, Rowland L, et al. A simplified model of screening questionnaire and home monitoring for obstructive sleep apnoea in primary care. Thorax 2011;66(3):213–9.
33. Wimms AJ, Kelly JL, Turnbull CD, et al. Continuous positive airway pressure versus standard care for the treatment of people with mild obstructive sleep apnoea (MERGE): a multicentre, randomised controlled trial - the Lancet Respiratory Medicine. Available at: https://www.thelancet.com/journals/lanres/article/PIIS2213-2600(19)30402-3/fulltext. Accessed January 31, 2020.
34. Bratton DJ, Gaisl T, Schlatzer C, et al. Comparison of the effects of continuous positive airway pressure and mandibular advancement devices on sleepiness in patients with obstructive sleep apnoea: a network meta-analysis. Lancet Respir Med 2015;3(11):869–78.
35. Sânchez-de-la-Torre M, Gozal D. Obstructive sleep apnea: in search of precision. Expert Rev Precis Med Drug Dev 2017;2(4):217–28.
36. Gagnadoux F, et al. Relationship Between OSA Clinical Phenotypes and CPAP Treatment Outcomes. Chest 149; 1:288–90.
37. Weaver TE. Novel aspects of CPAP treatment and interventions to improve CPAP adherence. J Clin Med 2019;8(12). https://doi.org/10.3390/jcm8122220.
38. Fields BG, Behari P, McCloskey S, et al. Remote ambulatory management of veterans with obstructive sleep apnea. Sleep 2016;39(3):501–9.
39. Weaver TE, Kribbs NB, Pack A, et al. Night-to-night variability in CPAP use over the first three months of treatment. Sleep 1997;20(4):278–83.
40. Hwang D, Chang JW, Benjafield AV, et al. Effect of telemedicine education and telemonitoring on continuous positive airway pressure adherence. the Tele-OSA randomized trial. Am J Respir Crit Care Med 2017;197(1):117–26.
41. Wozniak DR, Lasserson TJ, Smith I. Educational, supportive and behavioural interventions to improve usage of continuous positive airway pressure machines in adults with obstructive sleep apnoea. Cochrane Database Syst Rev 2014;(1):CD007736.
42. Murase K, Tanizawa K, Minami T, et al. A randomized controlled trial of telemedicine for long-term sleep apnea CPAP management. Ann Am Thorac Soc 2019. https://doi.org/10.1513/AnnalsATS.201907-494OC.
43. Kotzian ST, Saletu M, Schwarzinger A, et al. Proactive telemedicine monitoring of sleep apnea treatment improves adherence in people with stroke– a randomized controlled trial (HOPES study). Sleep Med 2019;64:48–55.
44. Bakker JP, Weaver TE, Parthasarathy S, et al. Adherence to CPAP: what should we be aiming for, and how can we get there? Chest 2019;155(6):1272–87.
45. Seyffert M, Lagisetty P, Landgraf J, et al. Internet-delivered cognitive behavioral therapy to treat insomnia: a systematic review and meta-analysis. PLoS One 2016;11(2). https://doi.org/10.1371/journal.pone.0149139.
46. Khawaja IS, Hurwitz TD, Herr A, et al. Can primary care sleep medicine integration work? Prim Care Companion CNS Disord 2014;16(no. 2). https://doi.org/10.4088/PCC.13br01593.

47. Espie CA, Kyle SD, Williams C, et al. A randomized, placebo-controlled trial of on-line cognitive behavioral therapy for chronic insomnia disorder delivered via an automated media-rich web application. Sleep 2012;35(6):769–81.
48. Holmqvist M, Vincent N, Walsh K. Web- vs telehealth-based delivery of cognitive behavioral therapy for insomnia: a randomized controlled trial. Sleep Med 2014; 15(2):187–95.
49. Bouchard S, Paquin B, Payeur R, et al. Delivering cognitive-behavior therapy for panic disorder with agoraphobia in videoconference. Telemed J E Health 2004; 10(1):13–25.
50. Frueh BC, Monnier J, Yim E, et al. A randomized trial of telepsychiatry for post-traumatic stress disorder. J Telemed Telecare 2016. https://doi.org/10.1258/135763307780677604.
51. Kryger MH, Walid R, Manfreda J. Diagnoses received by narcolepsy patients in the year prior to diagnosis by a sleep specialist. Sleep 2002;25(1):36–41.
52. Khosla S, Deak MC, Gault D, et al. Consumer sleep technology: an American Academy of Sleep Medicine Position Statement. J Clin Sleep Med 2018;14(05): 877–80.
53. Piwek L, Ellis DA, Andrews S, et al. The rise of consumer health wearables: Prom-ises and barriers. PLoS Med 2016;13(2). https://doi.org/10.1371/journal.pmed. 1001953.
54. Hanes CA, Wong KKH, Saini B. Diagnostic pathways for obstructive sleep apnoea in the Australian community: observations from pharmacy-based CPAP providers. Sleep Breath 2015;19(4):1241–8.
55. Hanes CA, Wong KKH, Saini B. Consolidating innovative practice models: the case for obstructive sleep apnea services in Australian pharmacies. Res Soc Adm Pharm 2015;11(3):412–27.

The Opportunities for Telehealth in Pediatric Practice and Public Health

C. Jason Wang, MD, PhD[a],*, Jasmin Ma, BS[b,1],
Barry Zuckerman, MD[c], Josip Car, MD, PhD[d,e,2]

KEYWORDS

- Telehealth • Telemedicine • Public health • Pediatrics • Applications • Limitations
- Review

KEY POINTS

- Telehealth can be delivered asynchronously, synchronously, or through remote patient monitoring. Terms related to telehealth include digital health, connected health, telemedicine, eHealth, and mobile health.
- The cost, use, and effectiveness of telehealth vary depending on the technology deployed and by specialty.
- Telehealth use requires patient and provider adaptability, and is driven by convenience, accessibility, and increased health services demand caused by longer life-expectancies and lower mortality.
- The adoption and expansion of telehealth are restricted by current state and federal policies, privacy and security concerns, and the lack of cost-benefit analyses.
- Current telehealth literature provides more consistent evidence of benefits for communication and counseling, and from remote patient monitoring of chronic conditions. However, research is still lacking, especially in cost analyses, and is often limited by study implementations.

This article originally appeared in Pediatric Clinics, Volume 67, Issue 4, August 2020.
[a] Center for Policy, Outcomes, and Prevention, Stanford University School of Medicine, 117 Encina Commons, Stanford, CA 94305, USA; [b] Center for Policy, Outcomes and Prevention, Stanford University School of Medicine, Stanford, CA, USA; [c] Department of Pediatrics, Boston University School of Medicine, 801 Harrison Avenue, Boston, MA 02118, USA; [d] Department of Primary Care and Public Health, Imperial College London, London, UK; [e] Centre for Population Health Sciences, Lee Kong Chian School of Medicine, Nanyang Technological University, Singapore, Clinical Sciences Building, 11 Mandalay Road, Singapore 308232, Singapore
[1] Present address: 117 Encina Commons, StanfordCA 94305.
[2] Present address: Clinical Sciences Building, 11 Mandalay Road, Singapore 308232.
* Corresponding author. 117 Encina Commons, Stanford CA 94305.
E-mail address: cjwang1@stanford.edu

Clinics Collections 10 (2021) 67–75
https://doi.org/10.1016/j.ccol.2020.12.007
2352-7986/21/© 2020 Elsevier Inc. All rights reserved.

INTRODUCTION

The US Department of Health and Human Services defines telehealth as "the use of electronic information and telecommunication technologies to support and promote long-distance clinical health care, patient and professional health-related education, public health, and health administration."[1] Digital health and connected health are broad terms that refer to the use of technology to access or to integrate health services.[2–4] Related terms that are often used in conjunction include telemedicine, a subset of telehealth that refers to the delivery of clinical health care at a distance[5]; eHealth, the delivery of health services using the Internet and related technologies[6]; and mobile health, the delivery of health services using mobile devices[5] (**Fig. 1**).

USES OF TELEHEALTH

Telehealth can be delivered asynchronously via store and forward communications to transmit patient data and remote assessments; synchronously using real-time audio and video consultation, known as virtual visits; and through remote patient monitoring (RPM) using sensors and monitoring devices.[7,8]

Asynchronous Applications

Asynchronous applications increase accessibility to specialist evaluations independent of time and location. Their use includes gap service coverage, such as nighttime radiology coverage.[5] Radiologic and retinal imaging can be read by radiologists and ophthalmologists remotely and delivered to the patient's primary care provider.[3] Teledermatology is another increasingly common asynchronous

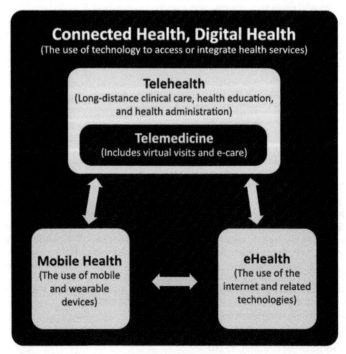

Fig. 1. The relationships between common terms associated with telehealth.

application where diagnoses are often made based on photos taken and uploaded from a patient's phone.[3] In pediatrics, common asynchronous applications include tele-echocardiography, teledermatology, and teleretinal screening.[9]

Synchronous Applications

Virtual visits have made health care more accessible generally and address some barriers for rural or underserved patients, who account for 20% of the United States' population according to the 2010 Census.[9,10] The use of scheduled virtual visits varies by specialty and includes routine follow-up, chronic condition management, medication updates, engagement of families in outpatient care, surgical preadmission testing, postoperative pain management, and postoperative follow-up.[11] Telehealth is also applicable in the improvement of coordination of care. For example, virtual visits can be used by children with chronic kidney disease for ongoing assessment of pre-transplant or established dialysis patients.[12]

Many emergency departments, urgent care centers, and intensive care units (ICUs) use virtual visits and large video consultations to improve the outcomes of acute or time-sensitive interventions (eg, stroke). Virtual visits also facilitate mandated services, such as the provision of health care to prison inmates.[5,7] Telehealth has improved outcomes in trauma incidents by allowing faster intervention during the critical period after a traumatic event.[7] For psychotherapy intervention and chronic disease management, a systematic review of 17 studies showed that the outcomes of videoconferencing groups are similar to those of in-person support groups. Thus, videoconferencing support groups may help overcome accessibility barriers such as mobility or distance.[13]

From a systematic review of pediatric telehealth, physicians made significantly fewer errors for patients who received a video consult compared with those who received a telephone consult or did not receive a consult at all. Physical examinations of neonatal ICU (NICU) patients performed and compared between on-site and off-site neonatologists showed good or excellent agreement for most assessments.[14]

Emergent new technologies

Robotic telepresence is a technology that allows face-to-face interactions between physicians and patients in the hospital without physical contact, thus decreasing risks of infection for vulnerable populations.[14] Certified bodies and frequent auditing are needed to incorporate appropriate trainings for such telehealth programs to ensure safety and efficacy.[15]

Virtual reality (VR) facilitates the user's perception of reality by creating a computer-generated environment using head-mounted displays, wall projectors, and touch-sensitive motors. VR has been explored for the treatment of a range of medical conditions, including anxiety, phobias, obesity, chronic pain, and eating disorders because of its capacity "to modulate subjective experience, offer respite from the confining nature of medical wards, or augment or replace analgesics in pain management."[16] In a randomized controlled trial that recruited 90 women with binge eating disorder at a rehab center, 44.4% of patients who used virtual reality were able to improve or maintain weight loss compared with 10.4% of patients in control conditions.[16] In the management of mental illness, VR-based cognitive and vocational training has been shown to improve cognitive outcomes.[17]

Moreover, simulated patients have been used in medical training.[15] Augmented reality (AR) refers to the enhancement of real-world experiences via the addition of computer-generated sensory information[18] and has been considered for real-time interactions with anatomy in surgical training and for consultations or mentoring with specialists independent of location.[18]

Remote Patient Monitoring and Remote Physiologic Monitoring

RPM uses mobile applications and sensory devices to collect community health care data or deliver real-time patient information to practitioners.[5] Expectations associated with remote patient monitoring include decreased hospital use, improved patient compliance, improved satisfaction with health services, and improved quality of life.

In addition to its usage in urgent services and ICUs for monitoring vitals,[5] RPM allows chronic diseases to be increasingly managed at home versus at a long-term-care facility. Physicians are able to monitor vitals and other patient data to prevent emergency room visits.[10] Improvements in chronic disease management' are especially significant in the United States, where "more than 70% of deaths are associated with chronic diseases and approximately 75% of annual health care expenses are used on persons with chronic conditions."[19] Based on findings from 58 systematic reviews, RPM has been shown to improve mortality and quality of life, and reduce hospital admissions.[20] A meta-analysis of 11 randomized controlled trials showed that telehealth exercise-based cardiac rehabilitation is at least comparable with center-based rehabilitation for reducing cardiovascular risk factors and improving functional capacity.[21]

RPM also improves health care engagement of patients and family members and shows promise in encouraging patients to achieve and maintain health goals.[19] It is specifically helpful for monitoring pediatric patients with type 1 diabetes via alerts during hypoglycemic or hyperglycemic incidences. For cardiac patients, cardiovascular implantable devices have been shown to decrease incidences of adverse cardiac events.[14] Findings based on 53 systematic reviews showed that telehealth-mediated self-management support for long-term conditions such as diabetes, heart failure, asthma, chronic obstructive pulmonary disease, and cancer is not consistently better than in-person support, although no reviews showed evidence of harm. Reviews more consistently showed reductions in mortality and hospital admissions for patients with heart failure and improvements in glycemic control for type 2 diabetics.[22] Furthermore, a meta-analysis comprising 25 studies showed evidence that telehealth-mediated dietary interventions for adults with chronic conditions improved diet quality, fruit and vegetable intake, and sodium intake.[23]

Starting from January 1, 2020, hospitals and health systems receive more Medicare reimbursements for RPM services. In its final rule on chronic care remote physiologic monitoring,[24] the Centers for Medicare & Medicaid Services (CMS) has allowed RPM to be furnished as a service "incident to" under general supervision, defined by CMS as service performed under the supervision of a qualified health care professional and billed to Medicare in the name of that professional. As such, CMS allows Current Procedural Terminology code 99457 to be billed for the first 20 minutes per month of RPM services and also added a new code 99458 for patients receiving an additional 20 minutes of mHealth services in a given month.

Overall

The cost, patient adherence, technology use, and effectiveness of telehealth vary depending on the technology and specialty.[14] Based on 58 systematic reviews that evaluated the impact of telehealth based on clinical outcomes, use, or cost, telehealth is most consistently beneficial when used for communication, counseling, or RPM of chronic diseases.[20] For example, a systematic review of 22 studies showed that telehealth interventions for cancer survivors minimizes disruptions to patients' lives and facilitates personalized care.[25] Uses of pediatric telehealth include acute-care visits, pretransport assessment and stabilization of those in critical condition, RPM, and specialty consultations.[26]

Cost of telehealth

Costs associated with the setup and maintenance of telehealth systems should also be considered, including use of telehealth personnel, costs of consultations, information technology support, equipment licenses, connectivity charges, and medical records management.[7]

An analysis of episode-level costs based on a cross-sectional retrospective study that included visits for the most common telehealth diagnoses (sinusitis, upper respiratory infections, urinary tract infections, conjunctivitis, bronchitis, pharyngitis, influenza, cough, dermatitis, nausea/vomiting/diarrhea, and ear pain) showed similar follow-up rates (with follow-up rate being a possible indication for misdiagnoses or treatment failure) between patients evaluated virtually and those evaluated traditionally; lower treatment cost per episode of care (defined as the initial visit plus the following 3 weeks) for virtual visits, which also depended on the condition; lower laboratory testing rates after virtual visits; and higher antibiotic prescription rates after virtual visits.[8]

Using claims and enrollment data from approximately 300,000 patients, net annual spending on acute respiratory illness increased $45 per telehealth user. Only an estimate of 12% of telehealth visits replaced visits to other providers, whereas 88% represented new use.[27]

Why telehealth works

Improved outcomes, preference, ease of use, cost savings, improved communication, travel time, and improved self-management were the most prevalent factors for choosing telehealth.[28] Specifically, time savings and increased accessibility were noted reasons for scheduled virtual visits.[11] The usage of mobile health and the market for mobile applications are increasing because of the convenience of size and mobility.[5,7] There is widespread interest in using phone and Internet-based telehealth among patients with chronic diseases.[29] With improvements in mortality for premature infants, patients with cancer, and patients with cardiovascular diseases, there is an increasing demand for health services. Management via telehealth encourages patients to participate in their own care and allows physicians to intervene as needed.[14,19,25]

Social adaptability, including patient and staff acceptance, will facilitate telehealth adoption. Patient acceptance and confidence in telehealth are highest for emergencies and higher for treatment than for diagnosis. Rural participants responded most positively and the scores within families tend to be similar.[7] The acceptance of telehealth for patients with chronic diseases increases with younger age, higher levels of education, familiarity, perceived usefulness, perceived ease of use, and satisfaction.[17] Among survey participants from telehealth users of scheduled video visits, 91.3% reported satisfaction. Among the dissatisfied, most cited technical issues. Ease of use was agreed on by 86.7%, 91.0% reported having had enough time with the provider, 82.7% perceived the same level of care as in in-person visits, and 87.6% perceived at least an hour of time saved.[11] Qualitative interviews conducted with patients who declined to participate in another telehealth study showed that major concerns include threats to identity, independence, and self-care; requirements of technical proficiency and the ability to operate equipment; and experiences of service disruptions.[17]

Equally important is staff acceptance, which is influenced by the staff's working environment, the manner of introduction, personal experiences, training, support, and the process of integration for routine care.[30,31] A common concern is the belief that the use of virtual visits will decrease patient-provider relationships.[7] Initial impressions of telehealth are an important factor. One study showed that nurses tended to be uncertain about the role of telehealth, which was intensified by the limitations and apparent contradictions of current research about its cost and clinical effectiveness. The adaptability of nurses was also affected by training on identifying suitable patients, effective monitoring and triage, duration of use, and the expected benefits and drawbacks.[30] A survey on implementation of robotic telepresence showed that NICU nurses thought that physicians were easily accessible via robotic telepresence, adequately involved, and supportive of both nurses and patients.[14]

Current problems
The success and availability of telehealth depends on the speed of data transmission, reliability, and security.[7] AR and VR are currently limited by computer power, battery life, the size of devices, and portability.[18] In order to successfully engage patients and improve communication, technologies must accommodate to the user's needs. Besides the patient's condition, the chosen platform should be based on the patient's age, education, interests, physical capabilities, familiarity, access to technology, the amount of support for self-care, and functional independence.[19]

Policy and regulations are often disjointed at the federal and state levels. In the United States, because states currently define their own policies, there is a wide range of telehealth definitions and reimbursement policies. Similarly, health care systems vary from country to country.[19] Although there is ongoing effort to increase telehealth use and reimbursement, health care providers continue to encounter conflicting or vague policies for the requirements for insurance claims, practice standards, and licensure,[10,26] and there is no consistent pattern of coverage and reimbursement for the variety of applications.[7,12,26] Lack of cost-benefit analysis also hinders the development of telehealth policies federally as well as the adoption and growth of telehealth programs.[19]

In terms of cost, further research is needed to confirm that higher follow-up visit rates do not occur as a result of unresolved symptoms or because telehealth is used before in-person visits.[8] In addition, within the United States, many payers do not yet "recognize the home as a reimbursable site of care."[19]

Considering the expansion of pediatric telehealth, a survey administered by the Supporting Pediatrics Research on Outcomes and Utilization of Telehealth program with 56 responses from mostly academic medical centers using pediatric telehealth identified barriers including licensing requirements, provider interest, and limitations of training resources.[26]

There is also a lack of quality monitoring for telehealth practices. There are concerns of whether physicians can provide accurate diagnoses without a physical in-person examination, whether patients receive appropriate laboratory testing after the visit, and whether antibiotics are overprescribed.[8] If data from RPM and other telehealth technologies are used to make clinical decisions, the physicians must be able to rely on the precision and accuracy of gathered data.[19] Most successful telehealth models require an extensive team to coordinate care to translate processed data from various devices into clinical action.[19]

Privacy and security concerns are also a major consideration in the deployment of telehealth. Privacy risks involve a lack of control on the collection, use, and disclosure of sensitive personal information.[32] Routine transmissions from a medical device may be collected and stored by the device or the app developer in addition to the health care provider. Security concerns depend on the platform. A patient participating in a video consultation may be concerned about the presence of others in the room, whereas someone using RPM technology may have concerns about the reliability of the device.[7] Specifically, in telehealth models where 1 end of the communication is the patient, no Health Insurance Portability and Accountability Act regulation or required safeguards are in place, magnifying existing concerns.[32] Patients may perceive security features as nuisances if they do not perceive some of their protected health information (PHI) to be sensitive.[33] At present, federal and state guidelines for telehealth security and privacy are not standardized, leaving considerable gaps.[34]

In addition, there are limitations of current literature. Past studies tend to consist of people who were already positively disposed to telehealth.[19] An analysis of 110 telehealth studies on chronic diseases, with 108 reporting positive outcomes, showed that the studies averaged a length of 6 months and there were few studies of cost-effectiveness.[19] Published literature is lacking, particularly in pediatrics, with previous studies largely focused on acceptability or patient characteristics rather than outcomes.[8] Other areas that require more extensive research include the management of serious pediatric conditions, triage in urgent or primary care, and teledermatology outcomes.

SUMMARY

Telehealth shows enormous potential as a new way for clinicians to reach patients remotely, often in the comfort of their homes. However, wider adoption of telehealth would require careful consideration of patient preferences, safety, effectiveness, medicolegal, and operational issues.

DISCLOSURE

The authors have nothing to disclose.

REFERENCES

1. Health Resources & Services Administration. Telehealth Programs. Available at: https://www.hrsa.gov/rural-health/telehealth/index.html. Accessed September 17, 2019.
2. WHO. Monitoring and Evaluating Digital Health Interventions: A Practical Guide to Conducting Research and Assessment.; 2016. doi:CC BY-NC-SA 3.0 IGO.
3. Kvedar J, Coye MJ, Everett W. Connected health: A review of technologies and strategies to improve patient care with telemedicine and telehealth. Health Aff 2014;33(2):194–9.
4. Caulfield BM, Donnelly SC. What is connected health and why will it change your practice? QJM 2013;106(8):703–7.
5. Weinstein RS, Lopez AM, Joseph BA, et al. Telemedicine, telehealth, and mobile health applications that work: Opportunities and barriers. Am J Med 2014;127(3): 183–7.
6. Eysenbach G. What is e-health? J Med Internet Res 2001;3(2):e20.
7. Sikka N, Paradise S, Shu M. Telehealth in emergency medicine: a primer. 2014.
8. Gordon AS, Adamson WC, DeVries AR. Virtual visits for acute, nonurgent care: A claims analysis of episode-level utilization. J Med Internet Res 2017;19(2):1–11.
9. Marcin JP, Shaikh U, Steinhorn RH. Addressing health disparities in rural communities using telehealth. Pediatr Res 2016;79(1–2):169–76.

10. Marcoux RM, Vogenberg FR. Telehealth: applications from a legal and regulatory perspective. P T. 2016;41(9):567–70.
11. Powell RE, Stone D, Hollander JE. Patient and health system experience with implementation of an enterprise-wide telehealth scheduled video visit program: Mixed-methods study. J Med Internet Res 2018;20(2):1–7.
12. Brophy PD. Overview on the challenges and benefits of using telehealth tools in a pediatric population. Adv Chronic Kidney Dis 2017;24(1):17–21.
13. van Galen LS, Wang CJ, Nanayakkara PWB, et al. Telehealth requires expansion of physicians' communication competencies training. Med Teach 2019;41(6): 714–5.
14. Banbury A, Nancarrow S, Dart J, et al. Telehealth interventions delivering home-based support group videoconferencing: Systematic review. J Med Internet Res 2018;20(2). https://doi.org/10.2196/jmir.8090.
15. Sasangohar F, Davis E, Kash BA, et al. Remote patient monitoring and telemedicine in neonatal and pediatric settings: Scoping literature review. J Med Internet Res 2018;20(12):1–9.
16. Dascal J, Reid M, Ishak WW, et al. Virtual reality and medical inpatients: a systematic review of randomized, Controlled Trials. Innov Clin Neurosci 2017;14(1): 14–21.
17. Lawes-Wickwar S, McBain H, Mulligan K. Application and effectiveness of telehealth to support severe mental illness management: systematic review. JMIR Ment Health 2018;5(4):e62.
18. Khor WS, Baker B, Amin K, et al. Augmented and virtual reality in surgery—the digital surgical environment: applications, limitations and legal pitfalls. Ann Transl Med 2016;4(23):454.
19. Dinesen B, Nonnecke B, Lindeman D, et al. Personalized telehealth in the future: A global research agenda. J Med Internet Res 2016;18(3). https://doi.org/10.2196/jmir.5257.
20. Totten AM, Womack DM, Eden KB, et al. Telehealth: mapping the evidence for patient outcomes from systematic reviews [Internet]. Rockville (MD): Agency for Healthcare Research and Quality (US); 2016. Available at: https://www.ncbi.nlm.nih.gov/books/NBK379320/.
21. Rawstorn JC, Gant N, Direito A, et al. Telehealth exercise-based cardiac rehabilitation: A systematic review and meta-analysis. Heart 2016;102(15):1183–92.
22. Hanlon P, Daines L, Campbell C, et al. Telehealth interventions to support self-management of long-term conditions: A systematic metareview of diabetes, heart failure, asthma, chronic obstructive pulmonary disease, and cancer. J Med Internet Res 2017;19(5). https://doi.org/10.2196/jmir.6688.
23. Kelly JT, Reidlinger DP, Hoffmann TC, et al. Telehealth methods to deliver dietary interventions in adults with chronic disease: A systematic review and meta-analysis1,2. Am J Clin Nutr 2016;104(6):1693–702.
24. Centers for Medicare & Medicaid Services. Document 2019-24086. Office of the federal register 2019. Available at: https://www.federalregister.gov/documents/2019/11/15/2019-24086/medicare-program-cy-2020-revisions-to-payment-policies-under-the-physician-fee-schedule-and-other. Accessed February 10, 2020.
25. Cox A, Lucas G, Marcu A, et al. Cancer survivors' experience with telehealth: A systematic review and thematic synthesis. J Med Internet Res 2017;19(1):1–19.
26. Olson CA, Mcswain SD, Curfman AL, et al. The current pediatric telehealth landscape. Pediatrics 2018;141(3). https://doi.org/10.1542/peds.2017-2334.

27. Ashwood JS, Mehrotra A, Cowling D, et al. Direct-to-consumer telehealth may increase access to care but does not decrease spending. Health Aff 2017;36(3): 485–91.
28. Kruse CS, Krowski N, Rodriguez B, et al. Telehealth and patient satisfaction: a systematic review and narrative analysis. BMJ Open 2017;1–12. https://doi.org/10.1136/bmjopen-2017-016242.
29. Edwards L, Thomas C, Gregory A, et al. Are people with chronic diseases interested in using telehealth? A cross-sectional postal survey. J Med Internet Res 2014;16(5):1–16.
30. Taylor J, Coates E, Brewster L, et al. Examining the use of telehealth in community nursing: Identifying the factors affecting frontline staff acceptance and telehealth adoption. J Adv Nurs 2015;71(2):326–37.
31. Koivunen M, Saranto K. Nursing professionals' experiences of the facilitators and barriers to the use of telehealth applications: a systematic review of qualitative studies. Scand J Caring Sci 2018;32(1):24–44.
32. Hall BJL, Mcgraw D. For telehealth to succeed, privacy and security risks must be identified and addressed. Health Aff (Millwood) 2014;33(2):216–21.
33. Wang CJ, Huang DJ. The HIPAA conundrum in the era of mobile health and communications. JAMA 2013;310(11):1121–2.
34. Tuckson RV, Edmunds M, Hodgkins ML. Telehealth. N Engl J Med 2017;377: 1585–93.

Child Health and Telehealth in Global, Underresourced Settings

Julianna C. Hsing, BA[a,b,*], C. Jason Wang, MD, PhD[b,c],
Paul H. Wise, MD, MPH[b,c]

KEYWORDS

• Telehealth • Child health • Developing countries • Nutrition • Global

KEY POINTS

• Childhood mortality continues to be a public health priority worldwide.
• The application of telehealth to pediatric health care settings may be important to improving child health in developing countries.
• Despite barriers, pediatric telehealth has been used to improve health communication, assist clinical consultations, promote task-shifting, and support risk-shifting.
• Successful integration of telehealth to improve child health in developing countries may require an approach that is family-centered, culturally sustainable, and long-term developed.

INTRODUCTION

Telehealth, also known as telemedicine, is defined as the use of any form of information and communication technologies to exchange health information and provide health care services across geographic, time, social, cultural, and political barriers.[1] Over the years, telehealth (including mobile health [mHealth]) has been used to improve health care delivery in several ways, including improving access to health care, enhancing the quality of service delivery, improving the effectiveness of public health and primary care interventions, and improving the global shortage of health professionals through collaboration and training.[2]

Despite an increase in the number of published articles on the concept of telemedicine, many of these studies have taken place in industrialized countries. Few studies to date have reported the integration of telehealth within the pediatric health care

This article originally appeared in Pediatric Clinics, Volume 67, Issue 4, August 2020.
[a] Department of Epidemiology and Population Health, Stanford University School of Medicine, 150 Governor's Lane, Stanford, CA 94305, USA; [b] Center for Policy, Outcomes and Prevention, Stanford University School of Medicine, 117 Encina Commons, Stanford, CA 94305, USA; [c] Department of Pediatrics, Stanford University School of Medicine, 291 Campus Drive, Stanford, CA 94305, USA
* Corresponding author. 117 Encina Commons, Stanford, CA 94305.
E-mail address: jchsing@stanford.edu

system, especially in the context of the developing world, or low- and middle-income countries. A reason for this may be relative lack of rigorous research data to demonstrate that telehealth is indeed improving the delivery of pediatric health care. Such barriers as high costs, the lack of technical expertise, and the obstacle of establishing the necessary operational infrastructure are challenges in low-resource countries.[3] The growth of telehealth is opening new avenues for efficient, effective, and affordable pediatric health care services worldwide. However, a clearer understanding of the current landscape of pediatric telehealth in a global setting is strongly needed. To assess this landscape and its barriers, this article (1) provides examples of the current uses of pediatric telehealth in a global setting, (2) discusses key aspects of how telehealth can become successfully integrated in underresource countries, and (3) reviews the challenges that telehealth faces in said countries.

PEDIATRIC TELEHEALTH IN GLOBAL SETTINGS: AN OVERVIEW

Through our review of the literature, we found that telehealth has been used to: (1) improve health communication, (2) assist clinical consultations, (3) promote task-shifting, and (4) support risk-shifting in developing countries. To help illustrate these uses, we showcase examples from the literature of various health care programs worldwide, including one that was initiated by our faculty at Stanford University's Center for Health Policy.

Telehealth to Improve Health Communication: Stanford University's Guatemala Rural Child Health and Nutrition Program

With the evolution of the Internet and mobile phones from basic (voice only) to smartphones (text, voice, video, Internet, and gaming capabilities), it is natural that global health programs have leveraged telehealth technologies to support clinical practices by enhancing communication and improving care coordination for patients.[4–6] This has intuitive appeal, because many mHealth tools enable specialized physicians to provide health services far from the clinical setting, in remote areas, and among hard to reach communities.

Guatemala is one of the poorest countries and has one of the highest malnutrition rates in the world, with around 50% of all malnourished children in Central America residing in Guatemala.[7] To mitigate this, the Guatemala Rural Child Health and Nutrition Program was initiated to address the high rates of malnutrition, stunting, and child mortality in San Lucas Toliman, Guatemala. This program is a collaboration led by Dr Paul Wise and researchers at Stanford University and the larger system of community health promoters in Guatemala who are trained in a variety of areas, including hygiene, family education, nutrition supplementation, and primary medical care. Currently serving around 15,000 people in 22 communities, the Guatemala Rural Child Health and Nutrition Program has made a unique impact in the delivery of care in Mayan Guatemalan communities through the incorporation of an innovative mobile application (app) platform in the nutrition program. In working closely with the health promoters in Guatemala, Wise and his team designed an app that fit into their existing workflow, including the process of uploading patient data on the server via the dedicated Internet access point at the lead promoter's home. Routine follow-up care was much easier with the mobile app, because predictive algorithms were incorporated that immediately notified a health care promoter of when a child may soon fall to a more severe grade of malnutrition, and if intensive intervention will be warranted. In addition, the app automatically plotted the weight and height onto growth charts, relieving health promoters from the burden of hand-plotting data onto growth charts.

Analysis of the pilot data from using the mobile app showed that training time for promoters was reduced from 3 years to less than 6 months, which has only positively contributed to the continual decrease in child mortality and stunting from severe malnutrition.

Using Telehealth Technologies to Assist Specialized Consultations in the Remote Clinic

Several telemedicine networks around the world deliver services to support children and families on a routine basis, many to low-income countries. Examples of these services include: acute-care visits at day care centers, pretransport assessment of critically ill children at community hospital, in-home remote monitoring, and subspecialty consultations (eg, cardiology, radiology, neurology, general surgery) that support primary care pediatricians in remote areas.[8–13]

- Case 1: Children's National Medical Center: the pediatric telecardiology program
  Live transmission of echocardiograms from remote sites to the Children's National Medical Center is one of the most commonly used applications among its many international telehealth programs.[14] Published reports of its use have shown that real-time guidance and immediate interpretation of echocardiograms is feasible and accurate, resulting in timely transport of critically ill children with heart disease and preventing unnecessary transport of children with normal hearts.[15] In addition to providing improvements to patient management, this method can also help local sonographic technicians perform higher quality echocardiograms. Since the program began in 1998, more than 6000 studies have been performed from 10 regional hospitals and several international partners, including Qatar, Morocco, Uganda, and Germany.[14] Today, live synchronous video transmission is used to address other medical problems, including those related to maternal and child health, malnutrition, and infectious disease prevention.

- Case 2: Medical Missions for Children: the telemedicine outreach program
  Medical Missions for Children (MMC) is a US nonprofit organization that operates a global videoconferencing network. It delivers expertise from medical specialists and technicians based in hospitals in the United States to children needing care in developing countries by using telemedicine.[16] The mission of MMC is to improve health care for children in medically underserved communities by using telemedicine.[16] Through its telemedicine outreach program, which is a distance medicine network that electronically connects physicians to patients in more than 100 remote countries, MMC partnered with the University Hospital in Brazil and donated two telemedicine units to this hospital so that they could have consultations with the tertiary care hospitals in the United States. Through this partnership, MMC has been able to facilitate teleconsultations for physicians and other local health professionals needing advice about clinical management for their patients, and also provide a valuable learning experience for all medical professionals involved in the process.[17]

Using Telehealth to Promote Task-Shifting from Physician to Community Health Workers

One of the main constraints in public health work is chronic shortage of well-trained health workers. Although this shortage is global, low- and middle-income countries, where such diseases as human immunodeficiency virus (HIV) and AIDS are a burden, feel this shortage the most. For instance, in Uganda, the shortage of health workers is so extreme that several districts have no physicians at all.[18] As a result, in 2006, the World Health Organization launched a task-shifting plan to strengthen and expand the pool of human resources for health. According to the World Health Organization, task-shifting is a process of delegation whereby tasks are moved, where appropriate, to less specialized health workers, and when combined with the tools used in telemedicine, the benefits are great.[18]

- *Case 1: Task-shifting in Uganda for HIV/AIDS antiretroviral therapy*
  In Uganda, task-shifting is currently the basis for providing antiretroviral therapy. Generally, providing antiretroviral therapy to 1000 individuals in settings in which resources are constrained requires an estimated one to two doctors, up to seven nurses, about three pharmacy staff, and a wide range of community workers. However, with only one doctor for every 22,000 patients and an overall health worker deficit of up to 80%, Uganda was forced to make task-shifting work. Nurses now undertake a range of tasks that were formerly the responsibility of doctors, whereas community health workers, who have training but not professional qualifications, are taking over tasks that were previously the responsibility of nurses. Examples of responsibilities that have been task-shifted to nurses include: managing coinfections in people with HIV, prescribing medication to prevent coinfection, determining clinical stage of people with HIV, and deciding eligibility for HIV therapy. Tasks that have been shifted to community health workers include: taking vital signs, HIV testing, counseling and education on antiretroviral therapy, monitoring and supporting adherence to therapy, and basic clinical follow-up.[19]

  However, having quality and supportive supervision and clinical mentoring when task-shifting antiretroviral therapy is important, especially in resource-constrained health settings where the health system is already weak and overwhelmed. Moreover, the complex referral process and subsequent consultation is still a frustrating challenge for patients and health care workers due to long waiting times, delays in and duplication of laboratory results, the cost of travel, and the time taken to consult a specialist.[20] Telemedicine can help address these problems by providing quality, clinical mentoring, timely access to a specialist, reducing the need and associated costs of travel, reductant consultation waiting times, and promoting home-based care.

- *Case 2: Task-shifting through community health promoters in Guatemala*
  A unique aspect of the nutrition program in Guatemala is the intentional task-shifting of roles from physicians to the community health promoters. They accomplish this by using a "train the trainer" approach where study staff and physicians provide extensive training locally and remotely to lead promoters. In turn, these lead promoters train other promoters and other trainees. As a result, community health promoters are not just focused on growth monitoring and providing supplements. Rather, they see their role as much larger where they can collectively work together to address larger community-level issues at hand. The promoter training curriculum also includes lessons on how to navigate and use the app, because they will eventually be the ones collecting data via the app's platform when Stanford physicians are not onsite.

Task-shifting expands the human resource pool rapidly and efficiently by building bridges among the health facility, its workers, the community, and patients.[18] When combined with telemedicine, training a new community health worker is completed in a much shorter period of time than it would usually take to train to be a licensed nurse. Task-shifting can also lead to the demographic reorganization of services and help them to move closer to the communities where they are needed. Local services provided by community health workers have been shown to bring positive benefits in an increased uptake of services, more timely detection and treatment, avoidance of overtreatment, and enhanced adherence to treatment.[18]

Use of Telehealth to Support Risk-Shifting in Developing Countries

Unstable governments and internal violence are common barriers in the developing world. However, telehealth can help overcome these barriers, because it is capable of putting specialized health care providers out of immediate risk. Telehealth can also offer the tools to provide support in response to disaster-based humanitarian need. Studies have shown that major medical and public health benefits can be provided even 3 to 6 months after disasters.[21]

- *Case 1: Delivering health services in areas of unstable governance and conflict through the Guatemala Rural Child Health and Nutrition Program*
  Rural areas, such as San Lucas Toliman, Guatemala, in developing countries are characterized by lack of resources and scarcity of communications infrastructure. These circumstances make it difficult to provide appropriate health care services. In Guatemala in particular, the 36-year-long civil war created a significant strain on health services and systems. However, innovative tools, such as telehealth, can be used for diagnosis and management to deliver patient care in underserved clinics and hospitals. Moreover, bringing external expertise through online consultation and the use of remote monitoring in areas of high demand may be valuable. Through the Guatemala nutrition initiative, Wise and his team at Stanford and other government officials have discussed efforts in discovering new technologies that can address the political barriers that exist in these areas. This is important so that in case of future internal conflicts, health care professionals and volunteer workers can take appropriate actions to protect themselves and reduce their risk of danger or being targeted.
- *Case 2: Telemedicine in the conflict, war-torn region of Somalia*
  Médecins Sans Frontières (MSF), also known as Doctors Without Borders, is an international, independent, medical humanitarian organization best known for its projects in conflict zones and countries affected by endemic diseases. In Somalia, MSF runs a district hospital supported by a limited number of Somali clinicians. Expatriate health care staff are no longer physically on site because they face high security risks because of kidnappings and direct threats to life. As a result, many Somali clinicians now have little opportunity for continuing education, poor technical knowledge, and lack of exposure to new medical developments. To address this, MSF introduced the new idea of telemedicine in Somalia, specifically implementing a real-time exchange of audiovisual information between the clinicians in Somalia and a specialist pediatrician in Nairobi. This exportation of expertise instead of experts to Somalia proved to be effective not only in pediatric care management, but also in pediatric outcomes and also showed to have added value to Somalian clinicians.[21] More than 85% of the Somalian clinicians surveyed noted that telemedicine was useful in helping to improve recognition of risk signs and to improve management protocols and prescription practices.[21] After sufficient training, all clinicians were eventually able to use the technology in an independent manner. Because they work under deprived and insecure circumstances in the world, Somalian doctors believed strongly that telemedicine brought a sense of proximity and closeness with their tele-colleagues in Kenya.

- *Case 3: The Haiti earthquake in 2010*
  Investment in telemedicine capabilities has also the potential to reduce the overall medical costs for deploying and supporting medical personnel to disaster areas. In many developing countries, such as Haiti, poor operational and communication infrastructure leaves thousands of individuals without access to basic health services. For instance, when an earthquake struck Haiti in 2010, the National Aeronautics and Space Administration was unable to support the victims of the earthquake because of the lack of resources and infrastructure.[22] Telephones, although vital for the coordination of relief efforts and for the dissemination of information to families, were poorly established.[23] Moreover, connectivity to Internet servers was almost nonexistent, and thus improvised. Satellites in Miami helped link a team in Florida to communicate requests for medical supplies and medications to specialist consultants. Physicians also used satellites for triage and video consultations, and because many patients had crush injuries, physicians on the ground in Haiti video conferenced with burn surgeons in Miami to discuss how best to treat the extremity wounds.[24]

Because many developing countries are areas where conflict or natural disasters makes it difficult to seek appropriate medical attention, telemedicine can help shift and reduce the risk for the health care professional by delivering care remotely.

INTEGRATING TELEHEALTH IN THE COMMUNITY CONTEXT OF RESOURCE-CONSTRAINED COUNTRIES

It is clear that developing countries have different health issues and needs than those of developed countries (eg, poverty, communicable diseases, maternal child health/infant mortality, workforce shortage, limited availability of broad-band Internet, high communication costs, low technological and educational literacy levels, language barriers).[1] What, then, allows certain telehealth programs to work in developing countries?

- *Centering care around family and from within the community:* The family unit is one of the most important aspects of many cultures. Therefore, it is important to consider telehealth as an enhancement to existing human and cultural relationships. This approach may be especially beneficial in pediatric health care settings, because care always involves the child and parent. In Guatemala, Wise and his team ensured that the foundation of the health promoters program was built on the family unit so that trust is established with the families they service. Moreover, the health promoters program empowers local community workers to play a larger role in the well-being of other community members through the "train the trainer" approach. Although the Stanford team has expert knowledge in implementing nutrition growth intervention in the area, they view community health workers as "key collaborators," who share insights for taking care of the local communities.
- *Using appropriate and culturally acceptable technologies:* Once the community has been understood, the appropriate technologies available are determined and become embedded into the local fabric of the community. This can become more apparent with the use of mobile phones for health-related concerns (eg, community announcements, appointment/check-up reminders) and with the gathering of health volunteers and workers who meet regularly to attending training sessions. During the mobile app development project, Stanford

researchers worked closely with many health promoters across 22 different Mayan communities to codesign a user interface that would be most useful for them and would make tracking nutrition faster, easier, and more accurate. Additionally, the hope of this codesign process was to lower the training requirements so that health promoters and the locals still support the service after the "foreign developer" (ie, Stanford) has left that area. Over time, the health workers slowly developed the confidence in the new skills they needed to learn to help others within the community.

- *Long-term collaboration and continuation of care:* By combining an mHealth approach with an established, 10-plus-year relationship among outside physicians, local clinicians, and the local health promoters of Guatemala, the nutrition program was not only able to increase the inflow of patients, but also provide seamless continuation of care. Health care promoters have taken over a large part of the role of routine follow-up care, health management, and coordinating with various nonprofits who offer assistance. It is important for future telehealth efforts to be put in the context of the critical health needs of Guatemala and to blend into its current and future health care system. Our hope is that through the Guatemala Rural Child Health and Nutrition Program and its efforts in using technological innovations, we can expand and enhance population health management, care coordination, and individualized care in the Highlands of Guatemala.

CURRENT CHALLENGES OF TELEMEDICINE IN A GLOBAL SETTING

Telehealth alters traditional concepts of what constitutes the patient-doctor relationship by imposing a physical distance between the doctor and its patient. Although it has been reported that most diagnoses can be made through history taking and with a proxy examination performed by the health worker in the room with the patient, the pivotal question remains: does telemedicine enhance or detract from the therapeutic relationship between doctor and patient?[25] Especially in certain cultures where family and community are highly valued, a modern concept like telemedicine may meet some resistance and can lead to compromises in the quality of care.[1,26,27] Moreover, the nuances of body language and nonverbal communication are frequently lost in telemedicine interactions. If the health care provider is too focused on the interpreter present in the room, which may draw the physician's attention away from the patient, he or she may miss important aspects of the patient's behavior that could impact the diagnosis. In cases when a family member serves as the interpreter, they may not understand certain medical terms being discussed, leading to important points getting lost in translation.

Currently, most telehealth programs in the developing world tend to narrowly focus on one disease (eg, telecardiology, teleradiology, telesurgery). However, the reality is that patients typically do not have "one disease," and those who do benefit from telesurgery or telecardiology are only a small fraction of the world's population. Therefore, solutions for the developing world need to be more pragmatic in addressing the specific needs and contexts of the developing world.

Although Internet connectivity and signal quality (eg, 2G to 3G to 4G) has improved dramatically over the years, it is inevitable for poorer, lower-resource areas to be left without connectivity because of their inability to have ready access and ability as quick as other developed areas. The lack of systems support and update may lead to higher levels of virus and worm infections of electronic patient data, potential breaches of security, or engagement of terrorist tactics to reach political ends. In addition to limited connectivity, resources to own a cell phone are not common, meaning may patients may share phones to receive messages from their health provider. However, with different health-related messages for different patients being sent to the same phone, they are bound to receive health-related messages for other people, which is a potential breach of personal health information.

SUMMARY

Telehealth has a unique position in the delivery of health care at a global setting. It can provide value, particularly when it is used in the right context to strengthen and support a local team. Although the place of telemedicine in direct patient care delivery remains to be established, currently it is important for training of local health care professionals. As technology availability and evidence-based telehealth models increase, it is hoped the barriers surrounding telehealth will begin to fall one by one. Until then, more high-quality, evidence-based studies on effectiveness and safety of pediatric telehealth practice are strongly needed, and the faster the trust relationships between remote doctors and physicians are established, the quicker telemedicine services can take hold in the relevant communities.

DISCLOSURE

The authors have nothing to disclose.

REFERENCES

1. Scott R, Mars M. Telehealth in the developing world: current status and future prospects. Smart Homecare Technol Telehealth 2015;25. https://doi.org/10.2147/shtt.s75184.
2. Ray Dorsey E, Topol EJ. State of telehealth. N Engl J Med 2016;375(2):154–61.
3. Olson CA, Mcswain SD, Curfman AL, et al. The current pediatric telehealth landscape. Pediatrics 2018;141(3). https://doi.org/10.1542/peds.2017-2334.
4. Piette JD, Datwani H, Gaudioso S, et al. Hypertension management using mobile technology and home blood pressure monitoring: results of a randomized trial in two low/middle-income countries. Telemed J E Health 2012;18(8):613–20.
5. Abdulrahman SA, Ganasegeran K. m-Health in public health practice: A Constellation of Current Evidence. In: Jude HD, Balas VE, editors. Telemedicine technologies: Big Data, Deep Learning, Robotics, Mobile and Remote Applications for Global Healthcare. Elsevier Inc; 2019. p. 171–82.
6. Ganasegeran K, Abdulrahman SA. Adopting m-Health in clinical practice: A Boon or a Bane?. In: Jude HD, Balas VE, editors. Telemedicine technologies: Big Data, Deep Learning, Robotics, Mobile and Remote Applications for Global Healthcare. Elsevier Inc; 2019. p. 31–41.
7. Chary A, Messmer S, Sorenson E, et al. The normalization of childhood disease: an ethnographic study of child malnutrition in rural Guatemala. Hum Organ 2013; 72(2):87–97.
8. Satou GM, Rheuban K, Alverson D, et al. Telemedicine in pediatric cardiology: a scientific statement from the American Heart Association. Circulation 2017;135. https://doi.org/10.1161/CIR.0000000000000478.
9. Kuhle S, Mitchell L, Andrew M, et al. Urgent clinical challenges in children with ischemic stroke: analysis of 1065 patients from the 1-800-NOCLOTS pediatric stroke telephone consultation service. Stroke 2006;37(1):116–22.

10. Otero AV, Lopez-Magallon AJ, Jaimes D, et al. International telemedicine in pediatric cardiac critical care: a multicenter experience. Telemed J E Health 2014; 20(7):619–25.
11. Heath B, Salerno R, Hopkins A, et al. Pediatric critical care telemedicine in rural underserved emergency departments. Pediatr Crit Care Med 2009;10(5):588–91.
12. McConnochie KM, Wood NE, Kitzman HJ, et al. Telemedicine reduces absence resulting from illness in urban child care: evaluation of an innovation. Pediatrics 2005;115(5):1273–82.
13. Mahnke CB, Jordan CP, Bergvall E, et al. The Pacific asynchronous teleHealth (PATH) system: review of 1,000 pediatric teleconsultations. Telemed J E Health 2011;17(1):35–9.
14. Alverson DC, Swinfen LR, Swinfen LP, et al. Transforming systems of care for children in the global community efforts should be aimed at improving. Pediatr Ann 2009;579–86. https://doi.org/10.3928/00904481-20090918.
15. Sable C, Roca T, Gold J, et al. Live transmission of neonatal echocardiograms from underserved areas: accuracy, patient care, and cost. Telemed J 1999; 5(4):339–47.
16. Children MM for. Global medicine and teaching networks. Available at: www.mmis-sions.org/index.html. Accessed August 29, 2019.
17. Ozuah PO, Renzik M. Medical Missions for Children: a global telemedicine and teaching network. In: Wootton R, Patil NG, Scott RE, et al, editors. Telehealth in the developing world. Royal Society of Medicine Press Ltd; International Development Research Centre; 2009. p. 101–8.
18. World Health Organization. Taking stock task shifting to tackle health worker shortages.; 2007.
19. Baine SO, Kasangaki A. A scoping study on task shifting: the case of Uganda. BMC Health Serv Res 2014;14(1):1–11.
20. Kiberu VM, Scott RE, Mars M. Assessing core, e-learning, clinical and technology readiness to integrate telemedicine at public health facilities in Uganda: a health facility-based survey. BMC Health Serv Res 2019;19(1):1–11.
21. Zachariah R, Bienvenue B, Ayada L, et al. Practicing medicine without borders: tele-consultations and tele-mentoring for improving paediatric care in a conflict setting in Somalia? Trop Med Int Health 2012;17(9):1156–62.
22. Nicogossian AE, Doarn CR. Armenia 1988 earthquake and telemedicine: lessons learned and forgotten. Telemed J E Health 2011;17(9):741–5.
23. Brauman R. Haiti earthquake: what priorities? Centre de Reflexion sur l'Action et les Savoirs Humanitaires (CRASH) Foundation Medecins Sans Frontieres. 2010. Available at: https://www.msf-crash.org/en/publications/natural-disasters/haiti-earthquake-what-priorities. Accessed September 6, 2019.
24. Louden K. Telemedicine connects earthquake-ravaged Haiti to the world 2010. Available at: https://www.medscape.com/viewarticle/717232. Accessed September 6, 2019.
25. Wootton R, Darkins A. Telemedicine and the doctor-patient relationship. J R Coll Physicians Lond 1997;31(6):6–7.
26. Gogia SB, Maeder A, Mars M, et al. Unintended consequences of tele health and their possible solutions. Contribution of the IMIA Working Group on Telehealth. Yearb Med Inform 2016. https://doi.org/10.15265/IY-2016-012.
27. Institute of Medicine. The role of telehealth in an evolving health care environment: workshop summary. Washington, DC: The National Academies Press; 2012.

Reducing Infant Mortality Using Telemedicine and Implementation Science

Clare Nesmith, MD[a], Franscesca Miquel-Verges, MD[b],
Tara Venable, MD[a], Laura E. Carr, MD[a], Richard W. Hall, MD[a],*

KEYWORDS

- Telemedicine • Perinatal regionalization • Infant mortality • Implementation science
- Infant • Premature

KEY POINTS

- Perinatal regionalization is an evidence-based strategy to lower infant mortality.
- Barriers to perinatal regionalization can be mitigated using implementation science.
- Telemedicine is a critical tool for the implementation of an optimal perinatal regionalization strategy.
- Telemedicine can be used effectively to engage and educate community providers and stakeholders aiming to lower infant mortality.
- Telemedicine can be used to support appropriate referral and back transport of preterm and sick neonates

INTRODUCTION

Perinatal regionalization is an evidence-based strategy to reduce infant mortality (IM). The inability to implement optimal perinatal regionalization results in preventable infant deaths for very low birthweight (VLBW, <1500 g) infants.[1,2] Perinatal regionalization is achieved by establishing systems designating where neonates are born according to the level of care needed, regardless of financial need, race, or ethnicity. Regionalized systems assign hospitals risk-appropriate levels, and ensure high-risk neonates are born in facilities with appropriate technology and specialized health care providers, such as maternal fetal medicine and neonatology specialists.[3] Nationally, health care payment systems and institutional prestige have led to a trend toward

This article originally appeared in Obstetrics and Gynecology Clinics, Volume 47, Issue 2, June 2020.
[a] Division of Neonatology, Department of Pediatrics, University of Arkansas for Medical Sciences, Slot 512 B, 4301 West Markham, Little Rock, AR 72205, USA; [b] 1 Children's Way Slot 512-5, Little Rock, AR 72202, USA
* Corresponding author.
E-mail address: hallrichardw@uams.edu

Clinics Collections 10 (2021) 87–98
https://doi.org/10.1016/j.ccol.2020.12.009

deregionalization, resulting in higher IM.[4] *This trend, which is under provider control, results in the deaths of thousands of neonates every year in the United States, and minorities share the burden disproportionately.* The United States lags behind 28 other industrialized nations in IM, and there are significant disparities in this country, in large part because of failure to implement optimal regionalization.[5] Implementation strategies consist of engaging stakeholders (providers, payers, parents, and advocates) as champions, harnessing telemedicine connectivity, and using academic rigor to implement optimal regionalization.

BENEFITS OF PERINATAL REGIONALIZATION

The American College of Obstetricians and Gynecologists (ACOG) and the American Academy of Pediatrics (AAP) classify levels of care into levels 1 to 4, with AAP and ACOG level 1 providing basic care and level 4 providing the most sophisticated care. The emphasis from regionalization advocates has been on the AAP levels of care guidelines, but in February 2015, ACOG published a consensus guideline for maternal levels of care that generally correspond to the AAP levels. Research demonstrates VLBW neonatal mortality is lower for infants born at level 3 or 4 centers compared with those born in non–level 3 centers. In addition, evidence also shows IM of VLBW neonates is much higher at low-volume neonatal intensive care units (NICUs). The relative risk of death in NICUs with fewer than 25 VLBW annual admissions is 2.2 compared with high-volume NICUs with more than 100 annual VLBW admissions.[6] However, not all studies have found a significant effect of volume on IM. Rogowski and colleagues[7] found that NICU volume contributed only 9% to the variance in IM mortality using data from the large Vermont-Oxford network. However, the Vermont-Oxford Network database, while including mortality as a data point, also includes transfer to another facility. Thus, if a neonatal patient is transferred to another higher-level facility (for example, to a children's hospital for surgical treatment of necrotizing enterocolitis), then dies, the death may not be recorded as a death in the transferring hospital's database. Using Department of Health data, volume in Arkansas was found to be a significant contributor to IM (**Fig. 1**). Clearly, local data for each state or region should be used to determine specific requirements for designating level of care.

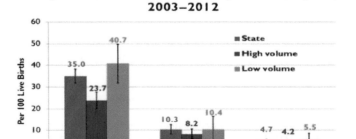

Fig. 1. Differences in infant mortality in Arkansas in low (<50 annual VLBW deliveries) versus high (>100 VLBW annual deliveries).

Intraventricular hemorrhage (IVH) causes significant adverse neuro-developmental sequelae for premature newborns.[8] IVH, as well as other morbidities associated with prematurity are lower when infants are delivered in a higher level of care hospital. Numerous studies have demonstrated that if infants are delivered where they are cared for after delivery, their risk for an IVH is less.[9,10] It is unclear whether the increased IVH rate is due to the transport itself or the difference in care at hospitals with lower levels of care. Regardless, to prevent adverse neurodevelopmental outcome, there is a significant benefit to delivering high-risk pregnancies in an appropriate-level hospital where their care can be continued until discharge or stable for back transport.

BARRIERS TO OPTIMAL REGIONALIZATION

Multiple barriers to regionalization exist. Regionalization requires complicated coordination and consensus among providers, hospitals, and patients.[11] In a study of adult clinicians and administrators in a variety of hospital settings, multiple barriers were identified. Barriers include those that affect the patient and the patient's family, the clinicians, and the hospitals. Traveling to a regional center puts an emotional and financial burden on the patient and family, particularly if the hospitalization is prolonged. One study found clinicians identified a loss of autonomy and income as barriers to regionalization and were concerned that reaching agreement among providers would be unlikely.[12] Further, regionalization has financial consequences for both the referring hospital as well as the accepting regional center. The same study also identified lack of a strong central authority and regulation in the area of regionalization as additional barriers.[12] In a subsequent national survey, adult intensivists proposed solutions to barriers to regionalization of care. These included the development of common information technology platforms across hospitals, using objective criteria to determine need for transfer, providing financial incentives to the referring hospitals and clinicians, and demonstrating through a clinical trial the benefits of regionalization.[13]

Similar barriers are found in regionalization of perinatal care. However, in the care of the mother and newborn, the coordination becomes more complicated and the burden to the family can be higher if the mother-newborn dyad is separated. Prestige and revenue are key barriers to transferring infants to hospitals with appropriate levels of care. The mean NICU charge for a baby weighing less than 1000 g at the Arkansas Perinatal Center was $124,171 in 2016 (Hall RW, 2016,unpublished data). Thus, transferring even one small neonate out of a smaller community hospital can seriously affect the referring hospital's financial viability. Further, in Arkansas, as in many other states, transferring a mother will cause the obstetric provider to lose 90% of the patient charge. Prestige is affected because some hospitals, providers, and patients interpret transferring patients as an indicator of poor performance of the community hospital, even though transferring to a higher level of care is a sign of best practice. Thus, even though data supporting regionalization of neonatal care are compelling, implementing that practice is challenging. **Table 1** summarizes barriers to perinatal regionalization and how they were addressed in Arkansas.

TELEMEDICINE HAS BEEN USED SUCCESSFULLY TO FACILITATE COOPERATION AMONG RURAL PROVIDERS

The benefits of telemedicine are highlighted when evaluating its ability to effect change in rural communities. These communities are important to the success of optimal perinatal regionalization because they are often classified at a lower level and low volume so they have to transfer infants out to achieve optimal neonatal

Table 1
Barriers to regionalization of neonatal care and methods of overcoming them

Barriers	Specific Issue	How Barriers Were Addressed
Loss of income	Loss of income for the referring provider and hospital	Back transport once patient stable Minimize patients needing referral out based on Arkansas infant mortality data Adopt slogan of "best care closest to home"
Loss of prestige	Perception of referral out meant inadequate local care	Data from Arkansas Department of Health shows improved outcome with appropriate referral Education of providers Peer pressure to "do the right thing"
Initial cost of telemedicine equipment	$162,000 (Telemedicine investment)	Initial funding from grant (National Institutes of Health) and local philanthropy Sustainable hospital investment over time because of ability to use the technology long term Infrastructure cost and support staff frequently estimated at $5000 annually
Connectivity	Inadequate bandwidth	Adequate bandwidth has become the norm in community hospitals
Community provider time	Local provider time for census rounds	Nurses participated in tele-nursery rounds (10 min 3 times wkly); physician participation needed only when specific questions or issues were raised
Perinatal provider time	Perinatal center provider time	Time needed was 1 h weekly Goodwill and enhanced communication made up for the slight drain on academic time
Lack of education	Education for community providers needed	Peds PLACE: wkly educational conferences connecting the perinatal center with community practices; community providers had input into lecture topics; free continuing medical education credits were offered

care. According to the US Census Bureau, as of December 2016, approximately 19.3% of the population live in rural areas, the equivalent of approximately 60 million people.[14] In Arkansas, approximately 42% of residents live in a rural county.[15] Rural communities have been well-labeled as health disparity populations, defined by the National Institutes of Health as a population in which there is "a significant disparity in the overall rate of disease incidence, prevalence, morbidity, or mortality in the specified population as compared with the general population."[16] These patients often have difficulty obtaining access to care as a result of the uneven distribution and relative shortage of medical care providers, issues that have persisted despite considerable efforts by both federal and state governments to address these health disparities.[17] As a result, rural patients find themselves with higher rates of disease and increased mortality, underscoring the need for easier, more readily available access to care, which can be addressed through the use of telemedicine. In fact, when implemented, telemedicine has proven to be valuable in facilitating cooperation among rural providers and specialists to decrease mortality and morbidity among certain patient populations. Developed by Dr Arora, Project ECHO (Extension for Community Healthcare Outcomes) demonstrated that the use of videoconferencing was successful in treating chronic hepatitis C infection in underserved, rural communities. His study compared treatment of patients at the University of New Mexico hepatitis C clinic with those treated by their primary care clinicians at specified ECHO clinic sites in rural areas and prisons in New Mexico. The primary endpoint was sustained virologic response, with the study showing that a total of 57.5% of patients treated at the University of New Mexico hepatitis C clinic and 58.2% of those treated at the ECHO sites had a sustained viral response.[18] These results are encouraging, revealing that when videoconferencing is used by rural providers to cooperate with specialists in the care of patients, telemedicine then becomes an effective way to treat disease in underserved communities. Telemedicine has similarly proven its value in rural communities, as demonstrated by Portnoy and colleagues[19] comparing asthma control between children seen at an in-person visit and those seen at a telemedicine session at a local, rural clinic using real-time equipment and a telefacilitator. A total of 34 in-person and 40 telemedicine patients completed all 3 visits, including an initial visit, a follow-up visit at 30 d, and a follow-up visit at 6 months. The results showed that all had a small, although statistically insignificant, improvement in their asthma control over time, and, most importantly, revealed that telemedicine was not inferior to in-person visits. It is not difficult, then, to see the many advantages that telemedicine can afford rural communities, particularly its ability to confer coordination of care among rural providers with specialists not readily available in-person. This coordination of care among rural providers via telemedicine has shown itself to be a promising vehicle for changing the landscape of disparate health care and related morbidity and mortality in rural America. Successful use of telemedicine is a key player in reducing IM by allowing for optimal perinatal regionalization and cooperation among rural health care providers and their urban specialists.

USE OF TELEMEDICINE IN OBSTETRICS

The ANGELS (Antenatal and Neonatal Guidelines, Education and Learning System) program has demonstrated how telemedicine can improve health care in a rural state like Arkansas. Telemedicine in Arkansas has allowed obstetricians to provide subspecialty care to rural areas for families with limited resources and has improved access to high-risk obstetrics for these families. In rural states such as Arkansas with remote areas, a high-risk center, through the use of telemedicine, can provide patients with the expertise of maternal fetal medicine specialists and geneticists. Through the use of teleultrasound technology, Health Insurance Portability and Accountability Act (HIPAA)-compliant broadband connections, and high-definition video, subspecialty expertise becomes available for complicated pregnancies in rural communities. For example, Fisk and colleagues[20] found that teleultrasound resulted in significantly fewer referrals to a specialist compared with those who did not have teleultrasound.

Because telemedicine provides real-time secure medical care, a plan for complicated pregnancies may be formulated allowing the family to ask questions and actively participate in the plan of care without traveling long distances. Barriers to subspecialty care, such as transportation, child care, time off work, and travel expenses, are addressed through consultation via telemedicine. Through virtually uniting patients, their local providers, and subspecialists, one study found changes to the management plan for 45.8% of the cases when a subspecialist comanaged via telemedicine with the generalist over management by a generalist alone. Patient satisfaction and the patient-physician relationship was not compromised, as 95% of the pregnant women in the study would highly recommend videoconferencing to others.1. Magann EF, Bronstein J, McKelvey SS, Wendel P, Smith DM, Lowery CL. Evolving trends in maternal fetal medicine referrals in a rural state using telemedicine. Archives of Gynecology & Obstetrics 2012;286:1383-92.

Using telemedicine, subspecialists can provide real-time interpretation of images and guide ultrasounds in rural areas. Through subspecialist-guided teleultrasound, the patient and generalist have access to real-time diagnosis and planning for delivery. Fetal diagnosis of congenital heart disease by telemedicine was found by McCrossan, and colleagues[21] to be 97% accurate. This accuracy affords communities with limited access to health care the advantage of subspecialists working with generalists to provide quality care. Arkansas used the existing educational interactive video network, then equipped rural hospitals with telemedicine equipment and broadband. This allowed a system used for education to also provide an avenue for consultation with specialists, genetic counselors, and ultrasounds available through the academic medical center. As these diagnoses are identified, a specific plan of care can be formulated by the family, the generalist, and the subspecialist to provide the best maternal and neonatal outcomes.

TECHNICAL REQUIREMENTS FOR TELEMEDICINE USE IN PERINATAL REGIONALIZATION

Generally, synchronous or live telemedicine is needed for this purpose because real-time interaction is needed for videoconferencing as well as neonatal assessment.[22] Sufficient audio-video quality is needed for appropriate patient assessment and provider communication. For example, an adequate assessment of respiratory distress in a neonate will require equipment capable of displaying respiratory effort, degree of nasal flaring, and degree of costal retractions. A single photo in time does not adequately portray respiratory effort in a neonate. Equipment required varies from software-based systems to turn-key videoconferencing units. Peripheral medical devices may be needed depending on the type of telemedicine being practiced. These devices can be hardwired or portable and include a stethoscope, otoscope, ophthalmoscope, pulse ox, or electrocardiogram.[23]

The American Telemedicine Association recommends a minimum of 640 × 360-pixel resolution at 30 frames per second transmission for video cameras. However, this is low definition, and the practical minimum standard should be high-definition video, with 1920 × 1080-pixel resolution recommended. The technology should support H.264 video compression standard or better, H.261 video compression compatibility, and G.711 audio compression standard or better to provide high-quality video and audio interaction.[22] Telemedicine also requires adequate bandwidth, as most use a high-speed Internet connection. A connectivity speed of 384 kbps for standard video and 1 mbps for high-definition video is recommended.[23] All technologies need to comply with legal, organizational, and regulatory requirements that will likely change as more technology develops.

Year-round information technology (IT) support is an essential part of telemedicine connectivity. Having someone available to ensure connectivity requires infrastructure capable of responding when there are technical issues. The IT personnel must be well trained in the equipment and be able to troubleshoot problems that may arise in the middle of the night.

TELEMEDICINE WAS USED EXTENSIVELY TO IMPLEMENT REGIONALIZATION OF NEONATAL INTENSIVE CARE IN ARKANSAS

In 2005, Arkansas was 1 of only 3 states in the United States without a formal system of perinatal regionalization. After evaluation of Arkansas Department of Health IM data linking delivery hospital to IM, the Arkansas Department of Health formed a Perinatal Advisory Committee to address the problem and provide solutions with the goal of lowering IM through perinatal regionalization[24] (**Fig. 2**). Telemedicine was used to provide clinical care and education in the following ways[2]:

- 24 hour/7 day obstetric consultation through telemedicine.
- 24 hour/7 day neonatal consultation through telemedicine.
- Weekly educational conference (Peds PLACE) emphasizing interaction with community providers.
- Telemedicine "census rounds" 3 times per week involving community hospital providers and the academic center to assess appropriate back transport candidates, and provide follow-up on those patients referred to higher level of care.
- Obstetric census rounds twice weekly to assess need for transport to a higher level of care.

Arkansas was successful in implementing regionalized NICU care, changing the pattern of neonatal deliveries in telemedicine-equipped hospitals, which resulted in significantly lower IM.[2] Formative evaluations were used throughout the implementation process of regionalization. The formative evaluation process began with a granular assessment of IM data related to birthing hospital. The Arkansas Department of Health provided unbiased rigorous statistical assessment to evaluate the statewide hospital data. The implementation strategies used in Arkansas were centered around monthly 90-minute stakeholder meetings. Stakeholders included academic and community providers (physicians and/or hospital administrators) from *all* level 3 hospitals, the Arkansas Department of Health, Arkansas Hospital Association, March of Dimes, Arkansas Medicaid, Arkansas Chapter of the AAP, and parent representatives. Other strategies included a physician champion, telemedicine to engage rural community providers, technical assistance, and education (Peds PLACE). The Children's Hospital CEO, who was perceived to be authoritative and unbiased, chaired the committee. Formative evaluation and these implementation strategies have been used successfully in other contexts to improve guideline adoption.[25,26] The process was organized conceptually around the 4 stages of the Simpson Transfer Model, which has been used in a variety of technology adaptations. Its use in Arkansas and how telemedicine was used to implement those strategies are described in **Table 2**.[27] The model was successful as judged by the increase in the maternal transfer of mothers expected to deliver VLBW neonates to appropriate hospitals (**Fig. 3**). Data on IM were supplied

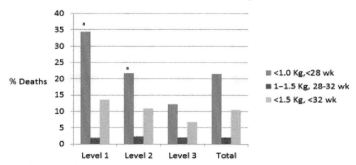

The Arkansas Story

Legend:
- <1.0 Kg,<28 wk
- 1–1.5 Kg, 28-32 wk
- <1.5 Kg, <32 wk

% Deaths (y-axis: 0–40)

Categories: Level 1, Level 2, Level 3, Total

Fig. 2. IM in designated nursery levels in Arkansas, 2001–2007. [a] $P<.001$. (Source: Arkansas Department of Health.)

Table 2
Utilization of Simpson transfer model

Stage	Methods	How Telemedicine Was Used
Exposure	Committee formed and exposed to the infant mortality (IM) data and place of delivery of very low birthweight neonates	Community neonatologists, pediatricians connected via telemedicine
Adoption	Intention to try a new approach to implementation of regionalization of care	Robust discussion over telemedicine by 2 groups adamantly opposed to outside control
Implementation	Exploratory evaluation of IM data, effects on census	Connectivity to the Department of Health, potential use in back transport
Practice	Frequent discussions over effects of regionalization	Frequent discussions regarding back transport candidates, clinical issues

by the Arkansas Department of Health. Without telemedicine, the committee would not have been able to engage the community partners on a regular basis, as they were all at least 2 hours' driving distance from the Perinatal Advisory meeting place. Community hospital stakeholder input throughout the process was essential for buy-in, especially because the hospitals and providers were being asked to give up patients (and revenue) to the larger perinatal centers. In addition, participation of all stakeholders throughout the process gave them the opportunity to review the data showing improved IM for the smallest infants at the larger perinatal centers. Peer pressure may have played a role in the ultimate acceptance of the perinatal guidelines.

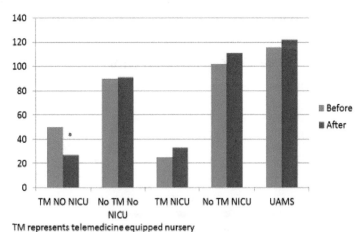

Change in number of deliveries before and after telemedicine intervention

TM represents telemedicine equipped nursery

Fig. 3. Differences in VLBW deliveries before versus after intervention in telemedicine-equipped hospitals. [a] $P = .0099$. Other values not significant.

Finally, the community hospitals asked and received data on IM and hospital of delivery as they requested it. Ultimately, the process proved successful statewide, with a significant reduction in IM (**Fig. 4**). In conclusion, telemedicine allowed the community hospitals and providers to participate fully in the process of regionalization without having to leave their own institution, saving time and money.

HOW CAN IMPLEMENTATION SCIENCE, USING TELEMEDICINE, BE USED IN OTHER STATES?

Widespread implementation of perinatal regionalization has not been achieved in many states, despite efforts by multiple groups such as respected national organizations and state health departments.[28] *Implementation science is the study of methods and strategies to promote the uptake of interventions that have proven effective into routine practice, with the aim of improving population health.* Using telemedicine technology, it was used to address the problem of perinatal regionalization. Although national guidelines provide an essential framework, implementation of optimal perinatal regionalization requires state-specific data. State and community-based support are essential for broad adoption of perinatal regionalization. Because states and communities have different cultures, ethnic groups, and laws, a "one-size-fits-all" approach is impractical. Although the literature is clear on the benefits of regionalization, there is little guidance on how to implement it. In Arkansas, telemedicine was used to initiate conversations with providers and stakeholders from rural communities regarding regionalization of care. The Arkansas implementation strategy package consisted of frequent telemedicine contacts (3 times weekly) with obstetric and pediatric providers in level 2 nurseries, a weekly pediatric educational conference with an emphasis on regionalization of care but with offerings related to other common pediatric problems, and 24/7 telemedicine consultation by maternal fetal medicine and neonatology providers at the perinatal center. The same strategy can be used by other states with telemedical connectivity.

Data provided by the Arkansas Department of Health were critical to the education of providers in Arkansas. Health department data can be used in other states because it is state-specific and trusted,. Thus, reliable evidence is essential to support regionalization of care in any state. The most difficult hurdle was that smaller rural nurseries

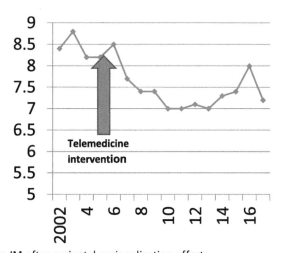

Fig. 4. Change in IM after perinatal regionalization efforts.

Table 3	
Strategies to optimize perinatal regionalization and lower infant mortality	
Process	**Specific Requirements**
Form stakeholder committee	Representatives from *all* community hospitals caring for very low birthweight neonates, American Academy of Pediatrics, American College of Obstetricians and Gynecologists, Medical Society, Hospital Association, March of Dimes, Health Department, academic institution, parent(s), administrative assistance.
Chair	Authoritative, unbiased.
Champion	Authoritative, unbiased (may or may not be the chair).
Telemedicine	*Connect all stakeholders, especially those in community hospitals. Local adaptation, understanding, and buy-in are essential.*
Technical assistance	Ability to troubleshoot telemedicine and connectivity issues.
Data acquisition	Reliable, unbiased. Granular assessment of data relating hospital of birth to infant mortality. Health Department data are ideal. Consider eliminating congenital anomalies, infants weighing less than 400 g.
Formative evaluation	Begin with granular data assessment, *focus* on infant mortality, process is data driven, encourage discussion of barriers from families, hospital chief executive officers, care providers, and families. Discuss how many infants can be saved; discuss effects of regionalization on all stakeholders; discuss various payment models; discuss quality indicators, such as volume.
Pilot testing	Test strategies to change delivery patterns, change in infant mortality.
Adapt strategies	Change strategies based on success or failure of pilot testing, assess fidelity to strategies.
Adopt strategies	Adopt successful strategies statewide, assess fidelity.

would have to give up some of their patients to the larger nurseries. Telemedicine helped to overcome that obstacle by disseminating the Department of Health data, providing education to all stakeholders, including hospital administrators, payers, nurses, and physicians. An aggressive back transport program, returning infants back to the referring hospital once they were stable, was seen as supporting local hospitals. Finally, trust was enhanced by the frequent contact. A suggested format for implementation strategies to optimize perinatal regionalization is summarized in **Table 3**.

SUMMARY

Perinatal regionalization is an effective way to lower IM. Despite the known advantages of perinatal regionalization, multiple barriers exist to its implementation. Implementation science, using telemedicine, can be used to overcome those barriers, enhancing the relationship between large perinatal centers and community hospitals.

DISCLOSURE

COBRE grant, NIGMS P20 103425.

REFERENCES

1. Lorch SA, Baiocchi M, Ahlberg CE, et al. The differential impact of delivery hospital on the outcomes of premature infants. Pediatrics 2012;130:270–8.

2. Kim EW, Teague-Ross TJ, Greenfield WW, et al. Telemedicine collaboration improves perinatal regionalization and lowers statewide infant mortality. J Perinatol 2013;33:725–30.

3. Hall-Barrow J, Hall RW, Burke BL Jr. Telemedicine and neonatal regionalization of care - ensuring that the right baby gets to the right nursery. Pediatr Ann 2009;38: 557–61.

4. Wall SN, Handler AS, Park CG. Hospital factors and nontransfer of small babies: a marker of deregionalized perinatal care? J Perinatology 2004;24:351–9.

5. Available at: www.cia.gov/library/publications/the-world-factbook/rankorder/2091rank.html.

6. Phibbs CS, Baker LC, Caughey AB, et al. Level and volume of neonatal intensive care and mortality in very-low-birth-weight infants. N Engl J Med 2007;356: 2165–75.

7. Rogowski JA, Horbar JD, Staiger DO, et al. Indirect vs direct hospital quality indicators for very low-birth-weight infants. JAMA 2004;291:202–9.

8. Bassan H, Limperopoulos C, Visconti K, et al. Neurodevelopmental outcome in survivors of periventricular hemorrhagic infarction. [see comment]. Pediatrics 2007;120:785–92.

9. Palmer KG, Kronsberg SS, Barton BA, et al. Effect of inborn versus outborn delivery on clinical outcomes in ventilated preterm neonates: secondary results from the NEOPAIN trial. J Perinatology 2005;25:270–5.

10. Towers CV, Bonebrake R, Padilla G, et al. The effect of transport on the rate of severe intraventricular hemorrhage in very low birth weight infants. Obstet Gynecol 2000;95:291–5.

11. Taylor JS, Shew SB. Impact of societal factors and health care delivery systems on gastroschisis outcomes. Semin Pediatr Surg 2018;27:316–20.

12. Kahn JM, Asch RJ, Iwashyna TJ, et al. Perceived barriers to the regionalization of adult critical care in the United States: a qualitative preliminary study. BMC Health Serv Res 2008;8:239.

13. Kahn JM, Asch RJ, Iwashyna TJ, et al. Physician attitudes toward regionalization of adult critical care: a national survey. Crit Care Med 2009;37:2149–54.

14. 2010 Census Urban and Rural Classification and Urban Area Criteria. 2010. Available at: https://www.census.gov/geo/reference/ua/urban-rural-2010.html.

15. Cartwright RD. Rural profile of Arkansas. University of Arkansas System Division of Agriculture; 2017. Available at: https://www.uaex.edu/publications/pdf/MP541.pdf.

16. Minority health and health disparities research and education act United States Public Law 106-525. Available at: https://www.govinfo.gov/content/pkg/PLAW-106publ525/pdf/PLAW-106publ525.pdf. 2000. p. 2498.

17. Hart LG, Salsberg E, Phillips DM, et al. Rural health care providers in the United States. J Rural Health 2002;18(Suppl):211–32.

18. Arora S, Thornton K, Murata G, et al. Outcomes of treatment for hepatitis C virus infection by primary care providers. N Engl J Med 2011;364:2199–207.

19. Portnoy JM, Waller M, De Lurgio S, et al. Telemedicine is as effective as in-person visits for patients with asthma. Ann Allergy Asthma Immunol 2016;117:241–5.

20. Fisk NM, Sepulveda W, Drysdale K, et al. Fetal telemedicine: six month pilot of real-time ultrasound and video consultation between the Isle of Wight and London. Br J Obstet Gynaecol 1996;103:1092-5.
21. McCrossan BA, Sands AJ, Kileen T, et al. Fetal diagnosis of congenital heart disease by telemedicine. Arch Dis Child Fetal Neonatal Ed 2011;96:F394-7.
22. Burke BL Jr, Hall RW, Section On Telehealth Care. Telemedicine: pediatric applications. Pediatrics 2015;136:e293-308.
23. Marcin JP. Telemedicine in the pediatric intensive care unit. Pediatr Clin North Am 2013;60:581-92.
24. Nugent R, Golden WE, Hall R, et al. Locations and outcomes of premature births in Arkansas. J Ark Med Soc 2011;107:258-9.
25. Naik AD, Lawrence B, Kiefer L, et al. Building a primary care/research partnership: lessons learned from a telehealth intervention for diabetes and depression. Fam Pract 2015;32:216-23.
26. Freed J, Lowe C, Flodgren G, et al. Telemedicine: Is it really worth it? A perspective from evidence and experience. J Innov Health Inform 2018;25:14-8.
27. Simpson DD. A conceptual framework for transferring research to practice. J Subst Abuse Treat 2002;22:171-82.
28. Kastenberg ZJ, Lee HC, Profit J, et al. Effect of deregionalized care on mortality in very low-birth-weight infants with necrotizing enterocolitis. JAMA Pediatr 2015; 169:26-32.

Implementing Telehealth in Pediatric Asthma

Tamara T. Perry, MD[a,b,*], Callie A. Margiotta, BS[b]

KEYWORDS

- Telemedicine • Asthma • Pediatrics

KEY POINTS

- Telemedicine can be used to deliver recommended asthma care in regions with inadequate access to specialists.
- Telemedicine can be used for pediatric asthma care to reduce travel burden for rural patients and families.
- Telemedicine can be used to reach patients in a variety of settings, including school-based and community settings.

PROBLEM TO BE SOLVED BY TELEMEDICINE

Asthma is one of the most frequent causes of pediatric health care use, with more than 1.8 million emergency department (ED) visits annually among children, and more than 13.8 million school days missed annually because of follow-up doctors' visits, acute illness, or uncontrolled symptoms.[1,2] Risk factors for poor asthma outcomes include increased exposure to environmental triggers,[3] financial barriers,[4] and reduced social support.[5] Uncontrolled asthma can lead to significant financial and social strain caused by costs associated with acute health care use[6]; time away from work for caregivers[7]; and travel, especially among patients living in rural regions who have to drive long distances to see their nearest asthma specialist.[8] Prior research has shown that guidelines-based care is more likely when asthma care is managed by a specialist,[9] and better outcomes are associated with guidelines-based care.[10] However, patients with the greatest need for asthma specialists often live in underserved areas, such as rural and low-income communities, where few asthma specialists exist.[11] Telemedicine should be used to remove or significantly reduce barriers to specialty care.

This article originally appeared in *Pediatric Clinics*, Volume 67, Issue 4, August 2020.
[a] Department of Pediatrics, University of Arkansas for Medical Sciences, 4301 West Markham Street, Little Rock, AR 72205, USA; [b] Arkansas Children's Research Institute, 13 Children's Way, Slot 512-13, Little Rock, AR 72202, USA
* Corresponding author. Department of Pediatrics, Allergy and Immunology Division, University of Arkansas for Medical Sciences, 13 Children's Way, Slot 512-13, Little Rock, AR 72202.
E-mail address: perrytamarat@uams.edu

Clinics Collections 10 (2021) 99–103
https://doi.org/10.1016/j.ccol.2020.12.010
2352-7986/21/© 2020 Elsevier Inc. All rights reserved.

CAN TELEMEDICINE BE USED TO IMPROVE ASTHMA CARE?

Asthma is a chronic condition with variability in symptoms over time caused by underlying severity, medication adherence, trigger exposure, and seasonal changes. National asthma guidelines recommend targeted asthma education and regular follow-up care as key aspects for monitoring disease control and asthma management.[10]

Because children spend most of their waking hours at school, prior investigations have assessed the use of school-based telemedicine (SBTM) interventions to improve asthma outcomes for underserved populations.[12] Perry and colleagues[13] implemented a randomized controlled trial in the rural Delta region of Arkansas to assess the effectiveness of an SBTM asthma education program compared with usual care among children enrolled in public schools. There was evidence of behavior change for intervention participants, with improvement in reported use of asthma medications and peak flow meter monitoring. However, no significant differences in the number of symptom-free-days (SFDs), compared with baseline, were found for either group. Investigators concluded that tele-education alone was insufficient to overcome the significant baseline morbidity among the study population.[13] Halterman and colleagues[14] implemented a comprehensive SBTM intervention that included directly observed therapy for daily preventive asthma medications as well as telemedicine follow-up care visits with the child's primary care provider. Children in the intervention group had more SFDs and reduced acute health care use compared with an enhanced usual-care group. Other investigators have proved feasibility for implementing SBTM interventions as well as their effectiveness in improving asthma outcomes, such as reduction in ED visits and improved quality of life.[15,16]

Asthma guidelines recommend that changes in medication therapy be guided by patient-reported symptoms and/or objective findings, such as lung function testing (or spirometry).[10] Spirometry with highly trained asthma specialists and respiratory therapists is particularly important among pediatric patients, who may need specific coaching and other techniques geared for children. For patients living in regions with poor access to specialty care, remote spirometry via telemedicine allows guidelines-based recommendations to monitor lung function. Berlinski and colleagues[17] reported the successful implementation of remote spirometry in rural settings with no adverse events and rates of interpretable spirometry data resembling rates of in-person spirometry.

Asthma guidelines address the importance of self-management through the use of a personalized asthma action plan[10] (AAP). Traditional paper AAPs are static, lack patient engagement,[18] and require patients to keep track of a paper document. To address these concerns, Perry and colleagues[19] implemented a randomized trial to compare the use and effectiveness of an interactive smartphone-based AAP with paper AAP among teens, a group at risk for poor asthma outcomes. Patients in the intervention group accessed their smartphone AAP more times per week compared with the paper AAP group. Intervention subjects with uncontrolled asthma at baseline showed improved Asthma Control Test scores after using the smartphone AAP for 6 months, whereas no improvements were seen in the control group. Findings suggest smartphone AAPs are a feasible method for improving self-management and asthma outcomes in this hard-to-reach pediatric population.

DIFFICULTIES AND BARRIERS TO IMPLEMENTATION OF TELEMEDICINE
Funding and Reimbursement

Financial sustainability is a significant barrier to establishing as well as maintaining a telemedicine program. The cost of technology proves to be a deciding factor, because of the need for significant investment in infrastructure when implementing telemedicine programs. Comprehensive telemedicine carts cost $10,000 to $35,000 for a single site,[20] plus there may be additional costs associated with the purchase of Health Insurance Portability and Accountability Act–compliant software. For rural telemedicine sites, high-speed Internet capabilities may be another added expense because these sites often lack the bandwidth to support the high-quality videoconferencing necessary for satisfactory telemedicine visits.[21]

In a national survey of pediatric telemedicine programs, lack of financial reimbursement is also cited as a main barrier to implementing telemedicine.[20] Parity in coverage and reimbursement is not currently federally mandated, and each state does not define and regulate telehealth in the same way, so states differ in the extent to which insurers reimburse.[22] To receive universal acceptance, there is a need for consistent state policy backing and increased government stakeholder support for implementing telemedicine programs.

Provider licensure and uptake
Another barrier includes licensure for physicians who want to provide remote care for patients across state lines. Regulations require provider licensure in the state of the originating site (patient's location), limiting providers' ability to see patients outside their home states, unless they are licensed in multiple states. The Interstate Medical Licensure Compact (IMLC) offers an expedited pathway for multistate licensure; however, IMLC is not available in all states. Another significant barrier to telemedicine is provider readiness and acceptability. Some providers are hesitant to implement telemedicine because of concerns that technology depersonalizes the patient-physician relationship.[23] However, current literature supports the use of telemedicine, with reports of high patient satisfaction because of the convenience, which enhances providers' ability to reach their patients.[8,24] Physicians need proper training to use the software and equipment because, with technology, there is always a possibility for technological glitches or lags that can further complicate the physician and patient experience. Physicians also must have a backup plan if the connection is lost as well as needing to set enough time before each visit to run tests, making sure there are no connectivity issues.[8] These extra steps for providing care outside of the traditional clinic setting can seem daunting if physicians are not properly informed of the added benefits of telemedicine. The health care industry is beginning to adapt to the ever-changing technological environment, albeit at a slower rate than technology is advancing. In light of this, physicians and the health care community should embrace these advances and integrate telemedicine into the medical school curriculum.

POTENTIAL FOR COST SAVINGS

Asthma is the third leading cause of hospitalizations in children younger than 15 years,[25] resulting in a significant health care cost burden. Acute health care use is dramatically reduced or avoided through proper asthma management.[26] Because outpatient care generally costs less for insurance companies than hospital-based inpatient care, conducting follow-up visits via telemedicine is a viable option to provide accessible and cost-effective preventive care. Bian and colleagues[15] report on the successful implementation of school-based telemedicine clinics that allowed students who needed immediate care during school hours to see pediatric clinicians. Clinicians were able to provide prompt clinical services to children as well as school nurse education on the proper administration of asthma medications. Investigators reported a 21% reduction in ED visits among the subsample of children with asthma.

According to a 2016 study, no-show rates of in-person visits in the United States exceed 20%.[27] Telemedicine can relieve this burden by making follow-up care more accessible. Portnoy and colleagues[28] reported that patients enrolled in telemedicine visits were more likely to complete all 3 of their follow-up asthma visits compared with usual in-person visits. This finding further encourages health care cost-saving opportunities by decreasing no-show rates and allowing specialists to see more patients.

SUMMARY

The nature of chronic disease management such as asthma in children calls for collaboration between patients, parents, educators, and physicians. Telemedicine has the potential to reach patients in a variety of settings, including school-based and community settings, thus providing more accessible care to patients who are at the highest risk. Inadequate access to specialists and travel burden for patients and families can lead to school/work absenteeism and poor compliance with treatment plans. Increased rates of cancellations and no-shows can lead to uncontrolled asthma outcomes requiring hospitalizations and acute health care use. Telemedicine provides an avenue for increasing convenient access to specialty care, leading to increased compliance with treatment plans. Current literature suggests that telemedicine is comparable with in-person asthma care. However, with continued implementation of larger-scale research designs, there is a call to further prove that these various telehealth models are not only equally effective but can improve patient satisfaction and chronic disease control long term. Technological advancements continue to increase the scope that medical practices reach, proving telemedicine to be beneficial for patients, providers, health care companies, and insurers. With the climate of the health care system and the difficulties clinicians now face, it is vital for telemedicine to be used as a solution to deliver convenient patient care to all.

DISCLOSURE

The authors have nothing to disclose.

REFERENCES

1. Zahran HS, Bailey CM, Damon SA, et al. Vital signs: asthma in children - United States, 2001-2016. MMWR Morb Mortal Wkly Rep 2018;67:149–55.
2. Johnson LH, Chambers P, Dexheimer JW. Asthma-related emergency department use: current perspectives. Open Access Emerg Med 2016;8:47–55.
3. Coleman AT, Rettiganti M, Bai S, et al. Mouse and cockroach exposure in rural Arkansas Delta region homes. Ann Allergy Asthma Immunol 2014;112:256–60.
4. Beck AF, Huang B, Simmons JM, et al. Role of financial and social hardships in asthma racial disparities. Pediatrics 2014;133:431–9.
5. Williams DR, Sternthal M, Wright RJ. Social determinants: taking the social context of asthma seriously. Pediatrics 2009;123(Suppl 3):S174–84.
6. Nurmagambetov T, Kuwahara R, Garbe P. The economic burden of asthma in the United States, 2008-2013. Ann Am Thorac Soc 2018;15:348–56.
7. Dean BB, Calimlim BM, Kindermann SL, et al. The impact of uncontrolled asthma on absenteeism and health-related quality of life. J Asthma 2009;46:861–6.
8. Taylor L, Waller M, Portnoy JM. Telemedicine for allergy services to rural communities. J Allergy Clin Immunol Pract 2019;7(8):2554–9.

9. Diette GB, Skinner EA, Nguyen TT, et al. Comparison of quality of care by specialist and generalist physicians as usual source of asthma care for children. Pediatrics 2001;108:432–7.
10. National asthma education and prevention program expert panel report 3: guidelines for the Diagnosis and Management of Asthma. National Heart Lung and Blood Institute; 2007. NIH Publication No. 07-4051. 2012.
11. Ownby DR. Asthma in rural America. Ann Allergy Asthma Immunol 2005;95:S17–22.
12. Perry TT, Turner JH. School-based telemedicine for asthma management. J Allergy Clin Immunol Pract 2019;7:2524–32.
13. Perry TT, Halterman JS, Brown RH, et al. Results of an asthma education program delivered via telemedicine in rural schools. Ann Allergy Asthma Immunol 2018; 120:401–8.
14. Halterman JS, Fagnano M, Tajon RS, et al. Effect of the school-based telemedicine enhanced asthma management (SB-TEAM) program on asthma morbidity: a randomized clinical trial. JAMA Pediatr 2018;172:e174938.
15. Bian J, Cristaldi KK, Summer AP, et al. Association of a school-based, asthma-focused telehealth program with emergency department visits among children enrolled in South Carolina Medicaid. JAMA Pediatr 2019. https://doi.org/10.1001/jamapediatrics.2019.3073.
16. Romano MJ, Hernandez J, Gaylor A, et al. Improvement in asthma symptoms and quality of life in pediatric patients through specialty care delivered via telemedicine. Telemed J E Health 2001;7:281–6.
17. Berlinski A, Chervinskiy SK, Simmons AL, et al. Delivery of high-quality pediatric spirometry in rural communities: A novel use for telemedicine. J Allergy Clin Immunol Pract 2018;6:1042–4.
18. Hynes L, Durkin K, Williford DN, et al. Comparing written versus pictorial asthma action plans to improve asthma management and health outcomes among children and adolescents: protocol of a pilot and feasibility randomized controlled trial. JMIR Res Protoc 2019;8:e11733.
19. Perry TT, Marshall A, Berlinski A, et al. Smartphone-based vs paper-based asthma action plans for adolescents. Ann Allergy Asthma Immunol 2017;118:298–303.
20. Olson CA, McSwain SD, Curfman AL, et al. The current pediatric telehealth landscape. Pediatrics 2018;141 [pii:e20172334].
21. Scott Kruse C, Karem P, Shifflett K, et al. Evaluating barriers to adopting telemedicine worldwide: A systematic review. J Telemed Telecare 2018;24:4–12.
22. Available at: https://www.cchpca.org/sites/default/files/2019-05/cchp_report_MASTER_spring_2019_FINAL.pdf. Accessed October 1, 2019.
23. Elliott T, Shih J, Dinakar C, et al. American College of Allergy, Asthma & Immunology position paper on the use of telemedicine for allergists. Ann Allergy Asthma Immunol 2017;119:512–7.
24. Utidjian L, Abramson E. Pediatric telehealth: opportunities and challenges. Pediatr Clin North Am 2016;63:367–78.
25. Available at: https://www.epa.gov/sites/production/files/2016-05/documents/asthma_fact_sheet_english_05_2016.pdf. Accessed October 1, 2019.
26. Rangachari P. A framework for measuring self-management effectiveness and health care use among pediatric asthma patients and families. J Asthma Allergy 2017;10:111–22.
27. Kheirkhah P, Feng Q, Travis LM, et al. Prevalence, predictors and economic consequences of no-shows. BMC Health Serv Res 2016;16:13.
28. Portnoy JM, Waller M, De Lurgio S, et al. Telemedicine is as effective as in-person visits for patients with asthma. Ann Allergy Asthma Immunol 2016;117:241–5.

Implementing Telehealth in Pediatric Type 1 Diabetes Mellitus

Jennifer L. Fogel, PhD[a], Jennifer K. Raymond, MD, MCR[a,b,*]

KEYWORDS

• Telehealth • Telemedicine • Type 1 diabetes mellitus • Pediatric endocrinology
• Chronic disease management

KEY POINTS

• Type 1 diabetes mellitus (T1D) is a lifelong disease requiring intensive glucose, insulin, food, activity, and lifestyle monitoring.
• Pediatric endocrinologists are geographically distributed unevenly, with some patients and their families spending extended time traveling to and from appointments on at least a quarterly basis.
• Telehealth technologies engage patients struggling to attend regular medical appointments.
• Telehealth technologies increase T1D patients' adherence to American Diabetes Association care guidelines and improve their quality of life.

Diabetes is and will remain a major health epidemic in the United States, with a projected increase of 54% to more than 54.9 million Americans living with diabetes between 2015 and 2030.[1] With the growing prevalence of diabetes, there is a reciprocal increase in demand for endocrinologists specializing in diabetes care. Although the Endocrine Society projects that there would be no gap in pediatric endocrinologist supply and demand,[2] there is a substantial uneven geographic distribution of pediatric endocrinologists across the United States, with ratios of children with diabetes to pediatric endocrinologists more than double in the Midwest (370:1), South (335:1), and West (367:1) compared with the Northeast (144:1).[3] Additionally, only 64.1% of US children have access to an endocrinologist within 20 miles, with the percentage going up to only 85.5% within 50 miles.[4] With most pediatric endocrinologists who manage diabetes located in large cities and academic centers, some patients in rural areas spend a significant amount of time traveling to appointments, with parents

This article originally appeared in *Pediatric Clinics*, Volume 67, Issue 4, August 2020.
[a] Division of Endocrinology, Department of Pediatrics, Children's Hospital Los Angeles, 4650 Sunset Boulevard, Los Angeles, CA 90027, USA; [b] Keck School of Medicine of the University of Southern California, 1975 Zonal Avenue, Los Angeles, CA 90089, USA
* Corresponding author. Division of Endocrinology, Department of Pediatrics, Children's Hospital Los Angeles, 4650 Sunset Boulevard, Los Angeles, CA 90027.
E-mail address: jraymond@chla.usc.edu

Clinics Collections 10 (2021) 105–108
https://doi.org/10.1016/j.ccol.2020.12.011
2352-7986/21/© 2020 Elsevier Inc. All rights reserved.

and patients missing up to a full day of work and school.[5,6] As with most chronic disease care, the American Diabetes Association recommends that children with type 1 diabetes mellitus (T1D) see their provider or other diabetes team members every 3 months, therefore significantly increasing the amount of time lost from work and school for patients and their families. Telehealth can change the current standard of care, allowing for increased access to providers and improved patient health outcomes in a cost-effective way.

Management of T1D lends itself well to telehealth because current technologies enable frequent communication between patients and their providers, and remote data sharing allows for review and adjustments in diabetes regimens. As with most chronic disease management, patients with T1D are required to have frequent appointments with their providers. With most patients with T1D diagnosed around late elementary or middle school age, telehealth technologies can be used to reach patients who are struggling to attend their quarterly medical appointments. As part of diabetes care management, physical examinations and vital signs likely are not critical for every visit; however, the care team can partner with a patient's primary care doctor if an examination or vital signs are needed, or patients can go to a local pharmacy for blood pressure checks. The required medical information—laboratory testing (eg, hemoglobin A_{1c}) and diabetes device data (from glucometers, insulin pumps, and continuous glucose monitors)—can be collected at a local laboratory and downloaded remotely, respectively, and then shared virtually with the provider.[5–7]

With the implementation of technology specializing in shared medical data, the comparison of telehealth versus in-person provider visits is minimal, with the main difference being the ability to perform a physical examination and take vital signs. Although there is minimal access to devices allowing for routine collection of vital signs via a telehealth appointment, providers have the ability to perform limited virtual physical examinations. Virtual physical examinations can include a general description of the patient, evaluation of work of breathing, skin findings, review of shot and pump sites, and so forth. There are certain telehealth tools that exist to allow for full physical examinations (eg, stethoscope and otoscope), but currently these are not options for routine home-based telehealth care. Another difference between in-person and telehealth appointments is the process for scheduling and connecting patients, which varies by platform.[5,7,8] In general, providers send emails or invitations for a visit. Patients then open and download any necessary apps onto computers or mobile devices. Most platforms allow for patients to enter a virtual waiting room prior to seeing the provider and/or can be seen and connected for a visit only when the provider opens the appointment.

There always are difficulties, challenges, and lessons learned when a new system of doing things is implemented, and telehealth is no different. Challenges arise with training patients and providers on how to use telehealth platforms, complete diabetes device downloads, and order and complete laboratory testing prior to provider appointments.[7,8] Therefore, having team members available for practice sessions prior to first appointments and being accessible to support the telehealth connection troubleshooting before and during visits are recommended. Providers have additional challenges in restructuring visits to ensure all required information is collected as well as addressing any anxiety or hesitation that may occur with implementing a new approach to medicine. Clinics will face their own technical, legal, financial, and documentation challenges that necessitate changes to scheduling, planning of laboratory integration prior to visits, online educational and onboarding resources for patients, new electronic medical record notes, and billing processes that can be slow to implement and require support from the entire hospital. Telehealth clinic visits should be completed in telehealth-only clinics and not mixed with in-person patients, because staying on time with telehealth clinics typically is easier than in-person clinics, due to elimination of the time required for rooming patients, no need to wait for vital signs, and no associated delays due to patients seeing multiple staff members. Additional challenges include ensuring that providers, patients, and their families have adequate Internet access and a private space for visits, that patients need to be within a provider's state of medical license at the time of their appointment, and that currently telehealth laws are different from state to state. Patience and appreciation are necessary for everyone involved while learning a new way to do medicine.

The use of telehealth for routine care has been shown to be equal to if not better than, in a variety of measurements, in-person care. Studies focused on patients with T1D demonstrated that telehealth allows for easier and more frequent contact with medical providers, increasing the population's adherence to American Diabetes Association guidelines and improving their retention in care, especially among young adults facing a challenging transitional period in their lives.[5,7,8] Additionally, telehealth appointments resulted in high rates of care satisfaction,[5–8] significant reduction in the amount of time off required from work and school,[7,8] increase in use of diabetes technologies,[6] and an indication of improved quality of life,[9] with no significant changes in cost.[9] Although these previous studies demonstrated these improvements occurred without a change in hemoglobin A_{1c} levels, Crossen and colleagues[8] recently reported an improvement in glycemic control and adherence to recommended outpatient care among high-risk pediatric patients with T1D participating in telehealth care visits.

Telehealth technology has been used and well accepted for its ability to reach patients struggling to attend routine medical care appointments, including pediatric patients with T1D. It is now time to develop manuals of procedures and best practices, train additional providers to slowly expand the use of telehealth, and adapt the model for implementation in low-socioeconomic-status populations as well as in racial/ethnic minority populations. Finally, telehealth should be considered for use with other alternative care models (such as shared medical appointments[10]) and expanded to care for patients with other endocrine disorders and with other chronic diseases currently managed in traditional medical appointments.

DISCLOSURE

Donaghue Foundation, ID# RGA011022.

REFERENCES

1. Rowley WR, Clement B, Arikan Y, et al. Diabetes 2030: insights from yesterday, today, and future trends. Popul Health Manag 2017;20(1):6–12.
2. Vigersky RA, Fish L, Hogan P, et al. The clinical endocrinology workforce: current status and future projections of supply and demand. J Clin Endocrinol Metab 2014;99(9):3112–21.
3. Lee JM, Davis MM, Menon RK, et al. Geographic distribution of childhood diabetes and obesity relative to the supply of pediatric endocrinologists in the United States. J Pediatr 2008;152(3):331–6.
4. Lu H, Holt JB, Cheng YJ, et al. Population-based geographic access to endocrinologists in the United States, 2012. BMC Health Serv Res 2015;15:541.
5. Wood CL, Clements SA, McFann K, et al. Use of telemedicine to improve adherence to american diabetes association standards in pediatric type 1 diabetes. Diabetes Technol Ther 2016;18(1):7–14.

6. Reid MW, Krishnan S, Berget C, et al. CoYoT1 clinic: home telemedicine increases young adult engagement in diabetes care. Diabetes Technol Ther 2018;20(5):370–9.

7. Raymond JK, Berget CL, Driscoll KA, et al. CoYoT1 clinic: innovative telemedicine care model for young adults with type 1 diabetes. Diabetes Technol Ther 2016; 18(6):385–90.

8. Crossen SS, Marcin JP, Qi L, et al. Home visits for children and adolescents with uncontrolled type 1 diabetes. Diabetes Technol Ther 2020;22(1):34–41.

9. Wan W, Nathan AG, Skandari MR, et al. Cost-effectiveness of shared telemedicine appointments in young adults with T1D: CoYoT1 trial. Diabetes Care 2019; 42(8):1589–92.

10. Bakhach M, Reid MW, Pyatak EA, et al. Home telemedicine (CoYoT1 Clinic): a novel approach to improve psychosocial outcomes in young adults with diabetes. Diabetes Educ 2019;45(4):420–30.

Telehealth Opportunities and Challenges for Managing Pediatric Obesity

Victor Cueto, MD, MS[a],*, Lee M. Sanders, MD, MPH[b]

KEYWORDS

- Pediatric obesity • Telehealth • mHealth

KEY POINTS

- Telehealth offers an acceptable and feasible approach for the treatment of pediatric obesity.
- Telehealth can address the unmet needs and common challenges of clinical care for pediatric obesity.
- Telehealth for pediatric obesity has the potential to improve access to care, engagement and satisfaction with care.

INTRODUCTION

The treatment and management of pediatric obesity is challenging. The cornerstone of medical treatment for pediatric obesity aims to promote lifestyle modification through the support of behavioral changes involving dietary and physical activity habits.[1-3] The most effective interventions are comprehensive behavioral programs that include multiple components, delivered by a multidisciplinary team, and involve a large amount of contact hours as well as a high frequency of visits between patients, families, and providers.[3] These comprehensive programs require considerable care coordination, and a significant investment of time, transportation, effort, and resources. Unfortunately, this model of care is often inconvenient, burdensome, and inaccessible, particularly for patients and families in underserved or rural communities.[4-7] Furthermore, the number of patients and families who need intensive behavioral therapy exceed the number of appropriately trained primary care providers and tertiary care centers available to offer services.[8,9] Ultimately, access to treatment is limited and programs suffer

This article originally appeared in *Pediatric Clinics*, Volume 67, Issue 4, August 2020.
[a] Division of General Internal Medicine, Department Internal Medicine, Rutgers New Jersey Medical School, 150 Bergen Street, Room H-251, Newark, NJ 07103, USA; [b] Division of General Pediatrics, Department Pediatrics, Stanford University School of Medicine, 1265 Welch Rd, 240x, Stanford, CA 94305, USA
* Corresponding author.
E-mail address: victor.cueto@rutgers.edu

from poor patient engagement and a high degree of attrition.[10,11] Telehealth holds significant promise for overcoming each of these challenges and has the potential to address geographic and logistical barriers, as well as improve access to primary care practices and tertiary care centers.

TELEHEALTH IN PRACTICE OF PEDIATRIC OBESITY

Telehealth is particularly well suited for pediatric obesity because the diagnosis, treatment, and ongoing management of this condition is not usually dependent on a physical examination or physical presence. Telehealth approaches to pediatric obesity are inclusive of a wide range of modalities, including human-to-human interactions via remote visits, interactive human-to-human text messaging, automated and algorithmic messaging independent of human contact, interactive mobile applications (apps), and multiple combinations of these and other emerging technologies.[12–20] Tradition has established the current practice of in-person visits and evaluations, yet there is arguably little in regard to the assessment and ongoing management of pediatric obesity that could not be accomplished using telehealth.

Telehealth Diagnosis and Assessment

Telehealth approaches may enhance the efficiency of obesity diagnosis and assessment. The initial evaluation of obesity is inclusive of a comprehensive history and thorough review of growth and weight trajectory, and an assessment of weight, height, blood pressure, and physical examination by well-trained professionals. Telehealth may be particularly well suited for the collection of important components of the initial evaluation, such as obtaining a family history, current and past medication use, past experience with self-directed or supervised weight management interventions, social history and home environment, sleep history, and an accurate record of usual dietary and physical activity habits.

Ongoing assessment of pediatric obesity through telehealth is made using reliable measurements of height and weight, and blood pressure, collected remotely at settings other than a clinic, such as at home or in a school health office. Bluetooth-enabled devices, such as scales and blood pressure cuffs, may transfer these measurements remotely to the medical record.

Telehealth may also aid the assessment of key physical examination findings pertinent to obesity and related comorbidities, such as acanthosis nigricans, hirsutism, intertrigo, or striae, which could be reliably ascertained through a telehealth format that incorporates synchronous video technology or asynchronous high-definition image technology. However, in-person visits may still be necessary to assess and monitor examination findings, such as lymphedema or joint tenderness, that require touch or advanced examination techniques.

Diagnostic evaluation for rare endogenous or exogenous causes of obesity and laboratory screening for common comorbid conditions, such as dyslipidemia, nonalcoholic fatty liver disease, polycystic ovarian syndrome, and metabolic syndrome, could also be accomplished using telehealth platforms that are integrated with electronic medical records.

Approach to Telehealth Treatment

The aim of medical treatment of pediatric obesity is to promote lifestyle modification and support behavior change. The essential components of effective interventions for pediatric obesity in primary care, specialty, and comprehensive behavioral programs involve providing education and information regarding diet and exercise behavior, while supporting ongoing self-monitoring, goal setting, and problem solving.[1–3] Clinical interventions may be delivered through individual or group sessions involving parents and children, separately or together. The components of the traditional in-person treatment model for pediatric obesity are entirely compatible with a telehealth approach, and may perhaps be more efficiently delivered using telehealth.

Beyond translating existing in-person treatment approaches to telehealth, the incorporation of additional established and emergent technologies into pediatric obesity care may serve to support and augment care. Specifically, the use of wearable devices (eg, smart wristbands, smart watches) and mobile apps (eg, health tracking software) may facilitate self-monitoring and improve personalization of treatment regimens.[12] These mobile technologies may also provide clinicians and patients with more continuous and richer data that can support individual behavior change and feedback, as well as assist clinicians with population health management.

Aside from medical treatment, the use of telehealth for pediatric obesity has also involved using telehealth modalities to support prebariatric and postbariatric surgery activities. Bariatric surgery is recommended and highly efficacious for adolescents and young adults who have not improved with lifestyle modification or suffer from severe obesity and comorbidities.[2,21] Telehealth has shown utility for delivering interventions and supporting the clinical care of patients before and after surgical procedures by facilitating treatment components, such as exercise and preventing regain of weight.[22,23]

Telehealth Treatment Models and Modalities

There have been limited published reports of telehealth modalities for the clinical treatment of pediatric obesity. However, the existing evidence from research studies and clinical practice have shown that a telehealth approach to treatment is feasible, well accepted, and comparable with traditional in-person care.[14–16] Studies and clinical practice models have incorporated multiple telehealth modalities including telephone, text messaging, and live video. These telehealth approaches have been heterogeneous in their involvement of staff, including physicians, specialists, dietitians, and health coaches. Similarly, treatment models have differed in that some have used direct telehealth, where a provider communicates with patients and families, whereas others have used teleconsultation, whereby a specialist supports care and provides consultation.

Studies highlighting different telehealth modalities and telehealth clinical models are presented in **Table 1**. These studies were selectively chosen as examples of the wide heterogeneity of technologies and staffing models used in treating obesity using telehealth. Additionally, these studies also showcase a few important findings and lessons learned in the implementation of telehealth for rural and urban populations, and the role of telehealth for improving access to services. These examples of telehealth implementation in the clinical practice of pediatric obesity underscore the utility of the approach, its potential benefits as compared with traditional care, and the unmet needs that motivate use.

Because of the geographic barriers to care and high prevalence of obesity in rural areas, a considerable proportion of telehealth studies in pediatric obesity have involved rural settings. A randomized controlled study of a rural population by Davis and colleagues[14] is notable for finding outcomes to be comparable between telemedicine visits from psychologists and traditional visits by primary care physicians. Another rural study by Irby and colleagues,[18] which showcases an obesity clinic innovation that adapted an existing tertiary clinical model to a telemedicine format, found that the telemedicine program considerably increased access to care while

Table 1
Selected studies highlighting telehealth modalities and models for pediatric obesity

Modality	Study/Setting	Care Model	Lessons Learned	Author
Tele-visits	RCT Rural	PCP visits vs psychologist tele-visits	Comparable attrition Telemedicine encounter similar to face-to-face per psychologists Comparable outcomes	Davis et al,[14] 2013
Tele-visits	Observational Rural	Specialist clinic visits vs specialist tele-visits	Increased access Comparable outcomes Comparable attrition	Irby et al,[18] 2012
Tele-visits	RCT, crossover Urban	PCP visits vs PCP visits + specialist tele-visit	Increased access Time saved for work/school Preference for tele-visits	Fleischman et al. Fleischman A, Hourigan SE, Lyon HN, et al. Creating an Integrated Care Model for Childhood Obesity: A Randomized Pilot Study Utilizing Telehealth in a Community Primary Care Setting. *Clin Obes.* 2016;6(6):380-388. doi:10.1111/ cob.12166
Tele-visits	Observational Survey Urban	Specialist clinic vs specialist tele-visits	No difference in satisfaction	Mulgrew et al,[16] 2011
Mobile app Tele-visits	Observational Retrospective cohort	Health coaches	High level of engagement Low level of attrition Change in weight status	Cueto et al,[17] 2019
Tele-visits Texting	RCT Urban	PCP + text vs PCP + text + health coach (tele/in-person)	Feasible and well accepted Comparable outcomes Greater satisfaction with health coaching	Taveras et al,[15] 2017

(continued on next page)

Table 1 *(continued)*				
Modality	Study/Setting	Care Model	Lessons Learned	Author
Tele-visits Texting GIS mapping	RCT Urban	PCP + text vs. PCP + text + health coach (tele/in-person)	High satisfaction Parents recommend video tele-visits Travel cost and time savings Tele-visits promoted face-face interaction	Bala et al,[13] 2019

Abbreviations: PCP, primary care provider; RCT, randomized controlled trial; GIS (geographic information system); tele, telehealth.

maintaining comparable engagement and clinical outcomes, as compared with the traditional program. Studies that have examined satisfaction with telehealth for pediatric obesity have either found no difference in satisfaction between traditional care and telehealth or improved satisfaction with telehealth.

A recent analysis by Bala and colleagues[13] of secondary data from a randomized controlled trial that used health coaching video visits, found video visits to be well received and accepted by families. The primary reasons reported for satisfaction with health coaching video visits included savings on travel costs and time, and the ability to have a face-to-face interaction. Overall, implementation of different telehealth modalities in clinical practice and clinical research interventions has been reported to be well accepted and satisfying for participants, increase access, save time and cost, and have comparable outcomes to traditional care.

Outside of clinical practice, the broader field of telehealth involving mobile devices and mobile health (mHealth) in pediatric obesity is fairly nascent. The bulk of pediatric studies have used text messaging and mobile apps as adjunctive or supportive elements of multicomponent interventions.[12] In a supportive role, text messaging and mobile devices have been shown to be feasible in aiding self-monitoring and promoting behavior changes related to pediatric obesity. Of note, the evidence for messaging technology, digital health, and mHealth is more robust for adults than pediatrics. Scalable and affordable evidence-based modalities in this field include unidirectional text messaging, bidirectional messaging, artificial intelligence enabled interactions, and fully automated approaches.[24,25] However, there is a lack of evidence for mHealth solutions as stand-alone modalities for treatment in pediatrics.[12] Similarly, research has shown that most mobile apps targeting pediatric obesity are commercially available, but not evidence-based or informed by expert recommendations.[26,27] This is an area of active research with ongoing studies and emerging research.[28–30]

Mobile devices have the potential to integrate multiple telehealth modalities, such as text messaging, telemedicine video visits, and mobile apps. This is evidenced in our study examining a commercial program consisting of multiple components including health coaching through video sessions, text messaging with health coaches, and self-monitoring through a mobile app platform, which found that participants maintained a high level of engagement, with a low degree of attrition, and a change in weight status associated with the number of coaching sessions received.[17] These findings suggest that mHealth solutions that integrate multiple modalities may emerge as an option for stand-alone treatment or a new avenue for providing clinical care for pediatric obesity using telehealth. The utility and role of multimodal mhealth platforms warrants further research.

Research Opportunities

Several ongoing controlled studies are testing the efficacy of telehealth modalities for obesity prevention and treatment.[28–30] Further clinical and population-based research is necessary to assess the utility and effectiveness of emerging telehealth innovation and treatment protocols. Comparative effectiveness studies should examine the relative contribution of different telehealth modalities to improve health outcomes (eg, blood pressure and adiposity) and comorbidities, and promote health behavior change (eg, dietary and physical activity). Potential research questions include the following:

- What is the utility of telehealth by provider type (eg, primary care, health coach, obesity specialist)?
- What is the comparative benefit of synchronous, asynchronous, and combined models of telehealth care?
- What is the relevant impact of different independent and combined telehealth approaches (eg, tele-visits, video coaching, text messaging, or mobile apps)?

Implementation science studies should explore models of telehealth in clinical practice that incorporate evidence-based protocols with different staffing patterns and treatment regimens with varying frequency of visits. Clinical intervention and population level studies should also examine the impact of telehealth on health disparities and underserved groups. A particular hypothesis to be explored is whether telehealth may be especially beneficial for low-income patients and families, for whom time away from work and school devoted to in-person visits may represent a disparate financial burden.

FUTURE OF TELEHEALTH IN PEDIATRIC OBESITY

The incorporation of telehealth in the care of pediatric patients with obesity is ongoing and evolving, with a significant degree of variability in clinical practice. The future of telehealth for pediatric obesity should include primary and tertiary care clinical settings. Health systems and clinicians should continue to explore the utility of telehealth to innovate and support in-person models, and inspire new models of care. The implementation of telehealth as a stand-alone model would take the field in a new direction. The redesign of existing clinical care practices and the creation of new programs must aim to align patient needs with access to care and workforce expertise. Ultimately, the economic viability of telehealth for pediatric obesity depends on the reimbursement of services and the relevant policies of insurers, individual states, and the federal government.[31] This is particularly true for federally qualified health centers, who provide care for the underserved, but are significantly influenced by and dependent on state Medicaid policies for expanding the scope and reach of telehealth services.[31] Telehealth implementation and reimbursement is an active focus of the Centers for Medicare and Medicaid Services, and recent guidance from Medicaid and new policies for Medicare have helped inform clinicians and health systems.[32,33] Presently all 50 state Medicaid programs provide some type of reimbursement for live video services.[34] However, federal statute, Medicaid rules, and state laws allow considerable flexibility regarding which telehealth services individual state Medicaid programs cover. Clinicians who provide pediatric obesity services for Medicaid beneficiaries should advocate for the establishment of a recognized and reimbursable treatment regimen similar to the intensive behavioral therapy program approved for adult Medicare beneficiaries.[35]

SUMMARY

Telehealth is well positioned to address the common challenges of providing high-quality care to children and adolescents with obesity. The potential benefits of telehealth for pediatric obesity are applicable across the full spectrum of care from diagnosis and assessment to ongoing management. Overall, telehealth models of care for pediatric obesity may improve access to care, are feasible and comparable with in-person programs, and are satisfying and engaging for patients and families.

REFERENCES

1. Barlow SE. Expert committee recommendations regarding the prevention, assessment, and treatment of child and adolescent overweight and obesity: summary report. Pediatrics 2007;120(Supplement 4):S164–92.
2. Styne DM, Arslanian SA, Connor EL, et al. Pediatric obesity-assessment, treatment, and prevention: an Endocrine Society clinical practice guideline. J Clin Endocrinol Metab 2017;102(3):709–57.
3. US Preventive Services Task Force, Grossman DC, Bibbins-Domingo K, Curry SJ, et al. Screening for obesity in children and adolescents: US Preventive Services Task Force recommendation statement. JAMA 2017;317(23):2417.
4. Dhaliwal J, Nosworthy NMI, Holt NL, et al. Attrition and the management of pediatric obesity: an integrative review. Child Obes 2014;10(6):461–73.
5. Skelton JA, Beech BM. Attrition in paediatric weight management: a review of the literature and new directions. Obes Rev 2011;12(5):e273–81.
6. Skelton JA, Irby MB, Geiger AM. A systematic review of satisfaction and pediatric obesity treatment: new avenues for addressing attrition. J Healthc Qual 2014;36(4):5–22.
7. Sallinen Gaffka BJ, Frank M, Hampl S, et al. Parents and pediatric weight management attrition: experiences and recommendations. Child Obes 2013;9(5):409–17.
8. Findholt NE, Davis MM, Michael YL. Perceived barriers, resources, and training needs of rural primary care providers relevant to the management of childhood obesity. J Rural Health 2013;29(Suppl 1):s17–24.
9. Lenders CM, Manders AJ, Perdomo JE, et al. Addressing pediatric obesity in ambulatory care: where are we and where are we going? Curr Obes Rep 2016;5(2):214–40.
10. Hampl S, Paves H, Laubscher K, et al. Patient engagement and attrition in pediatric obesity clinics and programs: results and recommendations. Pediatrics 2011;128(Supplement 2):S59–64.
11. Skelton JA, Goff DC, Ip E, et al. Attrition in a multidisciplinary pediatric weight management clinic. Child Obes 2011;7(3):185–93.
12. Turner T, Spruijt-Metz D, Wen CKF, et al. Prevention and treatment of pediatric obesity using mobile and wireless technologies: a systematic review. Pediatr Obes 2015;10(6):403–9.
13. Bala N, Price SN, Horan CM, et al. Use of telehealth to enhance care in a family-centered childhood obesity intervention. Clin Pediatr (Phila) 2019;58(7):789–97.
14. Davis AM, Sampilo M, Gallagher KS, et al. Treating rural pediatric obesity through telemedicine: outcomes from a small randomized controlled trial. J Pediatr Psychol 2013;38(9):932–43.

15. Taveras EM, Marshall R, Sharifi M, et al. Comparative effectiveness of clinical-community childhood obesity interventions: the connect for health randomized controlled trial. JAMA Pediatr 2017;171(8):e171325.

16. Mulgrew KW, Shaikh U, Nettiksimmons J. Comparison of parent satisfaction with care for childhood obesity delivered face-to-face and by telemedicine. Telemed J E Health 2011;17(5):383–7.

17. Cueto V, Wang CJ, Sanders L. Impact of a Mobile App-Based Health Coaching and Behavior Change Program on Participant Engagement and Weight Status of Overweight and Obese Children: Retrospective Cohort Study. JMIR MHealth UHealth 2019;7(11):e14458. https://doi.org/10.2196/14458.

18. Irby MB, Boles KA, Jordan C, et al. TeleFIT: adapting a multidisciplinary, tertiary-care pediatric obesity clinic to rural populations. Telemed J E Health 2012;18(3):247–9.

19. Coles N, Patel BP, Li P, et al. Breaking barriers: adjunctive use of the Ontario Telemedicine Network (OTN) to reach adolescents with obesity living in remote locations. J Telemed Telecare 2018. https://doi.org/10.1177/1357633X18816254.

20. Smith JD, Berkel C, Jordan N, et al. An individually tailored family-centered intervention for pediatric obesity in primary care: study protocol of a randomized type II hybrid effectiveness–implementation trial (Raising Healthy Children study). Implement Sci 2018;13. https://doi.org/10.1186/s13012-017-0697-2.

21. Kelly AS, Barlow SE, Rao G, et al. Severe obesity in children and adolescents: identification, associated health risks, and treatment approaches: a scientific statement from the American Heart Association. Circulation 2013;128(15):1689–712.

22. Baillot A, Boissy P, Tousignant M, et al. Feasibility and effect of in-home physical exercise training delivered via telehealth before bariatric surgery. J Telemed Telecare 2017;23(5):529–35.

23. Bradley LE, Forman EM, Kerrigan SG, et al. Project HELP: a remotely delivered behavioral intervention for weight regain after bariatric surgery. Obes Surg 2017;27(3):586–98.

24. Steinberg DM, Levine EL, Askew S, et al. Daily text messaging for weight control among racial and ethnic minority women: randomized controlled pilot study. J Med Internet Res 2013;15(11):e244.

25. Foley P, Steinberg D, Levine E, et al. Track: a randomized controlled trial of a digital health obesity treatment intervention for medically vulnerable primary care patients. Contemp Clin Trials 2016;48:12–20.

26. Schoeppe S, Alley S, Rebar AL, et al. Apps to improve diet, physical activity and sedentary behaviour in children and adolescents: a review of quality, features and behaviour change techniques. Int J Behav Nutr Phys Act 2017;14. https://doi.org/10.1186/s12966-017-0538-3.

27. Schoffman DE, Turner-McGrievy G, Jones SJ, et al. Mobile apps for pediatric obesity prevention and treatment, healthy eating, and physical activity promotion: just fun and games? Transl Behav Med 2013;3(3):320–5.

28. Healthy weight for teens - full text view - ClinicalTrials.gov. Available at: https://clinicaltrials.gov/ct2/show/NCT03939494. Accessed October 8, 2019.

29. Group telehealth weight management visits for adolescents with obesity - full text view - ClinicalTrials.gov. Available at: https://clinicaltrials.gov/ct2/show/NCT03508622. Accessed October 8, 2019.

30. Greenlight Plus Study: approaches to early childhood obesity prevention - full text view - ClinicalTrials.gov. Available at: https://clinicaltrials.gov/ct2/show/NCT04042467. Accessed October 8, 2019.

31. Uscher-Pines L, Bouskill K, Sousa J, et al. Experiences of Medicaid programs and health centers in implementing telehealth. RAND Corporation; 2019. https://doi.org/10.7249/RR2564.
32. Telemedicine | Medicaid. Available at: https://www.medicaid.gov/medicaid/benefits/telemedicine/index.html. Accessed January 14, 2020.
33. Telehealth Services | Medicare. Available at: https://www.cms.gov/Outreach-and-Education/Medicare-Learning-Network-MLN/MLNProducts/Downloads/TelehealthSrvcsfctsht.pdf. Accessed January 14, 2020.
34. State Telehealth Laws and Reimbursement Policies Report | CCHP Website. Available at: https://www.cchpca.org/telehealth-policy/state-telehealth-laws-and-reimbursement-policies-report. Accessed January 14, 2020.
35. Intensive Behavioral Therapy (IBT) for obesity | Medicare. Available at: https://www.cms.gov/Outreach-and-Education/Medicare-Learning-Network-   MLN/MLNMattersArticles/downloads/MM7641.pdf. Accessed January 14, 2020.

Clinical Applications of Telemedicine in Gynecology and Women's Health

Siwon Lee, MD, PhD, Wilbur C. Hitt, MD, FACOG FACOEM*

KEYWORDS

- Telemedicine • Telehealth • Gynecology • Well-woman visits

KEY POINTS

- Telemedicine is the practice of medicine using electronic information and telecommunication technologies from a distance.
- The use of telemedicine in gynecology is beneficial in screening, prevention, family planning, mental health, prescriptions, and procedures.
- Telemedicine will help patients and physicians in gynecology by increasing efficacy, extending the scope of practice, and improving outcomes.
- The future of telemedicine in gynecology is promising in terms of women's health care and gynecology surgery.

INTRODUCTION

Telemedicine and telehealth (TM/TH) are beneficial for patients living in remote and rural areas with limited medical resources. It is also practical for patients with rare or complex medical problems for which only subspecialists can recognize and treat. Local practitioners can get guidance and advice from a distant expert. The definition of telehealth is different from telemedicine because it contains a broader spectrum of distant health care services that involves remote "nonclinical" services.[1,2] For example, training health care providers, administrative meetings, medical education to providers and patients, in addition to clinical services, are examples of telehealth, whereas telemedicine only involves remote clinical services. The American Telemedicine Association and the World Health Organization (WHO) use the 2 terms interchangeably, focusing on the "remote" delivery of health care services as a critical factor.[1,2]

This article originally appeared in *Obstetrics and Gynecology Clinics*, Volume 47, Issue 2, June 2020.

Department of Obstetrics and Gynecology, Mount Sinai Medical Center, 4302 Alton Road, Suite 920, Miami Beach, FL 33140, USA

* Corresponding author.

E-mail address: Wchitt99@gmail.com

Clinics Collections 10 (2021) 119–130

https://doi.org/10.1016/j.ccol.2020.12.013

The history of telemedicine dates back to the 1950s. Telemedicine was first mentioned in a scientific article in 1974.[3,4] Telemedicine encompasses 3 methods of conveying information from a distant site: "store-and-forward," "real-time telemedicine," and "remote patient monitoring."[5] Store-and-forward involves acquiring medical information that is stored locally and subsequently sent to a specialist for interpretation later at a more convenient time. Real-time telemedicine provides real-time interactions between patients and physicians. Real-time interaction includes videoconferences, telephone, and online communications. In addition, the activities of history taking and physical examination can be done in an equivalent manner to the traditional on-site patient/physician interaction. With this method, the presence of both parties is required. With real-time interaction between the patient and physician, diagnosis and treatment can be offered to patients by virtual visits. Virtual visits permit patients with limited medical resources to access the care they need. Remote patient monitoring can be used for patients with chronic diseases, such as hypertension or diabetes. Examples of this type of monitoring include vital signs or blood glucose levels, which are transmitted to a provider electronically. This method can provide greater patient satisfaction as well as better health outcomes and is cost-effective.

Statistical data from the 2010 US County Census File for adult women (aged 15 years or older) and reproductive-aged women (15–44 years old) revealed that in the United States, there are 2.65 obstetrics and gynecology (OB-GYN) doctors for every 10,000 women and 5.39 OB-GYN doctors per 10,000 reproductive-aged women.[6] It is noteworthy that approximately 49% of all the US counties (3143) did not have a single OB-GYN doctor, and 8.2% of all US women lived in those predominantly rural counties.[7] Therefore, access to an OB-GYN specialist is challenging for the US population, especially in rural areas.

TM/TH can potentially improve access to general and specialty health services by reducing temporal and geographic barriers. With up-to-date technology, providers and patients will be able to communicate much more efficiently. Providers will have easier access to patient information, be able to conveniently update medical records, keep track of their patients, and write prescriptions. TM/TH will allow patients to check test results, request refills of prescriptions, review their medical record, view education materials, and even check in for appointments with mobile devices. The goal of TM/TH is to provide similar quality of care as the traditional physician/patient interaction but in a more economic and convenient manner. Patients do not have to miss work or travel great distances to have a physician/patient interaction. Remote patient monitoring should be able to detect problems earlier and result in fewer hospitalizations. All of these factors can result in a lower medical cost for both health care systems and patients.[1]

Unfortunately, some barriers and issues have kept TM/TH from expanding. TM/TH may disrupt the continuity of care because the patient might not be able to see the same health care provider every time. Sometimes diagnosis at a long distance will be difficult because some tests require additional equipment. Misdiagnosis because of distance or lack of information can lead to malpractice and legal problems. Finally, reimbursement for services can be an issue because there is no consensus about reimbursement between states and insurance companies, and this may be the biggest problem preventing TM/TH expansion.[1]

In gynecology, TM/TH can be used in many ways, including well-woman visits, preconception counseling (PCC), preventive care, infertility, psychiatry, family planning, teleradiology, and telesurgery.[5,8–11]

The purpose of this review is to summarize previously published literature on TM/TH applications to gynecology and women's health. The authors analyze the advantages and disadvantages of TM/TH in gynecology and suggest future applications to serve as a comprehensive source for new ideas.

WELL WOMAN'S VISIT AND PREVENTIVE CARE

Important features of a well-woman visit are a discussion of reproductive plans, care for women across her lifespan, and regular care for the perimenopausal and postmenopausal woman.

The well-woman visit consists of a screening for underlying medical conditions, maintenance of healthy life with preventive care, management of women at reproductive age with PCC, and referral to another specialist as needed. Indications for referral would include medical problems that require monitoring, history of pregnancy-related complications, and infertility. PCC is an excellent opportunity to counsel the patient on how to maintain a healthy lifestyle, improve her overall well-being, and provide preventive services.[8]

A head-to-toe physical examination was traditionally required during the well-woman visit. There are several instances whereby telemedicine can be a beneficial adjunct to the traditional physical examination. For example, the patient's history and review of system (ROS), follow-up of blood work, and additional screening tests are ideal for telemedicine.[8] A comprehensive history and ROS, including the gynecologic history, will give additional information to determine if the patient needs certain parts of the physical examination, such as a breast or pelvic examination. According to a recent American College of Obstetricians and Gynecologists (ACOG) committee opinion and a practice bulletin, pelvic and breast examinations are recommended only when indicated by medical history or symptoms.[12,13] A pelvic examination should be performed only after a thorough review of the patient's condition followed by a detailed discussion about risks and benefits of the examination between the health care provider and the patient.[12] There have been different opinions among the major groups that determine guideline recommendations for breast cancer screening.[14] ACOG's recommendations emphasize a shared decision making in choosing between the range of options recommended within different guidelines.[13]

The 2018 ACOG committee opinion on the annual well-woman examination recommended that the annual examination should include the woman's vital signs, body mass index (BMI), and assessment/management of the patient's health by screening, counseling, and immunizations based on the woman's age and risk factors.[8] OB-GYN doctors should be playing a critical role in engaging patients in shared decision making, encouraging healthy lifestyles, and counseling about effective preventive health practices.[8] Obtaining a family history is crucial in evaluating a patient's risk profile by identifying women at an increased risk for familial cancer. This early identification is important for optimal genetic testing and counseling; not uncommonly, there are some situations when it may not be possible to complete all of the recommended services in 1 visit or with 1 health care provider. TM/TH with team-based care, including the OB-GYN physicians, physician assistant (PA), nurse practitioner (NP), and other health care providers may facilitate meeting the needs of medical care for these women.

PRECONCEPTION COUNSELING

An important component of the well-woman visit for a reproductive-aged woman is a discussion about her life plan on reproduction. The patient can undergo screening and tests depending on her history, symptoms, and risk factors. This time is the ideal time when PCC, infertility assessment, health care related to sexually transmitted diseases, and a discussion on the full range of contraceptive options that are available can take place. The goal of PCC is not just to help a patient achieve pregnancy but to establish a favorable pregnancy outcome with a healthy mother and a baby.

PCC is an extension of a well-woman visit. A detailed discussion on lifestyle habits, body weight and nutrition, screening tests for antibody status that require vaccination as well as screening for a medical condition should be done in addition to routine gynecology testing. When something is detected or if the patient has known chronic medical conditions, these need to be addressed, controlled, and monitored. Reproductive history, including recurrent pregnancy loss (RPL), previous stillbirth, history of delivery of an infant with congenital anomalies, history of preterm labor, gestational diabetes, or preeclampsia, is meaningful information. Genetic counseling and screening can be offered to patients with increased risks of genetic disease.

Initial PCC using TM/TH can be either done with a general OB-GYN doctor, primary care physician (PCP), NP, or PA; then, if something abnormal is detected, the patient can be referred for specialist consultation using the TM/TH system. Ideal candidates for these consultations are women with known medical problems, for example, seizure disorders, blood clotting disorders, thyroid disease, chronic hypertension, diabetes, history of pregestational diabetes, poor obstetric history, and RPL. Assessment of body habitus can be done by calculating the BMI. Depending on BMI, the patient can be referred for counseling by a nutritionist and/or referral for bariatric treatment if appropriate.

TM/TH can be used not only for specialist consultation but also for general PCC. Lifestyle modifications, like smoking, alcohol, and recreational drug cessation, are a critical component of PCC and can be done using TM/TH.[15,16]

FAMILY PLANNING

Family planning is another essential component of the well-woman visit. When a woman reaches an age when contraception is important, it is crucial to counsel, educate, and provide the ideal form of contraception to each woman to maintain her optimal reproductive health. Nonetheless, getting an oral contraceptive (OCP) prescription has been the one of the greatest barriers to this population because of the difficulty in accessing physicians. According to a study in 2016, about 29% of women had difficulties in obtaining OCP prescriptions or refills.[9] The most common reasons were difficulty meeting a doctor, having no PCP or gynecologist, busy work schedule, and high medical costs.[9] Efforts to expand OCP prescription availability could be achieved by allowing a pharmacist to prescribe an OCP or making OCPs nonprescription drugs. Making OCPs nonprescription is realistically not possible because of the risks that could be caused by uncontrolled use of hormonal agents.[5,17] A newer effort to expand accessibility to OCPs is by using TM/TH to screen for medical conditions and provide a prescription. TM/TH has allowed a safe and effective way to provide education and prescription for contraception at an affordable cost with easier accessibility. Concerns have been voiced about the safety of using TM/TH to identify contraindications to the use of OCPs. Therefore, it is important to gather sufficient information using TM/TH to ensure that OCPS are safely prescribed.

INFERTILITY WORKUP

Team work is important for a comprehensive infertility workup. Reproductive endocrinology and infertility (REI) specialists, and PA, NP, embryologist, endocrine laboratory technician, nutritionist, psychiatrist, or psychologist are all part of the team that assists the women dealing with the physical and emotional aspects of infertility. Infertility treatment can involve multiple office visits, especially when patients are undergoing assisted reproductive technology. Currently, infertility management is generally not covered by most insurance carriers, which imposes a heavy burden in terms of time and money on the infertile couple. TM/TH can be helpful by reducing on-site visits when the physical encounter with the health care provider is not necessary.

Infertility management not only involves the general health management of the infertile woman but also may involve a genetic evaluation, mental illness counseling, detailed discussion about treatment options, laboratory tests, hysterosalpingography (HSG), ultrasound (US), and prescriptions for medications and injections before egg retrieval or embryo transfer procedures. One of the essential steps in the management of the infertility patient is the initial encounter between the physician and the patient. Usually, more than 30 minutes on average is necessary for a comprehensive history and ROS to understand the extent of what is involved in the couple's infertility.

Depression and anxiety are commonly present in many infertility patients. It has been reported that up to 40% of women with infertility have depression/anxiety, compared with a baseline rate of only 3% in the general population.[18] Although it is difficult to quantitate, stress appears to be a cause of infertility in some infertile women, and stress reduction has been shown to lead to an increased risk for a successful pregnancy.[10,19] Some previous studies have demonstrated that lifestyle modification programs and online psychoeducational support improved outcomes in patients with infertility by providing information and emotional support.[20–22]

In general, the initial infertility workup can be done by an OB-GYN generalist or another women's health care provider, but once an abnormal finding is identified, referral to an REI specialist is strongly recommended. Immediate referral to an REI specialist using TM/TH can reduce the overall medical cost, emotional stress, and time to conception.[23] At the initial evaluation, practitioners should make every effort not to order unnecessary tests. Usually, a full evaluation of a female patient begins from the onset of the menstrual period and needs a full menstrual cycle to complete. Once all female and male evaluations are completed, TM/TH consultation with REI specialist can be done to discuss the test results and the overall chance of achieving a healthy pregnancy and to set a realistic goal.

Currently, only psychoeducational support and teleradiology are actively used clinically in the TM/TH treatment of infertility. However, in the near future, using video conferencing with an REI specialist, medication prescription, and simple procedures that can be done under the guidance of a specialist will become possible. Video conferencing will result in fewer clinic visits and a reduction in the financial burden carried by infertility patients.

TELERADIOLOGY: ULTRASOUND

US is by far the safest, least invasive, and cost-effective imaging modality in gynecology. Conventional transvaginal 2-dimensional (2D) US is used to evaluate pelvic anatomy for suspected abnormalities in the uterus, fallopian tubes, and ovaries. Uterine leiomyoma, endometrial polyps, and ovarian or fallopian tube pathologic conditions can be detected with US. Recent advances in 3-dimensional and real-time 4-dimensional (3D/4D) US have added value to the evaluation of uterine anomalies or endometrial lesions. Telesonography has been used with obstetric US since 1997. Recent technology has made the assessment of the fetal heart remotely with real-time fetal echocardiogram using 4D spatiotemporal image correlation possible.[6] In gynecology, telesonography has had limited use. Although it may be early to incorporate TM/TH into routine clinical gynecologic practice, there has been a recent move toward using self-operated endovaginal telemonitoring and 3D/4D US for the assessment of the uterus in place of the traditional HSG in infertility patients. These studies have shown that using TM/TH technique was as accurate as the conventional in-person method, although more evidence-based studies need to be conducted to be applied in clinical practice.[24–26] Advantages of adding 3D/4D to 2D US are the ability to reconstruct an original image into any plane of choice, including the coronal plane, which is difficult with conventional 2D US. Other advantages of 3D/4D are no radiation exposure, easy accessibility, low cost, and the ability to operate from a long distance by another operator. these advantages are what makes the TM/TH system possible. TM/TH is an attractive option for assisting gynecologists in making diagnoses and making it easier for second opinions from specialists.

CERVICAL CANCER SCREENING AND COLPOSCOPY

Cervical cancer was the leading cause of cancer death for women in the Unites States. However, in the past 40 years, the number of cases and the number of deaths from cervical cancer have decreased significantly. This decline is the result of many women getting regular pap tests and human papillomavirus (HPV) testing, which can find a cervical precancerous lesion before it turns into cancer.[27,28] However, in developing countries with low medical resources, cervical cancer is still a major health challenge, with a high incidence and a high number of cancer-related deaths.[29–31] The problems in the developing countries are due to a lack in cervical cancer screening and follow up, problems with interpretation of the results of screening, and a lack of preventative education.

   Following screening for cervical cancer with pap smears and/or HPV testing, colposcopy with or without biopsy may be indicated in some patients. Colposcopy is a simple method to diagnose cervical pathologic condition with a low-power binocular microscope and a high-intensity light source that can magnify the cervix. The most common indications for colposcopy are positive pap smears, positive HPV testing, and/or persistent unsatisfactory results from cytology. Acetowhite changes after acetic acid or changes in color to yellow or pale after Lugol solution are generally indications for biopsy of those sites. One of the problems with colposcopy is that significant pathologic changes can often be misinterpreted because of low specificity and high interobserver and intraobserver variability, which can only be achieved by proper training and good quality control.[32–34] Currently, in the United States, colposcopy training is only done during residency, and the Council on Resident Education in Obstetrics and Gynecology does not monitor how many cases of colposcopies are done to ensure proficiency during training. Compared with the United Kingdom, in the United States, there is no written certification examination or no standard curriculum for training colposcopy during residencies. This set of challenges results in a shortage of gynecologists properly trained in colposcopy. Because of a shortage of well-trained colposcopists, patients in areas with no specialists may have to travel great distances when they need a colposcopic evaluation. As a solution, the American Society for Colposcopy and Cervical Pathology published colposcopy standards recommendations in 2017 to influence the practice and to try and warrant quality assurance of colposcopy.[35,36] Another way to solve this problem is to use traditional binocular colposcopy combined with digital colposcopy using the TM/TH system. Colposcopy can be connected to a camera, and a still image or video images can be obtained and sent to the specialist for review.[5,37] The expert will review the images and give an opinion on the diagnosis and management as needed.[37] Nowadays, real-time assessment is even possible for the expert to review using video-conferencing technology, which enables the patient and physician to interact before, during, and after the procedure just as is done in an office setting.[38] The specialist will help guide the local practitioner to take the biopsies in the appropriate areas of concern. In previous studies, in-person examinations, real-time telecolposcopy, and store-and-forward of digital images were compared and showed a similar rate in the detection of cervical cancer. However, biopsy rates were higher in the store-and-forward group compared with on-site colposcopy.[39–41] TM/TH for colposcopy has the potential for improving the quality and reliability of the colposcopy, which would result in better counseling and teleconsulting with a gynecology oncologist when necessary. TM/TH will help reduce medical cost, improve quality control, and possibly decrease the level of interobserver variability.[5,32,42,43] Future large randomized trials will be needed to validate the validity of TM/TH for colposcopy. Overall, TM/TH can help improve capacity for colposcopy in areas without specialists and will be beneficial for inexperienced colposcopists who would benefit from the expertise of a specialist at a distance. TM/TH will make it possible for a more standardized practice of colposcopy using optimization of the document of colposcopic findings and assessment of competence of trainees.

MEDICAL ABORTION

Another essential aspect of family planning is the termination of pregnancy (TOP). According to WHO, the first-trimester TOP can be achieved on an outpatient basis by midlevel providers and by having the patient self-administer the medication and self-assess the abortion completeness at home.[44,45] There are limited data on the safety of medical abortion using TM/TH, but that data showed reassuring safety outcomes.[46,47] ACOG defines a medical abortion as the TOP before 10 weeks of gestation using mifepristone and misoprostol.[48] The efficacy of this regimen is approximately 92% in women with a gestation up to 49 days.[48] The first medical abortion using telemedicine occurred in 2008 at the Planned Parenthood of the Heartland facility in Iowa.[49] Using telemedicine as a means of TOP has increased the proportion of medical abortions undertaken before 12 weeks of gestation. TOP before 12 weeks is more likely to result in a complete abortion.[48,50] Studies have reported that medical abortions via telemedicine are as likely to be successful and to have a similar risk for adverse events as procedures done on site.[46,49]

MENTAL ILLNESSES IN GYNECOLOGY

Mental illness in gynecology can benefit from the use of TM/TH.[51] The prevalence of depression/anxiety is common in infertile women. Infertile women have comparable levels of anxiety and depression to those with heart disease, human immunodeficiency virus, or metastatic cancer.[9,10,52,53] Interventions that have included emotional support have been well researched and have shown favorable outcomes in this population. Psychological interventions may be offered in many forms, including individual counseling and therapy. Programs for infertile women that have provided counseling, personal attention, and support have shown a reduction in depression/anxiety and an increase in the pregnancy rate.[54,55] Recently, psychological interventions offered online have become popular. Studies comparing patients who received psychoeducational support through the Internet with patients who received no intervention showed that the intervention group had lower levels of depressive/anxiety symptoms and improved pregnancy rates after the intervention. This finding suggests that TM/TH maybe helpful in treating for mental illness in gynecology.[20–22,56]

PREOPERATIVE COUNSELING, POSTOPERATIVE CARE, AND TELESURGERY

TM/TH is currently used for preoperative and postoperative consultations, education on surgical procedures to patients, and teleconferencing locations with limited medical resources,[11] which has enabled patients to be able to make decisions on site rather than having to be transferred to larger facilities for education and consultations.[6] Routine postoperative care, using telemedicine, has been reported to be safe and effective.[11] TM/TH has allowed patients to be seen by specialists in distant sites without traveling to those sites, saving significant time and expense and resulting in increased patient satisfaction and reducing overall total medical cost.[11,57,58] Telemedicine, using videoconferencing, could also help physicians to assess minor complications and reduce unnecessary hospital visits.

Telesurgery is broadly defined as performing surgery from a distance[3] and is accomplished by supervising the surgery from a distance using real-time video-conference or performing the surgery using a robot. The first method can be used in remote or underserved areas where a specialist is not available to perform the procedure. In addition, it can be used in patients with a rare disease that requires specialist consultation. Multiple surgeons from different parts of the world can collaborate by a network to provide the best possible treatment for the individual patient, allowing not only the best care for the patient but also the exchange of ideas between physicians from anywhere in the world.[3,59] The second method involves robotic and telesurgical technology with minimally invasive gynecologic surgery. This method also enables the exchange of surgical techniques between the physicians and allows standardization of surgical training and better patient outcomes.[3] In gynecology, robotic-assisted surgery can be used in benign gynecology, gynecology oncology, reproductive endocrinology, and urogynecology. In a study comparing laparotomy with laparoscopy and robotic-assisted laparoscopy, the outcomes of wound complications (infectious and lung-related morbidity), postoperative ileus, and hematoma formation were compared between groups. There were more complications reported in the laparotomy group compared with the laparoscopy and robotic-assisted laparoscopy groups. No differences were noted between robotic-assisted and simple laparoscopic procedures, which could enable people in rural areas to have these surgeries using TM/TH.[60–62]

SUMMARY

With the rapid evolution of the Internet and information technology, TM/TH has evolved as a technology that is becoming more and more a part of the everyday practice of medicine in delivering high-quality health care.[11,63] Goals of TM/TH are not only improving the quality of medical care but also increasing convenience, increasing efficacy, and decreasing cost. TM/TH can be used as a cost-effective method of using medical resources and can lead to quick and reliable decisions. TM/TH is no longer a future medicine. Incorporating modern medicine into traditional in-person medicine is unavoidable. Now is the time for the health care providers to make changes in the mode of managing their patients. Telemedicine is one of the most rapidly growing areas in modern medicine, and many physicians see it as a method to increase efficiency, extend the scope of their practice, and improve outcomes. An important benefit of TM/TH is building a virtual community of physicians, thus facilitating discussion of their experiences, ideas, and cases in real time.

In gynecology, there is no doubt that TM/TH will play a crucial role in well-woman care. Although TM/TH looks very promising, some barriers require attention. For example, lack of in-person human interactions, misdiagnosis and malpractice insurance issues and legal issues, reimbursement and billing, problems with current state-specific medical licensing, and security of patient information are very important issues to be addressed and worked on before expansion of TM/TH. Although high-quality, large studies are still necessary to validate its efficacy and usefulness, TM/TH has validated its value and advantages, especially in areas with limited medical resources.

DISCLOSURE

The authors have nothing to disclose.

REFERENCES

1. American Telemedicine Association. About telemedicine: the ultimate frontier for superior healthcare delivery. Available at: http://www.americantelemed.org/about-telemedicine. Accessed November 15, 2017.

2. World Health Organization. Telemedicine: opportunities and developments in member states. 2010. Available at: http://www.who.int/goe/publications/goe_telemedicine_2010.pdf. Accessed November 15, 2017.

3. Senapati S, Advincula A. Telemedicine and robotics: paving the way to the globalization of surgery. Int J Gynaecol Obstet 2005;91(3):210–6.

4. Zundel KM. Telemedicine: history, applications, and impact on librarianship. Bull Med Libr Assoc 1996;84(1):71.

5. Greiner AL. Telemedicine applications in obstetrics and gynecology. Clin Obstet Gynecol 2017;60(4):853–66.

6. Bullard TB, Rosenberg MS, Ladde J, et al. Digital images taken with a mobile phone can assist in the triage of neurosurgical patients to a level 1 trauma centre. J Telemed Telecare 2013;19(2):80–3.

7. Rayburn WF, Klagholz JC, Murray-Krezan C, et al. Distribution of American Congress of Obstetricians and Gynecologists fellows and junior fellows in practice in the United States. Obstet Gynecol 2012;119(5):1017–22.

8. Well-Woman visit. ACOG Committee opinion No. 755. American College of Obstetricians and Gynecologists. Obstet Gynecol 2018;132(4):e181–6.

9. Grindlay K, Grossman D. Prescription birth control access among US women at risk of unintended pregnancy. J Womens Health 2016;25(3):249–54.

10. Domar AD, Clapp D, Slawsby EA, et al. Impact of group psychological interventions on pregnancy rates in infertile women. Fertil Steril 2000;73(4):805–11.

11. Asiri A, AlBishi S, AlMadani W, et al. The use of telemedicine in surgical care: a systematic review. Acta Inform Med 2018;26(3):201.

12. The utility of and indications for routine pelvic examination. ACOG Committee Opinion No. 754. American College of Obstetricians and Gynecologists. Obstet Gynecol 2018;132:e174–80.

13. Breast cancer risk assessment and screening in average-risk women. Practice Bulletin No. 179. American College of Obstetricians and Gynecologists. Obstet Gynecol 2017;131:e1–16.

14. Center for Disease Control. Breast cancer screening guidelines for women. U.S. Preventive Services Task Force. 2016. American Cancer. Society. 2015. American College. Available at: https://www.cdc.gov/cancer/breast/pdf/BreastCancerScreeningGuidelines.pdf. Accessed November 15, 2017.

15. Gunatilake RP, Perlow JH. Obesity and pregnancy: clinical management of the obese gravida. Am J Obstet Gynecol 2011;204(2):106–19.

16. Vergel R, Sanchez L, Heredero B, et al. Primary prevention of neural tube defects with folic acid supplementation: Cuban experience. Prenat Diagn 1990;10(3): 149–52.

17. Gomez AM. Availability of pharmacist-prescribed contraception in California, 2017. JAMA 2017;318(22):2253–4.

18. Chen T-H, Chang S-P, Tsai C-F, et al. Prevalence of depressive and anxiety disorders in an assisted reproductive technique clinic. Hum Reprod 2004;19(10): 2313–8.

19. van Dijk MR, Koster MP, Willemsen SP, et al. Healthy preconception nutrition and lifestyle using personalized mobile health coaching is associated with enhanced pregnancy chance. Reprod Biomed Online 2017;35(4):453–60.

20. Sexton MB, Byrd MR, O'Donohue WT, et al. Web-based treatment for infertility-related psychological distress. Arch Womens Ment Health 2010;13(4):347–58.

21. Cousineau TM, Green TC, Corsini E, et al. Online psychoeducational support for infertile women: a randomized controlled trial. Hum Reprod 2007;23(3):554–66.

22. Hämmerli K, Znoj H, Berger T. Internet-based support for infertile patients: a randomized controlled study. J Behav Med 2010;33(2):135–46.

23. VanderLaan B, Karande V, Krohm C, et al. Cost considerations with infertility therapy: outcome and cost comparison between health maintenance organization and preferred provider organization care based on physician and facility cost. Hum Reprod 1998;13(5):1200–5.

24. Saravelos SH, Jayaprakasan K, Ojha K, et al. Assessment of the uterus with three-dimensional ultrasound in women undergoing ART. Hum Reprod Update 2017;23(2):188–210.

25. Pereira I, von Horn K, Depenbusch M, et al. Self-operated endovaginal telemonitoring: a prospective, clinical validation study. Fertil Steril 2016;106(2):306–10.e1.

26. Wang Y, Qian L. Three- or four-dimensional hysterosalpingo contrast sonography for diagnosing tubal patency in infertile females: a systematic review with meta-analysis. Br J Radiol 2016;89(1063):20151013.

27. National Institutes of Health. Cervical cancer. NIH Consens Statement 1996; 14(1):1–38.

28. U.S. Cancer Statistics Working Group. U.S. Cancer statistics data visualizations tool, based on November 2018 submission data (1999-2016). Altlanta (GA): U.S. Department of Health and Human Services, Centers for Disease Control and Prevention and National Cancer Institute; 2019. Available at: www.cdc.gov/cancer/dataviz.

29. Stewart B, Wild CP. World cancer report 2014. Lyon (France): National Agency for Research on Cancer; 2014.

30. International Agency for Cancer Research. Globocan 2012—estimated cancer incidence, mortality and prevalence worldwide in 2012. Population fact sheets 2012. Available at: http://globocan.iarc.fr/Pages/fact_sheets_population.aspx#. Accessed October 28, 2015.

31. Linde DS, Andersen MS, Mwaiselage JD, et al. Text messages to increase attendance to follow-up cervical cancer screening appointments among HPV-positive Tanzanian women (Connected2Care): study protocol for a randomised controlled trial. Trials 2017;18(1):555.

32. Schaedel D, Kuehn W. The role of new information and communication technologies in gynecological diagnosis of cervical cancer. J Turk Ger Gynecol Assoc 2006;7(4):280–1.

33. Hopman EH, Voorhorst FJ, Kenemans P, et al. Observer agreement on interpreting colposcopic images of CIN. Gynecol Oncol 1995;58(2):206–9.

34. Etherington I, Luesley D, Shafi M, et al. Observer variability among colposcopists from the West Midlands region. BJOG 1997;104(12):1380–4.
35. Wentzensen N, Massad LS, Mayeaux EJ Jr, et al. Evidence-based consensus recommendations for colposcopy practice for cervical cancer prevention in the United States. J Low Genit Tract Dis 2017;21(4):216–22.
36. Mayeaux JE, Novetsky AP, Chelmow D, et al. ASCCP colposcopy standards: colposcopy quality improvement recommendations for the United States. J Low Genit Tract Dis 2017;21(4):242–8.
37. Hitt WC, Low GM, Lynch CE, et al. Application of a telecolposcopy program in rural settings. Telemed J E Health 2016;22(10):816–20.
38. Louwers J, Kocken M, Ter Harmsel W, et al. Digital colposcopy: ready for use? An overview of literature. BJOG 2009;116(2):220–9.
39. Hitt WC, Low G, Bird TM, et al. Telemedical cervical cancer screening to bridge Medicaid service care gap for rural women. Telemed J E Health 2013;19(5): 403–8.
40. Etherington IJ. Telecolposcopy—a feasibility study in primary care. J Telemed Telecare 2002;8(2_suppl):22–4.
41. Ferris DG, Bishai DM, Litaker MS, et al. Telemedicine network telecolposcopy compared with computer-based telecolposcopy. J Low Genit Tract Dis 2004; 8(2):94–101.
42. Ricard-Gauthier D, Wisniak A, Catarino R, et al. Use of smartphones as adjuvant tools for cervical cancer screening in low-resource settings. J Low Genit Tract Dis 2015;19(4):295–300.
43. Spitzer M. The era of "digital colposcopy" will be here soon. J Low Genit Tract Dis 2015;19(4):273–4.
44. Endler M, Lavelanet A, Cleeve A, et al. Telemedicine for medical abortion: a systematic review. BJOG 2019;126(9):1094–102.
45. World Health Organization. Health worker roles in providing safe abortion care and post-abortion contraception. Geneva (Switzerland): World Health Organization; 2015.
46. Grossman D, Grindlay K. Safety of medical abortion provided through telemedicine compared with in person. Obstet Gynecol 2017;130(4):778–82.
47. Aiken AR, Digol I, Trussell J, et al. Self reported outcomes and adverse events after medical abortion through online telemedicine: population based study in the Republic of Ireland and Northern Ireland. BMJ 2017;357:j2011.
48. Medical management of first-trimester abortion. Practice Bulletin No 143. American College of Obstetricians and Gynecologists. Obstet Gynecol 2014;123: 676–92.
49. Grossman D, Grindlay K, Buchacker T, et al. Effectiveness and acceptability of medical abortion provided through telemedicine. Obstetrics Gynecol 2011; 118(2):296–303.
50. Grossman DA, Grindlay K, Buchacker T, et al. Changes in service delivery patterns after introduction of telemedicine provision of medical abortion in Iowa. Am J Public Health 2013;103(1):73–8.
51. Douglas MD, Xu J, Heggs A, et al. Assessing telemedicine utilization by using Medicaid claims data. Psychiatr Serv 2016;68(2):173–8.
52. Domar AD, Broome A, Zuttermeister PC, et al. The prevalence and predictability of depression in infertile women. Fertil Steril 1992;58(6):1158–63.
53. Domar AD, Zuttermeister P, Friedman R. The psychological impact of infertility: a comparison with patients with other medical conditions. J Psychosom Obstet Gynaecol 1993;14:45–52.

54. Domar AD, Rooney KL, Wiegand B, et al. Impact of a group mind/body intervention on pregnancy rates in IVF patients. Fertil Steril 2011;95(7):2269–73.

55. Terzioglu F. Investigation into effectiveness of counseling on assisted reproductive techniques in Turkey. J Psychosom Obstet Gynaecol 2001;22(3):133–41.

56. Clifton J, Parent J, Worrall G, et al. An internet-based mind/body intervention to mitigate distress in women experiencing infertility: a randomized pilot trial. Fertil Steril 2016;106(3):e62.

57. Costa MA, Yao CA, Gillenwater TJ, et al. Telemedicine in cleft care: reliability and predictability in regional and international practice settings. J Craniofac Surg 2015;26(4):1116–20.

58. Urquhart AC, Antoniotti NM, Berg RL. Telemedicine—an efficient and cost-effective approach in parathyroid surgery. Laryngoscope 2011;121(7):1422–5.

59. Rafiq A, Merrell RC. Telemedicine for access to quality care on medical practice and continuing medical education in a global arena. J Contin Educ Health Prof 2005;25(1):34–42.

60. Cho J, Shamshirsaz A, Nezhat C, et al. New technologies for reproductive medicine: laparoscopy, endoscopy, robotic surgery and gynecology. A review of the literature. Minerva Ginecologica 2010;62(2):137–67.

61. Stark M, Benhidjeb T, Gidaro S, et al. The future of telesurgery: a universal system with haptic sensation. J Turk Ger Gynecol Assoc 2012;13(1):74.

62. Haidegger T, Sándor J, Benyó Z. Surgery in space: the future of robotic telesurgery. Surg Endosc 2011;25(3):681–90.

63. World Health Organization, Region Office for Europe. From innovation to implementation eHealth in the WHO European Region. Available at: http://www.euro.who.int/_data/assets/pdf_file/0012/302331?From-Innovation-to-Implementation-eHealth-Report-EU.pdf. Accessed March 18, 2018.

Telehealth in Maternity Care

Haywood L. Brown, MD[a],*, Nathaniel DeNicola, MD, MSHP[b]

KEYWORDS

- Telehealth • Prenatal and postpartum care • Licensing • Credentialing
- Reimbursement

KEY POINTS

- Telehealth and telemedicine can be employed in obstetric practice to facilitate prenatal and postpartum care using various platforms that include videoconferencing and e-medicine.
- Telehealth is governed by the same physician-patient relationships that would be used with a face-to-face encounter, and Internet-based platforms must provide transfer of information that is Health Insurance Portability and Accountability Act compliant.
- The obstetrician-gynecologist and other obstetric providers must address and overcome potential barriers to adopting a telemedicine program, such as connectivity, licensure, legal, credentialing, and reimbursement requirements of states to ensure quality and safe telehealth delivery.

INTRODUCTION

Telehealth involves using digital information and communication technologies, such as computers and mobile devices, to manage health and well-being. Telehealth, also called e-health or mobile health (m-health), includes a variety of health care services. The Centers for Medicare & Medicaid Services define telemedicine as "the use of medical information exchanged from one site to another via electronic communications to improve a patient's health." Telemedicine now is generally thought of as 1 component of telehealth. The World Health Organization defines telehealth as, "The delivery of health care services, where distance is a critical factor, by all health care professionals using information and communication technologies for the exchange of valid information for diagnosis, treatment and prevention of disease and injuries, research and evaluation, and for the continuing education of health care providers, all in the interests of advancing the health of individuals and their communities."[1]

This article originally appeared in *Obstetrics and Gynecology Clinics*, Volume 47, Issue 3, September 2020.

[a] Diversity, Department of Obstetrics and Gynecology, University of South Florida, 13101 Bruce B. Downs Drive, MDC- 3rd Floor, Tampa, FL 33612, USA; [b] Department of Obstetrics and Gynecology, The George Washington University, 2511 I Street Northwest, Washington, DC 20037, USA
* Corresponding author.
E-mail address: haywoodb@usf.edu

Clinics Collections 10 (2021) 131–136
https://doi.org/10.1016/j.ccol.2020.12.014
2352-7986/21/© 2020 Elsevier Inc. All rights reserved.

The goal of telehealth is better facilitating care coordination and collaboration, improving quality of care and compliance, fewer hospital admissions and readmissions, fewer face-to-face office visits and cancellations, and improving rural access to care and follow-up in medical and surgical postoperative and postpartum care. Electronic-visits can save patients and doctors time compared with face-to-face office visits. It is of great benefit for those with an established physician-patient relationship and for follow-up care.

One important consideration for telehealth is the use of synchronous versus asynchronous interventions. Synchronous, or real-time, interventions include audiovisual consultations that allow an obstetrician-gynecologist to perform clinical counseling remotely in place of an in-person visit. Real-time audio-visual communication also has been used for clinical scenarios like peer-to-peer consultation, ultrasound imaging review, and directed physical examinations. In other scenarios, the use of asynchronous or store-and-forward telehealth interventions may be more applicable. Some examples of these could include remote monitoring of patient-generated data, such as maternal weight gain and blood glucose, and certain symptom or medical screening questionnaires.[2]

Telehealth is rapidly being adopted into obstetrics and gynecology practice.[2] Telehealth can be helpful especially for obstetric and postpartum care in rural areas and for those who do not have easy access to transportation. Prenatal, intrapartum, and postpartum care in the United States is fragmented between providers and health care facilities that provide obstetric services. This is further compounded by the maldistribution of obstetric providers in the United States.[3] Approximately 6% of the nation's obstetricians and gynecologists practice in rural communities, yet 15%, or approximately 46 million people, live in rural communities. Furthermore, fewer than half of rural women live within a 30-minute drive to the nearest facility providing obstetric services.[4,5]

Access and fragmentation of care for the US obstetric population is further challenged by the fact that 50% of all US hospitals provide care for 3 or fewer deliveries per day. In these situations, identification of risk, team training, and readiness are necessary to address preventable maternal morbidity and mortality.

TELEMEDICINE IN MATERNAL CARE

An example for telemedicine in prenatal care is the program, Text4baby, which utilizes the health belief model by sending cues for positive behavioral and attitude change while providing salient information.

Text4baby is an initiative that seeks to help pregnant women and new mothers increase their knowledge about caring for personal health and giving the infant the best possible start in life.[6] The National Healthy Mothers, Healthy Babies Coalition launched Text4baby, the first free health text messaging service in the United States, in February 2010. Messaging includes information on alcohol and tobacco cessation as well as taking prenatal vitamins and seeking prenatal care. Higher levels of text message exposure changed attitudes and beliefs and predicted lower self-reported alcohol consumption postpartum (odds ratio [OR] 0.212; 95% CI, 0.046–0.973; $P = .046$). The Text4baby program found 40% of enrollees were from underserved zip codes. Additionally, 82% were from households where the yearly income was less than $20,000 per year.[6]

A systematic review of 47 articles that included low-risk and high-risk obstetric, family planning, and general gynecology patient encounters suggests benefit with telehealth interventions, including text messaging and remote monitoring. Text messaging and remote monitoring decrease the number of unscheduled visits.[7]

In 2014, Babyscripts began a program of remote prenatal encounters geared toward transforming how doctors and pregnant women think of and use technology to improve prenatal care. Two landmark studies and partnerships with General Electric, March of Dimes, StartUp Health, and relationships with many of the leading hospitals, health systems, and medical practices around the country have proved to be of benefit in replacing face-to-face prenatal visit encounters for low-risk obstetric patients by monitoring and transmitted blood pressure and weight measurements directly to the prenatal providers, who can incorporate these measurements into the patients' records.[8,9] Remote monitoring for high risk pregnancies with gestational diabetes mellitus also has been included in the platform by providing glucose monitoring and follow-up to providers.

There is a shortage and maldistribution of obstetricians in the United States, particularly in rural communities. Team training is important to provide for readiness to manage preventable morbidity from hemorrhage and for management of hypertension. Through telehealth, regionalized obstetric care relationships and partnerships can be tightened between health centers (clinics), hospitals, and all obstetric care providers: obstetricians, family physicians, advanced practice nurse practitioners, and midwives.

Most recently, through legislation, the state of Texas, in collaboration with the American College of Obstetricians and Gynecologists, established a partnership—Levels of Maternal care verification program.[10] The Maternal Health Compact, published by Mann and colleagues,[11] can be adopted by every facility and community providing obstetric care. The Compact addresses readiness by formalizing relationships between lower-resource hospitals, which may be in rural access communities, to promote the transfer of a pregnant woman who requires a higher level of maternity care. Through telehealth and teleconsultation, the lower-level facility can be connected to the higher-level facility for immediate consultation for an obstetric emergency or anticipated complications, thereby averting the potential for severe morbidity or mortality. For example, a woman diagnosed with placenta previa or invasive placenta disorder would benefit from transfer to a facility capable of dealing with the potential hemorrhage. A woman with a preterm or term preeclampsia with severe features could be transferred when medically stable from a lower-resource facility to a higher-level facility, where hypertension management protocols can be implemented to prevent potential hypertension-related morbidity and cerebral hemorrhage. This communication and support to the clinicians and facilities on the transfer and receiving end of obstetric care define the maternal levels of care that, if universally adopted by all states and facilities, can be an intervention that would lead to reduction in maternal morbidity and mortality.[12]

Emergency obstetric care could be adapted from programs, such as those by Avera e-Care, based in Sioux Falls, South Dakota, for tele-ICU and e-Emergency care throughout the Avera e-Care network of facilities in South Dakota and neighboring states in the network. Emergency obstetrics (tele-Obstetrics) could assist in management of obstetric emergency, such as hemorrhage (pharmacologic and balloon insertion), evaluation of fetal monitoring tracings, and complicated deliveries by nonobstetrician delivery providers (family physicians and midwives) in rural settings, such as those communities in South Dakota where distance and weather can have an impact on immediate transfer of an obstetric patient at risk for morbidity and mortality to a tertiary center.[11]

Postpartum lactation counseling and follow-up can be facilitated through telehealth video encounters, especially for women in rural communities where access to follow-up and resources is challenging. Text communications and Web-based platforms focused on breastfeeding have showed improvement in breastfeeding exclusivity and continuation rates postpartum.[7] These types of encounters can lead to improvement in the disparity in breastfeeding continuation in minority women. Women who are experiencing problems with breastfeeding in the first several weeks postpartum are less likely to continue with exclusive breastfeeding for the recommended weeks and are more likely to discontinue breastfeeding in favor of formula feeding. Connecting with a professional particularly in lactation can provide the encouragement that a woman needs for both maternal and newborn benefit.[7,13]

Telemedicine, specifically telepsychiatry, has been practiced in this country since at least the mid-1960s. In 1964, the Nebraska Psychiatric Institute received a grant from the National Institute of Mental Health to link the Institute with Norfolk State Hospital, more than 100 miles away, by closed-circuit television. Telepsychiatry uses technology to facilitate psychiatric care at a distance and can be used specifically in follow-up for women screened and diagnosed with postpartum depression. Case studies from Australia evaluated the effectiveness of telemedicine as a strategy for providing a broad range of services related to child and adolescent mental health and to improve the accessibility of rural and remote health to specialist child and adolescent mental health consultation and support.[14]

With regard to postpartum depression follow-up, telehealth overcomes the barrier of having to travel to see a specialist and allows for screening in the weeks and months after childbirth to prevent the exacerbation of depressive symptoms. Videoconferencing can be used for check-in visits with a nurse, obstetrician, or other obstetric service provider or with a psychiatric physician or psychotherapist, who can adjust medications as necessary without having the woman travel to an office for a face-to-face encounter.

CHALLENGES IN IMPLEMENTATION OF TELEHEALTH

One of the essential challenges to implementation of telehealth is overcoming network, connectivity, and equipment requirements and expenses required for initiation of a telehealth program. This can be especially of concern in rural clinical and hospital settings where services are most needed to improve access and follow-up. It is important for telehealth providers and facilities to be familiar with the hardware, software, and security requirements to provide quality, safe, and Health Insurance Portability and Accountability Act–compliant care.

Box 1
Telehealth and the physician-patient relationship

Patient-physician relationship
- A patient-physician relationship generally is formed when a physician affirmatively acts in patient care by examining, diagnosing, treating, or agreeing to do so.
- Once a physician consensually enters into relationship with a patient in any of these ways, a legal contract is formed.
- The physician owes a duty to that patient to continue to treat or properly terminate the relationship.

Liability
- Duty of care for patient
- Where is medicine practiced (states)?
- Where is practitioner licensed (states)?
- Is physical contact require?
- Is standard of care applied (patient or doctor)?

Licensing, credentialing, and privileging for telehealth depend on the state(s) and facilities where the services are being provided. Telemedicine parity refers to the equivalent health insurance reimbursement for similar in-person and telehealth services.[15] Thirty-five states have enacted telemedicine parity laws defining reimbursement for fee for services.[16] Rules for patient encounters, documentation, and treatment guidelines should be the same as for face-to-face enounters that govern the physician-patient relationship. Liability insurance policies should cover telemedicine across all states where a physician is providing services (**Box 1**).

SUMMARY

Telehealth and enhanced technology for clinical care and education augment the fragmented model of current prenatal, intrapartum, and postpartum obstetric practice and will enhance quality and safety issues in maternity care. Telehealth is critical to full implementation of Levels of Maternal Care and the Alliance for Innovation on Maternal Health safety bundles to improve quality and safety in care delivery, especially in rural access communities.

Innovation in health care delivery through telemedicine/telehealth is evolving at a rapid speed.

Teleconsultation for inpatient, outpatient, and emergency management is rapidly becoming a modality to improve access and the quality of care in rural and urban settings for all specialties, including obstetrics and gynecology.

Obstacles to implementation of a robust telemedicine program include available technology in many rural settings, cost and reimbursement, and liability concerns.

Postpartum follow-up for all women can be facilitated by embracing technology and telehealth through various platforms and to provide health promotion.

DISCLOSURE

H.L. Brown: Merck for Mother Advisory Board and Up to Date contributor. N. DeNicola has nothing to disclose.

REFERENCES

1. WHO. A health telematics policy in support of WHO's Health-For-All strategy for global health development: report of the WHO group consultation on health telematics, 11–16 December, Geneva, 1997. Geneva (Switzerland): World Health Organization; 1998.

2. Implementing Telehealth in Practice. ACOG Committee opinion number 798 presidential task force on Telehealth. The American College of Obstetricians and Gynecologists 2020;135(2):e73–9.

3. Phelan ST, Wetzel L. Maternal death in rural America. Contemp Ob Gyn 2018;17(8).

4. Marsa L. Labor pains: the ob gyn shortage. AAMC News 2018.

5. Kozhimannil KB, Hung P, Henning-Smith C, et al. Association between loss of hospital-based obstetric services and birth outcomes in rural counties in the US. ACOG guidance: emergency treatment for severe hypertension in pregnancy. JAMA 2018;319(12):1239–47.

6. Whittaker R, Matoff-Stepp S, Meehan J, et al. Text4baby: development and implementation of a national text messaging health information service. Am J Public Health 2012;102(12):2207–13.

7. DeNicola N Grossman D, Marko K, Somalkar S, et al. Telehealth interventions to improve obstetric and gynecologic health outcomes: a systematic review. Obstet Gynecol 2020;135:371–82.
8. Marko KI, Krapf JM, Meltzer AC, et al. Testing the feasibility of remote patient monitoring in prenatal care using a mobile app and connected devices: a prospective observational trial. JMIR Res Protoc 2016;5(4):e200.
9. Marko KI, Ganju N, Krapf JM, et al. A resource and cost analysis on the impact of reduced visits for prenatal care. Obstet Gynecol 2016. https://doi.org/10.1097/01.AOG.0000483884.36730.d5.
10. Texas Levels of Maternal Care Verification Program. Available at: https://www.acog.org/About-ACOG/ACOG-Departments/LOMC/Texas-Levels-of-Maternal-Care-Verification-Program?IsMobileSet=falseBarriers to Breastfeeding in the United States. https://www.ncbi.nlm.nih.gov/books/NBK52688/. Accessed March 29, 2020.
11. Mann S, McKay K, Brown H. The maternal health compact. N Engl J Med 2017; 376:1304–5.
12. Obstetric care consensus No. 2. Levels of maternal care. Obstet Gynecol 2015; 125:502–15.
13. dos Santos LF, Borges RF, de Azambuja Zocche DA. Telehealth and breastfeeding: an integrative review. Telemed J E Health 2019. https://doi.org/10.1089/tmj.2019.0073.
14. Mitchell JM, Robinson PJ, McEvoy M, et al. Two case studies of telehealth technologies used for the delivery of professional development for health, education and welfare professionals in remote mining towns. J Telemed Telecare 2001;7: 174–80.
15. ACOG committee opinion number 798. Implementing Telehealth in Practice. Obstet Gynecol 2020;135:E73–9.
16. Center for Connected Health Policy. State Telehealth Laws and Reimbursement Policies Report. Available at: http://www.cchpca.org/state-laws-and-reimbursement-policies. Accessed March 29, 2020.

Child and Adolescent Telepsychiatry Education and Training

Shabana Khan, MD[a],*, Ujjwal Ramtekkar, MD, MBA, MPE[b]

KEYWORDS

- Telemedicine • Telepsychiatry • Telemental health • E-health • Telehealth
- Training and education • Child psychiatry

KEY POINTS

- Telepsychiatry education and training are important to ensure successful implementation and sustainability of pediatric telepsychiatry services.
- Limited literature exists on telepsychiatry education and training and the vast majority does not address considerations unique to practicing telepsychiatry with children and adolescents.
- Future directions include developing an evidence-based pediatric telepsychiatry curriculum for trainees and practicing child and adolescent psychiatrists.

INTRODUCTION

Recent data estimate that approximately 11% of children and adolescents in the United States have a serious emotional disturbance with significant functional impairment,[1] and approximately half of adults with psychiatric illness receive their diagnosis before age 15.[2] Despite the availability of effective treatments, a significant percentage of youth with mental health disorders do not receive needed treatment and for those who do, there often is a significant delay from symptom onset to diagnosis and treatment initiation.

One reason for the lack of or delays in treatment is the significant shortage and maldistribution of child and adolescent psychiatrists. These access issues have a disproportionate impact on children and adolescents living outside major metropolitan areas

This article originally appeared in *Psychiatric Clinics*, Volume 42, Issue 4, December 2019.
Disclosure Statement: The authors have nothing to disclose.
[a] Department of Child and Adolescent Psychiatry, Hassenfeld Children's Hospital at NYU Langone Health, One Park Avenue, 7th Floor, New York, NY 10016, USA; [b] Partner for Kids (ACO), Division of Child and Adolescent Psychiatry, Nationwide Children's Hospital/Ohio State University, 700 Children's Drive, T4 Suite A.007, Columbus, OH 43025, USA
* Corresponding author.
E-mail address: Shabana.Khan@nyulangone.org
Twitter: @ShabanaKhanMD (S.K.); @UjjRam (U.R.)

Clinics Collections 10 (2021) 137–144
https://doi.org/10.1016/j.ccol.2020.12.015
2352-7986/21/© 2020 Elsevier Inc. All rights reserved.

and in inner-city communities.[3] There are approximately 8200 practicing child and adolescent psychiatrists in the United States,[4] and more than 15 million youth in need of the special expertise of a child and adolescent psychiatrist.[5]

Telepsychiatry, the use of videoconferencing to provide psychiatric evaluation, consultation, supervision, education, and treatment, has potential benefits on both ends of the connection. Studies demonstrate that the clinical outcomes of care delivered via telepsychiatry are comparable to that of in-person care.[6] In some cases, care provided by telepsychiatry may be better than in person. Patients with certain diagnoses, such as posttraumatic stress disorder, autism spectrum disorder, or anxiety disorders, may prefer telepsychiatry due to feelings of control, safety, and distance created by this modality.[7] Despite the increasing use of telepsychiatry for children and adolescents, formal clinician training continues to be limited.

On the patient end, telepsychiatry can address access issues in pediatric behavioral health, limit unnecessary travel, reduce school absences and parental time off from work, bring specialty care to local communities, and improve outcomes by reducing delays in diagnosis and treatment. Children have grown up around technology and are comfortable seeing their doctor by video. Additionally, children and families in smaller, rural communities may be more willing to seek psychiatric care at a distance due to enhanced feelings of confidentiality, because it is less likely that they will run into their telepsychiatrist, who may be physically located hundreds of miles away from them.

On the practitioner end, telemedicine, including telepsychiatry, can enhance physician satisfaction with the ability to reach populations that are otherwise unreachable, streamline clinical workflows, allow better continuity of care, facilitate collaboration among virtual care teams, allow for greater flexibility in work schedules, reduce feelings of isolation, offer conveniences such as eliminating the need to commute to an office or between sites, and improve the health and well-being of physicians. When done right, the use of technology in medicine can help mitigate physician burnout. These benefits increase the likelihood of recruiting and retaining child and adolescent psychiatrists.

To ensure successful implementation and sustainability of telepsychiatry, education and training are important not only for psychiatrists but also for the entire team of health care professionals who are actively involved with the practice of telepsychiatry, including telepresenters, nurses, medical assistants, social workers, psychologists, medical students, and postgraduate trainees. Patients and guardians also should be provided with information on telepsychiatry and given the opportunity to ask questions about the care they will receive through this modality.

This article reviews the current literature on telepsychiatry education and training, provides resources including best practices and guidelines, provides an overview of considerations unique to the practice of telepsychiatry with children and adolescents, and discusses future directions to advance education and training in child and adolescent telepsychiatry.

REVIEW OF THE LITERATURE ON TELEPSYCHIATRY EDUCATION AND TRAINING

Limited literature exists on telepsychiatry education and training and the vast majority does not address considerations unique to practicing telepsychiatry with children and adolescents. Furthermore, the main focus of the evidence base is on postgraduate medical education without addressing education and training for actively practicing child and adolescent psychiatrists, who would also benefit significantly from access to reliable resources to help guide their telemedicine practice. Psychiatrists may be resistant to integrating telepsychiatry into their practice without relevant education, clinical experience, and exposure to the technology.

A majority of current medical students and postgraduate trainees are digital natives who are comfortable with technology and consider it to be an integral and necessary part of their lives. Despite the rapid expansion of technology in health care, most medical schools do not include telemedicine education and training as a required part of their curriculum. The integration of telemedicine-based lessons, ethics case studies, clinical rotations, and teleassessments offer great value for medical schools and their students.[8] Because psychiatry is one of the most common uses of telemedicine, telepsychiatry often is the first clinical exposure medical students have to telemedicine at academic medical centers. This uniquely positions our field to lead telemedicine education and training. Early training in and exposure to the use of innovative technology in medicine may help recruit medical students into child and adolescent psychiatry.

Currently, the Accreditation Council for Graduate Medical Education (ACGME), the accrediting body for psychiatry residency programs in the United States, does not require telepsychiatry training in psychiatry residencies.[9] The American Academy of Child and Adolescent Psychiatry (AACAP) and the American Psychiatric Association (APA) strongly support the inclusion of telepsychiatry education and training into graduate medical education.

A survey of psychiatry residency programs across the United States found that few programs offered a curriculum in telepsychiatry and most programs reported an interest in a sample curriculum.[10]

A literature review on telepsychiatry in graduate medical education identified 20 publications describing training psychiatry residents in telepsychiatry.[11] The majority of the literature was primarily descriptive, and the investigators concluded that a more evidence-based approach to telepsychiatry training is needed, including an assessment of residents' learning needs, use of multiple learning modalities, and evaluations of educational curricula.

Crawford and colleagues[12] used an assessment of resident learning needs to identify specific skills required for the practice of effective telepsychiatry and to provide an evidence base to guide the development of telepsychiatry curricula in postgraduate psychiatry training. The specific domains of competency identified were technical skills; assessment skills; relational skills and communication; collaborative and interprofessional skills; administrative skills; medicolegal skills; community psychiatry and community-specific knowledge; cultural psychiatry skills, including knowledge of indigenous cultures; and knowledge of health systems. Hilty and colleagues[13] proposed a framework for telepsychiatric training and e-health for trainees and clinicians, with competencies organized using the ACGME framework.

More data are needed on what core skills should be required for telepsychiatry training. To date, there are no published studies assessing telepsychiatry education and curriculum development in child and adolescent psychiatry fellowship programs in the United States.

TELEHEALTH FOR EDUCATION, CONSULTATION, AND MENTORING IN CHILD PSYCHIATRY

The benefits of telehealth extend beyond direct patient care. Videoconferencing can be used to provide telesupervision to medical trainees across a wide variety of settings and specialties, including child and adolescent psychiatry, particularly in rural and other underserved areas in the United States and internationally with limited access to local supervision.

Project Extension for Community Healthcare Outcomes (ECHO) uses telehealth technology to provide education, consultation and mentoring. It was originally established at the University of New Mexico to provide education to primary care providers (PCPs) on the management of hepatitis C. In the past decade, the model has expanded across a variety of specialties, including child and adolescent psychiatry, to provide didactic training and case-based interactive consultation to PCPs and allied health professionals. This model has been shown effective in improving patient outcomes and provider knowledge.[14]

Project ECHO is a case-based, interactive, learning collaborative model with a hub-and-spoke structure. It is designed to reduce access-to-care barriers for populations in underserved communities by using telehealth technologies to link a centrally located multidisciplinary team of specialists at a hub with PCPs in spoke communities. The hub team in psychiatry typically includes a psychiatrist, psychologist, clinical pharmacist, social worker, information technology support specialist, and program coordinator. Some hub teams may include a PCP, parent, and/or teacher to include their perspectives. The hub team specialists do not provide direct patient care to patients at spoke sites; they serve as a resource for PCPs. The facilitated discussion typically includes diagnostic guidance, suggestions for further evaluation and psychosocial support, and nonpharmacologic and pharmacologic treatment. Academic programs serving as hubs often use the program to train their psychiatry trainees in teleconsultation skills.

The Project ECHO model has been successfully used for general psychiatry as well as specialty areas, such as child and adolescent psychiatry, autism, addiction, and systems of care models like collaborative care.

Project ECHO can be used for professional development using the current criteria of continued professional development: participation, satisfaction, learning, competence, performance, patient, and community health. The model also aligns with current best practice recommendations for continued medical education.[15]

SPECIAL CONSIDERATIONS FOR TELEPSYCHIATRY WITH CHILDREN AND ADOLESCENTS

Children and adolescents in the digital age are accustomed to being connected through the use of electronics, such as social media, video games, and interactive videoconferencing applications on mobile devices (eg, FaceTime). Pediatric outcomes studies indicate that adolescents are more comfortable with telepsychiatry and treatment outcomes are comparable to in-person visits.[16,17] It is important for psychiatrists to effectively translate basic tenets of in-person interactions to psychiatric assessments conducted via telepsychiatry.

Telepsychiatry with children requires intentional actions to overcome the physical separation. In order to engage and instantly build rapport with a child, a psychiatrist can comment on curious actions, such as children making faces at the camera while watching their own image in a picture-in-picture view, or comment on children's clothing, toys, or objects they are carrying. In addition to reinforcing that a child is visible to the psychiatrist, this provides an opportunity to discuss the novel experience of a video visit before addressing clinical matters. When children are moving around due to hyperactivity, exploratory behaviors, agitation, or other reasons, however, it is important to ensure that they are in the camera frame for uninterrupted observation. Using a remotely controlled, pan-tilt-zoom camera, therefore, may be preferred in telepsychiatry with children over the integrated, stationary cameras used with adults or older adolescents. For younger children, parents can have children sit on their laps during the session if needed. For older adolescents with a parent or other individuals present, the camera may need appropriate adjustment to accommodate 2 or more individuals in the frame. Involving the adolescent and their family in this process of setting up can foster a sense of engagement and make the interaction collaborative from the beginning of the session.

Appropriate lighting and nondistracting surroundings are essential for reliable observation and assessment of any involuntary motor movements, facial expression, and subtleties of affect. Ample, indirect lighting and a clutter-free background on both ends of the connection are key for best viewing. These technical aspects of the camera and lighting assist in enhancing the quality and comfort of telepsychiatry sessions. Educators can teach these rapport-building technical considerations to residents and child and adolescent psychiatry fellows conducting telepsychiatry. Simulations using camera recordings of trainees during mock telepsychiatry sessions can serve as an excellent tool for practicing these technical aspects and skills.

Nonverbal communication plays a crucial role in creating an authentic experience through expression of empathy, professionalism, and therapeutic intentions. This is especially important when typical physical interactions like shaking hands have to be replaced by gestures on screen. With children and adolescents as the primary audience, the psychiatrist must ensure good eye contact and communicate with an exaggerated tone of voice, facial expressions, and energetic hand gestures. The psychiatrist should use appropriate camera placement to convey natural eye contact. Leaning forward can express empathy and leaning back can show interest in hearing more. Using high fives or thumbs-up on camera with youth also serve as good alternatives for verbal encouragers like "good job" and can help share more information. It is important to identify and practice nonverbal gestures, including facial expressions on camera in advance to ensure that those are visible in the camera frame during telepsychiatry sessions. Educators and supervisors can teach the basic tenets of being an empathetic listener through a deliberate emphasis on nonverbal communication in telepsychiatry.

Training in child and adolescent telepsychiatry includes staying up-to-date on the constantly evolving reimbursement, legal and regulatory environment, and new models of delivery. Key administrative, ethical, and clinical aspects, including emergency management, also must be learned.

OTHER TECHNOLOGIES

Apart from the traditional live, interactive, audio-video communication, other forms of technology also are becoming mainstream in health care; these include mobile technology integrated in phones, wearable devices, and standalone remote devices, collectively referred to as mHealth. With more than 70% of teens connected to the Internet and mobile devices, these tools are becoming important sources of data collection as well as interventions through Web-based and app-based platforms. More recently, artificial intelligence has been used to develop modalities using mobile text or conversational agents (chatbots) for cognitive-behavioral therapy interventions. The literature on these applications of technology, however, is still emerging. Educators should consider using technology curricula to better equip child and adolescent psychiatry trainees to understand the current landscape, provide guidance on how to evaluate these technologies, provide an overview of current research on feasibility and outcomes, and discuss different digital tools that can be utilized in daily practice for assessment, patient communication, treatment, and monitoring of health outcomes.[18]

PEDIATRIC TELEPSYCHIATRY EDUCATION AND TRAINING RESOURCES

Some academic medical centers provide formal orientation, education, and training in telepsychiatry to their postgraduate trainees and/or faculty; however, there is great variability in the breadth and quality of educational content, training, and clinical exposure. Large health care systems, such as the Department of Veterans Affairs and the Department of Defense, also provide telepsychiatry orientation and training to their staff.

Individual psychiatrists without access to such resources may obtain education by review of relevant scientific literature and through telepsychiatry presentations or workshops online or in-person, such as those offered through the AACAP, APA, and the American Telemedicine Association (ATA). There is no formal, nationally recognized certification in telepsychiatry. Some psychiatrists start providing clinical telepsychiatry services without baseline education or training and learn through clinical experience and consultation with colleagues.

The 2017 AACAP "Clinical Update: Telepsychiatry with Children and Adolescents"[19] reviews the use of telepsychiatry to deliver psychiatric, mental health, and care coordination services to youth across settings as direct service and in collaboration with other clinicians. The update presents procedures for conducting telepsychiatry services and optimizing the clinical experience.

The AACAP, in partnership with the APA, developed an online Child and Adolescent Telepsychiatry Toolkit[20] in 2019 to address issues unique to practicing telepsychiatry with children and adolescents. The toolkit consists of a series of video series that cover topics in telepsychiatry related to the history, training, practice and clinical issues, reimbursement, and legal issues from leading child and adolescent psychiatrists. This toolkit was developed to complement the APA's Telepsychiatry Toolkit by adding pediatric-specific considerations.

The 2017 ATA "Practice Guidelines for Telemental Health with Children and Adolescents"[21] provides a clinical guideline for the delivery of child and adolescent mental health and behavioral services by a licensed health care provider through real-time videoconferencing.

The APA and ATA released the "Best Practices in Videoconferencing-Based Telemental Health" guide[22] in 2018 to assist practitioners in providing effective and safe medical care founded on expert consensus, research evidence, available resources, and patient needs.

The telepsychiatry committees of the AACAP and ATA regularly provide up-to-date resources on telepsychiatry. **Table 1** summarizes key online resources for pediatric telepsychiatry.

FUTURE DIRECTIONS

This article provides an overview of the current literature on telepsychiatry education and training and preliminary guidance on developing education and training resources specific to pediatric telepsychiatry. Additional research is needed to assess the current state of telepsychiatry education and training in child and adolescent psychiatry fellowship programs. Future opportunities include developing an evidence-based pediatric telepsychiatry curriculum for trainees and practicing child and adolescent psychiatrists. Ongoing efforts are under way in the development of a curriculum in pediatric telebehavioral health to improve training nationally and address workforce shortages and geographic maldistribution. Future educational initiatives should address training not only for child psychiatrists but also for the entire multidisciplinary team of health care professionals who will be actively involved with the practice of

Table 1
Pediatric telepsychiatry resources and useful Web sites

Resource	Web Site
AACAP Telepsychiatry Resource Page	https://www.aacap.org/AACAP/Clinical_Practice_Center/Business_of_Practice/Telepsychiatry/Telepsych_Home.aspx
APA Telepsychiatry Toolkit	https://www.psychiatry.org/psychiatrists/practice/telepsychiatry/toolkit
Joint AACAP-APA Child and Adolescent Telepsychiatry Toolkit	https://www.psychiatry.org/psychiatrists/practice/telepsychiatry/toolkit/child-adolescent
Center for Telehealth and e-Health Law	https://ctel.org/
Center for Connected Health Policy	https://www.cchpca.org/
National Consortium of Telehealth Resource Centers	https://www.telehealthresourcecenter.org/
ATA	https://www.americantelemed.org/

All Web sites were accessed May 15, 2019.

telepsychiatry, including telepresenters, nurses, medical assistants, social workers, psychologists, and medical students.

ACKNOWLEDGMENT

A special thanks to the AACAP Telepsychiatry Committee, and Drs. Kathleen Myers, Sandra DeJong, and David Pruitt.

REFERENCES

1. Williams NJ, Scott L, Aarons GA. Prevalence of serious emotional disturbance among U.S. children: a meta-analysis. Psychiatr Serv 2018;69(1):32–40.

2. Jones PB. Adult mental health disorders and their age at onset. Br J Psychiatry Suppl 2013;54:s5–10.

3. Flaum M. Telemental health as a solution to the widening gap between supply and demand for mental health services. In: Myers K, Turvey C, editors. Telemental health: clinical, technical and administrative foundation for evidence-based practice. London: Elsevier Insights; 2013. p. 11–25.

4. American Medical Association. Physician masterfile. 2017. Available at: https://www.ama-assn.org/practice-management/masterfile/ama-physician-masterfile. Accessed March 1, 2019.

5. AACAP resources for primary care: workforce issues. Available at: https://www.aacap.org/aacap/resources_for_primary_care/Workforce_Issues.aspx. Accessed April 15, 2019.

6. O'Reilly R, Bishop J, Maddox K, et al. Is telepsychiatry equivalent to face-to-face psychiatry? Results from a randomized controlled equivalence trial. Psychiatr Serv 2007;58(6):836–43.

7. Shore JH, Savin DM, Novins D, et al. Cultural aspects of telepsychiatry. J Telemed Telecare 2006;12(3):116–21.

8. Waseh S, Dicker AP. Telemedicine training in undergraduate medical education: mixed-methods review. JMIR Med Educ 2019;5(1):e12515.

9. Accreditation Council for Graduate Medical Education (ACGME). Program requirements for graduate medical education in psychiatry 2017. Available at: https://www.acgme.org/Portals/0/PFAssets/ProgramRequirements/400_psychiatry_2017-07-01.pdf. Accessed April 15, 2019.

10. Hoffman P, Kane JM. Telepsychiatry education and curriculum development in residency training. Acad Psychiatry 2015;39(1):108–9.

11. Sunderji N, Crawford A, Jovanovic M. Telepsychiatry in graduate medical education: a narrative review. Acad Psychiatry 2015;39(1):55–62.

12. Crawford A, Sunderji N, Lopez J, et al. Defining competencies for the practice of telepsychiatry through an assessment of resident learning needs. BMC Med Educ 2016;16:28.

13. Hilty DM, Crawford A, Teshima J, et al. A framework for telepsychiatric training and e-health: competency-based education, evaluation and implications. Int Rev Psychiatry 2015;27(6):569–92.

14. Zhou C, Crawford A, Serhal E, et al. The impact of project ECHO on participant and patient outcomes: a systematic review. Acad Med 2016;91(10):1439–61.

15. Arora S, Kalishman SG, Thornton KA, et al. Project ECHO: a telementoring network model for continuing professional development. J Contin Educ Health Prof 2017;37(4):239–44.

16. Elford R, White H, Bowering R, et al. A randomized, controlled trial of child psychiatric assessments conducted using videoconferencing. J Telemed Telecare 2000;6(2):73–82.

17. Myers K, Vander Stoep A, McCarty C, et al. Child and adolescent telepsychiatry: Variations in utilization, referral patterns and practice trends. J Telemed Telecare 2010;16:128.

18. Gipson SY-MT, Kim JW, Shin AL, et al. Teaching child and adolescent psychiatry in the twenty-first century. Child Adolesc Psychiatr Clin N Am 2017;26(1):93–103.

19. American Academy of Child and Adolescent Psychiatry (AACAP) Committee on Telepsychiatry and AACAP Committee on Quality Issues. Clinical update: telepsychiatry with children and adolescents. J Am Acad Child Adolesc Psychiatry 2017;56(10):875–93.

20. AACAP-APA child and adolescent telepsychiatry toolkit. 2019. Available at: https://www.psychiatry.org/psychiatrists/practice/telepsychiatry/toolkit/child-adolescent. Accessed April 15, 2019.

21. Myers K, Nelson EL, Rabinowitz T, et al. American telemedicine association practice guidelines for telemental health with children and adolescents. Telemed J E Health 2017;23(10):779–804.

22. Shore JH, Yellowlees P, Caudill R, et al. Best practices in videoconferencing-based telemental health April 2018. Telemed J E Health 2018;24(11):827–32.

Recommendations for Using Clinical Video Telehealth with Patients at High Risk for Suicide

Meghan M. McGinn, PhD[a,b,*], Milena S. Roussev, PhD[a],
Erika M. Shearer, PhD[c], Russell A. McCann, PhD[b,c],
Sasha M. Rojas, MS[a,d], Bradford L. Felker, MD[a,b]

KEYWORDS

• Telemedicine • Suicide • Mental health services • Access to health care

KEY POINTS

• Clinical video telehealth (CVT) has the potential to deliver much-needed mental health services to individuals at risk for suicide who face access barriers.
• None of the literature, professional guidelines, and laws pertaining to the provision of mental health services via CVT suggest that high-risk patients should be excluded from this modality.
• Best practices for assessment and management of suicide risk can be feasibly performed by mental health professionals via CVT.
• Mental health professionals delivering services via CVT to high-risk patients would benefit from a multidisciplinary network of CVT providers for referral and consultation.

There is a growing body of evidence supporting the safe and effective use of clinical video telehealth (CVT) in the provision of mental health services,[1,2] and the benefits of using this modality, including increasing access and reducing rates of hospitalization, have been widely cited.[3–5] At the same time, there remains concern among many

This article originally appeared in *Psychiatric Clinics*, Volume 42, Issue 4, December 2019.
Disclosure: The authors have no relationships with any commercial company that has a direct financial interest in the subject matter or materials discussed in this article or with a company making a competing product. The views expressed in this article are those of the authors and do not necessarily reflect the position or policy of the Department of Veterans Affairs or the United States government.
[a] VA Puget Sound Health Care System, S-116-MHC, 1660 South Columbian Way, Seattle, WA 98108, USA; [b] Department of Psychiatry and Behavioral Sciences, University of Washington School of Medicine, 1959 NE Pacific St, Seattle, WA, USA; [c] VA Puget Sound Health Care System, A-116-VIP, 9600 Veterans Drive Southwest, Tacoma, WA 98493, USA; [d] University of Arkansas, Fayetteville, AR, USA
* Corresponding author. VA Puget Sound Health Care System, S-116-MHC, 1660 South Columbian Way, Seattle, WA 98108.
E-mail address: meghan.mcginn@va.gov

Clinics Collections 10 (2021) 145–153
https://doi.org/10.1016/j.ccol.2020.12.016

providers about the use of CVT, particularly for those patients considered at high risk for suicide.[6] This concern creates a juxtaposition such that the patients who are most in need of access to mental health services are often excluded from using CVT because of provider perceptions that the modality is not appropriate for high risk patients.

The current article (1) reviews the body of published studies, professional guidelines, and laws that pertain to the use of CVT with patients at high risk for suicide, and (2) provides practical recommendations for how to adapt best-practice guidelines for assessing and managing suicide risk when treating high-risk patients for the CVT modality. The authors are providers with extensive experience in the provision of mental health treatment via CVT within the Veterans Administration (VA) health care system, and case examples are included to show the recommended adaptations for using this modality in the assessment and management of individuals at high risk for suicide.

RESEARCH EVIDENCE FOR THE USE OF CLINICAL VIDEO TELEHEALTH WITH HIGH-RISK PATIENTS

There is strong evidence to suggest the equivalency of mental health services delivered via CVT compared with in-person delivery; however, many clinical trials have excluded participants who were considered high risk.[1,2,7] There is not 1 randomized control trial (RCT) that examines the effects of CVT, compared with in-person treatment, on clinical risk outcomes among high-risk populations. Secondary analysis from a recent RCT suggests individuals who presented with greater levels of hopelessness at baseline were likely to improve more if they completed in-person treatment compared with CVT, although both groups did improve after treatment.[8] It is clear that the field would benefit from research that is more inclusive of high-risk individuals and that directly studies risk outcomes.

At the same time, the literature to date does provide evidence that emergency situations that arise in the context of therapy can be successfully managed via CVT,[9] and CVT has been effectively used in the assessment and treatment of psychiatric emergency patients[10] as well as persons in rural shelters after experiencing domestic violence.[11] Furthermore, in a study examining clinical outcomes of patients enrolled in CVT services between 2006 and 2010, Godleski and colleagues[3] found a 25% decrease in hospitalizations among veterans receiving care via CVT, and, among those who were admitted, they observed a decrease in days of psychiatric hospitalization. There is also evidence outside the VA system that CVT can help reduce rehospitalization within a 12-month period and increase treatment adherence in rural patients following psychiatric hospitalization.[12] In summary, although there is a lack of clinical trial data that specifically target high-risk patients, there are observable benefits of this modality and a precedent for how to manage risk safely.

Some investigators have speculated that CVT offers some unique benefits for suicide assessment compared with care as usual, which is often telephone-based risk assessment. For example, Godleski and colleagues[13] note that CVT (1) offers visual cues about the patients' emotional states, (2) allows for suicide assessments in remote areas where providers may not be available, (3) can reduce the need for hospitalization when effective treatments can be provided via CVT, and (4) can allow culturally sensitive care to be delivered, particularly where language barriers might be present. Pruitt and collegues[5] reviewed clinical benefits of CVT to the home, in which veterans received mental health services directly into their homes. They argue that CVT may enhance safety for both patients and practitioners, such that collaboratively establishing a safety plan with the patient may in itself offer therapeutic benefits.

PROFESSIONAL GUIDELINES REGARDING THE USE OF CLINICAL VIDEO TELEHEALTH

Practice standards and guidelines relevant to providing CVT services to high-risk patients have been published by various professional associations, including the National Association of Social Workers[14] and American Psychological Association (APA),[15] as well as a joint taskforce comprising the American Psychiatric Association and American Telemedicine Association (ATA).[16] None of these guidelines identify a circumstance in which using the CVT modality in practice would always be contraindicated. Instead, these guidelines focus on offering various considerations that may affect the determination of whether CVT would be clinically appropriate for patients.

Identified factors to consider when determining the appropriateness include patients' cognitive capacity, history of cooperation, history of substance use, history of violence or self-injurious behavior, and nearby community resources (eg, hospitals, clinics, laboratories). In addition, patients should understand that CVT could be discontinued at any time, and that they may need to present in person to a clinic as part of the services offered (eg, physical examination, laboratory services). Collectively, these considerations are less salient when patients are seen via CVT while seated in a supervised setting (eg, at a rural clinic with medical support staff). Such sites may have ample medical resources that clinicians can leverage to support their patients. The aforementioned considerations for determining appropriateness of patients may carry more importance when patients are seen in nonclinic locations, such as their homes, vehicles, places of work, or other unsupervised locales. When clinical resources are not available during the encounter to conduct physical examinations and laboratory tests, and staff are not nearby to assist with emergency interventions, the importance of patient cooperativeness, such as their willingness to engage in suitable clinical alternatives and follow safety plans, becomes paramount.

These professional associations' guidelines separately address discipline-specific topics that are relevant to working with high-risk patients. For example, the 2018 APA/ATA guidelines speak to the prescription of controlled substances via CVT[16] and the 2013 APA guidelines discuss the use of test and assessment instruments over this modality.[15] However, there are also common themes across guidelines, such as the importance of a patient-specific emergency plan and the acknowledgment that patients' appropriateness for CVT may change over time.[14–16]

LAWS AFFECTING PROVISION OF CLINICAL VIDEO TELEHEALTH TO HIGH-RISK INDIVIDUALS

On a federal level, the Ryan Haight Act[17] affects psychiatric care for all patients by restricting the prescribing of controlled substances via CVT in certain contexts. A detailed overview of the Ryan Haight Act is beyond the scope of this article, and although there are additional exceptions, the Ryan Haight Act generally requires that providers prescribing a controlled substance via CVT either must have previously seen their patients once in person or their patients must be physically located at a Drug Enforcement Administration (DEA)–registered facility at the time of the prescription event. The Ryan Haight Act is not specific to care for high-risk patients; however, it does make it so psychiatric providers may be unable to prescribe in the same way via CVT as they might in person, creating a situation in which caring for high-risk patients via CVT could be affected such that it would be preferable to meet in person, or at least via another, legally tenable CVT arrangement that allows patients to receive the appropriate level of care (eg, while the patient is located at a DEA-registered clinic). It seems that the Ryan Haight Act's impact on CVT will soon change. In October 2018, the Substance Use–Disorder Prevention that Promotes Opioid Recovery and Treatment (SUPPORT) for Patients and Communities Act[18] was signed into law, which will require the United States Attorney General to implement a process for providers to register as exempt from restrictions put forth by the Ryan Haight Act, effectively enabling them to practice via CVT in a manner more consistent with in-person care. The Attorney General has until October 2019 to put this registration process into effect. The authors think that implementation of the SUPPORT Act will better enable providers to work with more varied clinical presentations via CVT, including those with higher risk.

State law also affects working with high-risk patients via CVT. Each state has laws that regulate the provision of CVT to patients physically located in the respective state. In general, providers need to be licensed in each state they support via CVT. Some states require that providers seek full licenses to practice via CVT, whereas some states offer CVT-specific licenses, and still other states have various mechanisms designed to both encourage and regulate providers from out of state serving patients in their area. Under a recent amendment to its medical regulations,[19] the VA health care system has ruled that providers are able to engage in interstate CVT practice without being licensed in more than 1 location; however, regardless, all providers may still be held liable to the laws of the state where their patients are seated. Providers may also be held liable to states where they are physically located as well.[13] Practically speaking, if providers are only licensed in 1 state and provide CVT within that same state, they need only to become familiar with that state's laws related to both mental health care broadly and CVT. If providers are licensed and practicing via CVT in multiple states, they need to be fully aware of the legal differences that exist between states, and adjust their practices accordingly. For example, providers might follow a certain process for getting patients involuntarily committed in one state, and be required to follow still a different commitment process in another state. If laws for providers' locations are not congruent, providers might be wise to proceed cautiously. The implications of varied state law have a major impact on working with high-risk patients.

ADAPTING BEST-PRACTICE GUIDELINES FOR WORKING WITH HIGH-RISK PATIENTS TO CLINICAL VIDEO TELEHEALTH DELIVERY

The literature, professional guidelines, and laws discussed earlier may heavily inform the provision of CVT to high-risk patients, but none of them suggest that CVT services should not be offered for such clinical presentations. As such, the second aim of this article is to discuss how to adapt best-practice guidelines for working with high-risk patients to CVT delivery of these services. Through a collaborative effort, the Department of Defense (DOD) and the VA developed the Clinical Practice Guideline for the Assessment and Management of Suicide Risk.[20] This guideline provides evidence-based recommendations and a structured framework for assessing suicide risk and facilitating hospitalization when warranted. The VA/DOD defines high-acute risk for suicide as individuals with persistent suicidal ideation, strong suicidal intention or plan, poor impulse control, or a recent suicide attempt or preparatory behavior, and identifies hospitalization as the first-line recommended treatment of such high-acute–risk individuals. Although there is not a CVT application analogous to inpatient care, providers may encounter patients at high risk for suicide via CVT during the assessment phase or after discharge. A discussion of how to adapt the VA/DOD recommendations to the CVT modality when working with high-risk patients is presented later (in bulleted points), accompanied by case examples from the authors' clinical experiences and informed by the extant literature and the professional guidelines mentioned earlier for use of CVT.

Assessment

The recommendations in the VA/DOD's Clinical Practice Guideline for the Assessment and Management of Suicide Risk[20] include the completion of a comprehensive assessment of suicide risk by a behavioral health provider. As in the case of in-person treatment, suicide risk assessment via the CVT modality may include data from several sources; for example, routinely administered screening measures as a part of measurement-based care (eg, Patient Health Questionnaire); visual cues that may indicate depressed mood; collateral reports from loved ones; and the patients' own verbal reports.

Although many elements of the assessment will be the same via CVT as in person, consider the following adaptations:

- To ensure patient safety, obtain the patients' location at the start of the interaction to allow for enacting an emergency plan.
- Consider HIPAA (Health Insurance Portability and Accountability Act)-compliant options for sending and receiving written questionnaires (eg, secure messaging, postal mail, patient holding completed measure up to the screen).
- If the patient is located out of state, familiarize yourself with the laws of that state, such as for involuntary commitment and abuse reporting.

Hospitalization

When a comprehensive risk assessment via CVT reveals that hospitalization is indicated, there are a few CVT-related considerations for facilitating this process:

- Remain connected with the patient via CVT throughout the process of coordinating hospitalization. If the connection is lost, try to reconnect via CVT or call the patient on the phone.
- While maintaining the CVT call, either the provider or the patient can call emergency services by telephone to coordinate involvement of emergency services for transport, if necessary.
- Use the support of other staff to assist with patient care coordination during the CVT call (eg, use the phone, pager, or internal instant messaging system to connect with suicide prevention coordinators, colleagues, or other support staff). Secondary support staff may be able to assist with contacting emergency departments or emergency services, or simply provide consultation in real time allowing the provider to document peer concurrence with the steps taken to ensure patient safety.
- Work with other individuals present in the home as needed.

Case Example: Assessment and Hospitalization via Clinical Video Telehealth

During a home-based CVT appointment, a 33-year-old divorced male veteran stated that he "just can't take it anymore" and discussed his concerns related to suicide. Through assessment, it was deemed that the veteran was at imminent risk for suicide and that his risk level warranted a higher level of care. The veteran was amenable to hospitalization. Because the veteran was at home, did not have a support person nearby to drive him to the hospital, and was not able to drive himself, the decision was made to contact emergency services for immediate evaluation and transport to the local hospital emergency department. The veteran was given the option of either calling the 911 himself or having his provider call 911, both while maintaining CVT connection with this provider. The veteran opted to call 911 himself. He maintained the CVT connection while he called 911 so that this provider could continue to observe and hear the interaction. While waiting for emergency services to arrive, the veteran continued with his provider and was able to engage in grounding techniques and discuss coordination of care related to the hospitalization.

When emergency services arrived, the veteran was able to introduce his provider to emergency services personnel via CVT, and together they discussed the clinical situation. The veteran was voluntarily hospitalized because of acute suicidal risk.

Determining the Appropriate Setting and Modality of Care After Discharge

The VA/DOD clinical practice guideline states that once an individual no longer has suicidal intent, has obtained a level of psychiatric stability (eg, is no longer intoxicated or acutely psychotic), and is willing and able to perform a safety plan, the patient should be moved to a less restrictive setting of care.[20] For individuals with access barriers, CVT is an appealing option as a less restrictive setting for outpatient care. However, because CVT is only a modality of care and not a specific treatment in itself, consider the following:

- First, consider what level of care and type of treatment is clinically indicated for the patient. For example, if substance use is a strong risk factor, consider referral to a substance use disorders program, or, if borderline personality disorder is the underlying disorder contributing to risk, consider referral to a full dialectical behavioral therapy (DBT[21]) program.
- Once referred to the appropriate clinical setting, then consider the appropriateness for delivering treatment via CVT in this setting. At a minimum, the patients need to be willing to follow through on a CVT-specific safety plan, meaning they must be willing to provide a location at each session so that the provider may activate the emergency plan as needed. The safety plan may also include limiting access to means during sessions to ensure that it is a safe setting for treatment.
- Note that not every high-risk patient is appropriate for CVT. Providers are encouraged to consider each high-risk patient on a case-by-case basis, and consult with colleagues when making this determination.

Case Example: Determining Appropriateness for Outpatient Treatment via Clinical Video Telehealth

A rurally located, 80-year-old veteran was referred for anger management. The veteran requested CVT to home, because he reportedly never leaves his house because of fear that he will end up hurting someone. He described to the referring provider, a primary care mental health provider at the community-based outpatient clinic, that he carries a loaded weapon with him at all times and that once in the past month he pointed the weapon at his own head when experiencing high distress. He did not have active suicidal ideation, plan, or intent at the time of referral, but he described having low frustration tolerance, and acknowledged that technology failure is a trigger for distress. The veteran also expressed that he did not want to work on learning skills that will help him to manage his anger and be able to leave his home, but rather wanted therapy that would allow him to "vent." Because of his belief that it keeps him safer to carry a weapon, he was unwilling to restrict access to his weapon during sessions. The details of this referral were discussed with the CVT team. Because technology failure, a trigger for the veteran's distress, is a common occurrence during CVT sessions and the veteran described a history of impulsive suicidal behavior (eg, holding a gun to his head) in the context of distress, it was determined that the CVT modality may put him at greater risk. The team recommended that the referring provider consider referral to a residential program or other in-person treatment, or, if the patient is truly unwilling to leave the house, consider whether telephone may be a more appropriate modality because it is less prone to technology failure.

Ongoing Management of Patients at Risk for Suicide in an Outpatient Setting

The VA/DOD clinical practice guideline for managing patients at risk for suicide suggests that the first goal of treatment with high-risk patients should be to secure patient safety by addressing the following: patient and family education, limiting access to lethal means, safety planning, addressing psychosocial risk factors, and documenting a rationale and treatment plan.[20] As is the case for assessment, most patient management via the CVT modality is congruent with the in-person modality, but the following adaptations should be considered:

- Suggest inviting family members to a video visit with the patient to provide family education. If they are already present in the home, this may be more easily accomplished via CVT.
- Include creating a safe space for treatment in discussion of access to lethal means. Use the ability for patients to show you their environment to help set up a safe space.
- A copy of the safety plan can be mailed/sent via secure messaging or a blank safety plan provided ahead of time for the patient to fill out.
- Include in informed consent that CVT may be discontinued if it is determined to be an unsafe or ineffective modality for the patient.

Other best-practice recommendations for managing high-risk patients include addressing psychosocial risk factors, offering evidence-based therapies that target suicide risk, considering pharmacotherapies that have been shown to reduce suicide risk in the case of specific underlying disorders, and increasing engagement with strategies such as case care management.[20] These recommendations are most efficiently performed with a team approach to treatment of high-risk patients, providing these patients with access to multiple disciplines (social workers, psychiatrists, psychologists, nurse care-managers) and providers with different areas of expertise. As such, the authors recommend:

- In large systems of care, train full interdisciplinary teams in the use of telehealth technologies in order to provide patient access to multiple resources and team support for the providers managing risk remotely.
- For providers operating independently, it is prudent to network with others who provide telemental health to ensure the availability of case consultation with peers who also have experience using the modality and the ability to refer to appropriate treatment if the patient's treatment needs change.
- If medications are indicated, consider implication of Ryan Haight Act[17] and eventually the SUPPORT Act.[18]
- Consider augmenting or following up treatment via CVT with telephone care management or electronic symptom monitoring.

Case Example: Ongoing Management of Risk via Clinical Video Telehealth Following Inpatient Discharge

A 47-year-old partnered male veteran was discharged from a 72-hour hospitalization following a recent suicide attempt. He was discharged back to his home-based CVT provider with whom he been engaged in biweekly treatment of posttraumatic stress disorder (PTSD). The veteran was unsure regarding whether he had suicidal intent because he had been so intoxicated that he could not remember whether his intention was to commit suicide or to serve as a cry for help. The veteran's distance from the VA as well as his lack of driver's license because of a previous conviction for driving under the influence made access to in-person treatment difficult. His substance use and abuse were assessed and it was determined that his alcohol use had increased dramatically and warranted additional treatment beyond his current provider's expertise. The veteran's home-based CVT provider consulted with the local VA addictions treatment center (ATC) regarding coordinating care. A plan was made for the veteran to meet with a provider on the ATC team for home-based treatment via CVT in addition to his PTSD treatment to increase the level of care because of his recent hospitalization as well as to provide alcohol use disorder treatment. The ATC provider was able to coordinate with a community-based outpatient clinic to collect urinalysis as necessary. Ultimately, after some work with the veteran, he was amenable to engaging in residential treatment of alcohol use disorder and PTSD. On discharge from the residential programs, he resumed home-based treatment with both his ATC and PTSD providers via CVT.

SUMMARY AND FUTURE DIRECTIONS

The present article summarizes the literature, professional guidelines, and laws pertaining to the delivery of mental health services to patients at high risk for suicide. Although more research is still needed, these sources are generally supportive of caring for high-risk patients via CVT. Many of the existing clinical practice guidelines for assessing and managing suicide risk can feasibly be performed with minor modification.

Future research should specifically address the effectiveness of interventions delivered via CVT at reducing suicide risk factors. Likewise, to our knowledge, CVT delivery of several of the recommended treatment options for suicide risk and underlying disorders (eg, DBT for borderline personality disorder[21]) have not yet been implemented and evaluated. However, existing research does provide evidence that providers can effectively manage acute emergencies remotely and that many patients benefit from treatments delivered via CVT.

Provider concerns about CVT with high-risk patients are still prevalent,[6] and thus it is important to consider how to support providers in managing risk remotely. The VA health care system, because of the larger quantity of trained providers, can provide some models for this type of support that could be applied to non-VA settings. For example, every VA medical center hires suicide prevention coordinators who are available to assist other staff in the case of an emergency. In addition, there are national and local provider-led consultation groups for those who provide CVT services. Although some resources exist outside the VA system (eg, the national suicide hotline), it would be helpful for professional organizations or individual states to develop similar support systems in the form of networks of providers for consultation, referral, and coordinated care. These systems would allow providers to confidently offer evidence-based care to those most at risk and in need of the services.

REFERENCES

1. Hilty DM, Ferrer DC, Parish MB, et al. The effectiveness of telemental health: a 2013 review. Telemed J E Health 2013;19(6):444–54.

2. Hubley S, Lynch SB, Schneck C, et al. Review of key telepsychiatry outcomes. World Psychiatry 2016;6(2):269–82.
3. Godleski L, Cervone D, Vogel D, et al. Home telemental health implementation and outcomes using electronic messaging. J Telemed Telecare 2012;18(1):17–9.
4. Lyketsos CG, Roques C, Hovanec L, et al. Telemedicine use and the reduction of psychiatric admissions from a long-term care facility. J Geriatr Psychiatry Neurol 2001;14:76–9.
5. Pruitt LD, Luxton DD, Shore P. Additional clinical benefits of home-based telemental health treatments. Prof Psychol Res Pract 2014;45(5):340–6.
6. Gilmore AK, Ward-Ciesielski EF. Perceived risks and use of psychotherapy via telemedicine for patients at risk for suicide. J Telemed Telecare 2017;25(1):59–63.
7. Turgoose D, Ashwick R, Murphy D. Systematic review of lessons learned from delivering tele-therapy to veterans with post-traumatic stress disorder. J Telemed Telecare 2018;24(9):575–85.
8. Pruitt LD, Vuletic S, Smolenski DJ, et al. Predicting post treatment client satisfaction between behavioral activation for depression delivered either in-person or via home-based telehealth. J Telemed Telecare 2019;25(8):460–7.
9. Gros DF, Veronee K, Strachan M, et al. Managing suicidality in home based telehealth. J Telemed Telecare 2011;17(6):332–5.
10. Sorvaniemi M, Ojanen E, Santamaki O. Telepsychiatry in emergency consultations: a follow-up study of sixty patients. Telemed J E Health 2005;11:439–41.
11. Thomas CR, Miller G, Hartshorn JC, et al. Telepsychiatry program for rural victims of domestic violence. Telemed J E Health 2005;11(5):567–73.
12. D'Souza R. Improving treatment adherence and longitudinal outcomes in patients with a serious mental illness by using telemedicine. J Telemed Telecare 2002; 8(2):113–5.
13. Godleski L, Nieves JE, Darkins A, et al. VA telemental health: suicide assessment. Behav Sci Law 2008;26:271–86.
14. National Association of Social Workers, Association of Social Work Boards, Council on Social Work Education, & Clinical Social Work Association. NASW, ASWB, CSWE & CSWA standards for technology in social work practice. 2017. Available at: https://www.socialworkers.org/includes/newIncludes/homepage/PRA-BRO-33617.TechStandards_FINAL_POSTING.pdf. Accessed February 26, 2019.
15. American Psychological Association, Joint Task Force for the Development of Telepsychiatry Guidelines for Psychologists. Guidelines for the practice of telepsychology. Am Psychol 2013;68(9):791–800.
16. Shore JH, Yellowlees P, Caudill R, et al. Best practices in videoconferencing-based telemental health April 2018. Telemed J E Health 2018;24(11):827–32.
17. Ryan haight online pharmacy consumer protection act of 2008, 21 U.S.C § 802 (54).
18. H.R. 6 , 115th Cong. (2018) (enacted).
19. Department of Veterans Affairs. Authority of health care providers to practice telehealth. FR Doc. 2018–10114, Filed 5–10–18.
20. Department of Veterans Affairs & Department of Defense. VA/DOD clinical practice guideline for assessment and management of patients at risk for suicide. The Assessment and Management of Risk for Suicide Working Group, Office of Quality Safety and Value, VA, Washington DC. & Quality Management Division, United States Army MEDCOM; 2013. p. 1–190.
21. Linehan MM. Cognitive behavioural therapy of borderline personality disorder. New York: Guilford; 1993.

Clinician-Delivered Teletherapy for Eating Disorders

Laura Elizabeth Sproch, PhD, Kimberly Peddicord Anderson, PhD*

KEYWORDS

- Teletherapy • Telepsychotherapy • Telepsychology • Eating disorder
- Telemedicine • Videoconferencing • Telemental health • Psychotherapy

KEY POINTS

- Videoconferencing (VC) psychotherapy is a means of improving access to evidence-based ED care for those in need.
- Research suggests that the application of evidence-based protocols using teletherapy formats leads to significant improvement of ED symptoms and associated problems; however, additional research is necessary.
- Specific administrative considerations, including legal issues, patient environment, and technology access, exist for ED teletherapy and require close examination before implementing such treatment.
- Therapeutic alliance, satisfaction, and safety issues are comparable between ED in-person and VC therapy, with notable exceptions. Recognition of the clinical benefits specific to teletherapy, and counterindications, is essential.
- The importance of therapist training before the application of VC psychotherapy cannot be overstated.

INTRODUCTION

The mental health field has progressed and evolved to accommodate for its clinical population, the ever-changing culture, and advancing scientific knowledge. The turn to evermore specialist care is one example of such adaptation. Time has shown that distinct clinical issues often require distinct evidence-based treatment and specialized training. The treatment of eating disorders (EDs) is no exception. In fact, evidence-based ED treatment particularly highlights the importance of specialist

This article originally appeared in *Psychiatric Clinics*, Volume 42, Issue 2, June 2019.

Disclosures: The authors have no disclosures of relationships with a commercial company that has a direct financial interest in subject manner or materials discussed in this article or with a company making a competing product.

Department of Psychology, The Center for Eating Disorders at Sheppard Pratt, 6535 North Charles Street, Suite 300, Baltimore, MD 21204, USA

* Corresponding author.

E-mail address: KAnderson@sheppardpratt.org

care requiring mandatory education, training, supervision, and experience.[1–3] One obvious barrier to implementing ED-specialized psychotherapy is that in large pockets of North America, access to well-trained ED therapists can seem impossible. This produces two critical issues: EDs treated by providers not well-trained in evidence-based treatment, and lack of initiation of care by those in need because services are not easily identified and accessed. Research shows that for the most part, EDs go untreated. Individuals instead receive treatment of other mental health conditions or obesity and from providers (eg, primary care physicians) without requisite training in ED treatment protocols.[4–6] Sparked by the technology boom and its never-ending quest for staying current, the mental health field has recognized this accessibility issue and started using technology to disseminate treatment. Behavioral health treatment delivered through the Internet allows clinicians to offer face-to-face treatment with patients remotely located. This article informs clinicians of the utility, feasibility, and special considerations of using teletherapy for ED-specialized care.

First, we must focus the terminology used in this article because the term "teletherapy" is broad. In previous work, teletherapy has included videoconferencing (VC), telephone services, email therapy, text therapy, smartphone applications, virtual reality, and guided and unguided self-help (through software and online programs). Numerous recent reviews have been conducted that outline a combination of a variety of these teletherapy services for EDs.[7–11] This article focuses exclusively on therapist-delivered psychotherapy for clinical EDs via VC and exclude alternate forms listed previously. We have selected this mode in particular because we believe it to be the most duplicative of in-person protocols for clinical EDs with an established strong evidence base. Self-help treatment is an exception to this statement because the efficacy of this treatment of particular ED presentations is clear and is well reviewed in another article of this issue (See Heng Yim and Ulrike Schmidt's article, "Self-help Treatment of Eating Disorders," in this issue).

EVIDENCE FOR TELETHERAPY
General Psychotherapy

Within the past 15 years, substantial implementation and evaluation of teletherapy in general clinical populations has occurred. In their review, Hilty and colleagues[12] concluded that for the most part, teletherapy is comparable with in-person treatment of adult depression and anxiety. According to Backhaus and colleagues,[13] therapist-delivered VC psychotherapy in particular tends to be feasible, can reduce burden, is satisfactory for patients, and leads to clinical symptom reduction in nonrandomized controlled clinical trials. Randomized controlled studies suggest that cognitive-behavioral therapy (CBT) for childhood depression,[14] psychiatric treatment including brief supportive counseling for adult depression,[15] family counseling for epilepsy,[16] anger management CBT group therapy for adults,[17] and CBT group therapy for post-traumatic stress disorder[18] produces similar clinical symptom change between in-person and VC psychotherapy.

Specialized Eating Disorder Treatment

One randomized controlled trial of therapist-delivered teletherapy for ED-specialized care has been conducted. Mitchell and colleagues[19] randomly assigned 128 adults diagnosed with either bulimia nervosa or ED not otherwise specified (with binge eating or purging at least once per week) to VC or in-person CBT. In the in-person condition, CBT therapists traveled to the participant's local community to provide therapy, whereas in the VC condition, participants received services via computer at a local health care facility. Results showed no statistically significant between-group differences in attrition; abstinence rates of objective binge eating, purging, and combined binge eating/purging; ED restraint and weight concern; self-esteem; and quality of life. Compared with the VC condition, participants in the in-person condition had significantly less frequent binge eating and purging episodes. That is, at baseline, VC participants endorsed 19.1 objective binge eating episodes over the course of 28 days, which decreased to 6.2 at end of treatment. In the in-person condition, episodes decreased from 21.9 to 3.7 during the same timeframe. For purging episodes, VC participants decreased from 36.8 to 11.1 episodes in a 28-day period, whereas those in the in-person condition decreased from 35.6 to 5.6. Of note, at 12-month follow-up, binge eating frequency was found to be no longer significant between conditions; however, purging frequency differences were significant in that VC participants' number of episodes was 19.4 compared with the in-person condition, which was 8.2. Response to treatment measured by reduction in bingeing and purging frequency occurred more rapidly in the in-person condition compared with the VC condition, which had a more gradual response. Results indicated that there were significant group differences (ie, participants receiving in-person treatment scoring at lower levels) at 12-month follow-up on shape concerns, at 3-month follow-up on eating concerns, and at treatment end on depression symptoms. Despite these findings, the authors summarize that the treatments were "roughly equivalent" because of minimally significant differences. In follow-up studies, results indicated that, compared with the in-person condition, the VC condition was associated with the benefit of lower costs.[20] Additionally, predictors of treatment response differences were found between conditions, suggesting earlier symptom change in the VC condition, compared with the in-person condition.[21] Also, although therapists' ratings of therapeutic alliance were lower in earlier stages of treatment, patients' reports of therapeutic alliance were similar in the VC and in-person conditions.[22]

A few studies have evaluated VC psychotherapy for EDs without control conditions. Family-based treatment of adolescents was found to be feasible and acceptable and led to increased weight, decreased eating pathology, and decreased depressive symptoms from baseline to end of treatment and to 6-month follow-up.[23] VC application of CBT for EDs has been shown to be satisfying for patients and has led to decreased ED symptoms, decreased depression, and improved nutritional knowledge.[24–26]

TELETHERAPY CONSIDERATIONS FOR EATING DISORDER CARE
Administrative Considerations

Teletherapy laws, regulations, consent, and licensure
In the United States, current federal law dictates Medicare coverage of teletherapy at the same rate as in-person treatment.[27] Certain restrictions apply, such as the requirement that patients are seen at an originating site (eg, local clinic setting, community health center, and hospital) and that a patient can only receive telemental health care if located within a health professional shortage area or outside a metropolitan statistical area. State law controls regulations for Medicaid and private insurers. As of 2018, telehealth parity laws have been adopted in 36 states requiring managed care companies to cover teletherapy at the same rate as in-person treatment. Specific coverage and training/documentation requirements vary depending on insurance provider and state regulations. If teletherapy is not a covered benefit within an insurance plan but access to ED-specialized care is not readily available, at times special approvals are made to cover such services. Because of the special considerations

required for teletherapy services, a separate consent form is recommended. Close review of the consent form by a provider with the patient is likely necessary to ensure agreement and understanding. Many of the topics reviewed in this article could be specifically included in a consent form (**Box 1**).

Regarding licensure, consultation with a therapist's professional board may help to ascertain where a clinician or patient needs to be located and licensed in order for services to be rendered. For example, in Maryland, a psychologist needs to be licensed in the state where a patient is physically located during a session to provide covered services. The Association of State and Provincial Psychology Boards' Psychology Interjurisdictional Compact (PSYPACT) is an interstate agreement created to facilitate treatment across state lines.[28] This agreement allows psychologists in PSYPACT-enacted states to treat patients located in states in which they are not licensed.

Teletherapist training

Training on specific considerations for the implementation of teletherapy is paramount. There are multiple telemedicine professional organizations on an international and national level that offer expert resources. In particular, the American Telemedicine Association is the leading American telehealth association that, among other contributions, offers a variety of educational opportunities, including courses, webinars, and trainings on telemedicine topics for providers. The American Telemedicine Association's *Practice Guidelines for Videoconferencing-Based Telemental Health*[29] and the

---

Box 1
Consent form topics recommended for teletherapy for EDs

Intention and purpose of teletherapy

Explanation of differences between teletherapy and in-person care

Eligibility criteria for teletherapy services

Specific minimum technology requirements

Limits of confidentiality in electronic communication

Technology backup plan

Establishment of a private therapy space

Privacy issues (eg, use of mobile devices for sessions or alerting provider if someone else is present)

Limits of session location based on state policy

Communication plan related to location changes

Safety management and identification of an emergency management plan

Identification of a support person

Medical management plan

Situations in which a teletherapy session would be discontinued

Appropriateness of session recordings

Risks and benefits

Alternatives to teletherapy

Circumstances in which teletherapy would not be warranted and plan for in-person services

American Psychological Association's *Guidelines for the Practice of Telepsychology*[30] provide practical considerations for teletherapy implementation. Additionally, state- and regional-level telemedicine organizations and resource centers support providers with particular needs related to their geographic area. ED-specific organizations, such as the Academy for Eating Disorders, can offer additional support on the topic of teletherapy within the area of EDs.

Patient environment
There are two versions of teletherapy that affect the environment in which a patient receives care. In some forms of VC teletherapy, the patient travels to an originating site where the individual uses a VC-connected office space to receive therapy services by a clinician remotely located. There are many benefits of this type of arrangement. Most importantly, is the availability of the originating site's staff members in case of an emergency, and the capability to manage paperwork and billing needs and to coordinate with a general practitioner on medical issues. The alternative setup is to have a patient use their own technology (eg, personal computer) to receive services in their personal environment. Obvious benefits of this variation include convenience for the patient and the clinician in that no additional relationship needs to be established with an office distantly located. In this version of teletherapy, special consideration may need to be given to the patient's chosen physical environment during a session. Private and confidential locations are required (eg, private office spaces or homes) where a patient believes that they can speak freely without the risk of someone overhearing therapy material. It should be made clear that patients should not have anyone else present in the session, unless discussed as a part of a treatment plan. The confidentiality of the space may need to be reevaluated regularly and problem solving conducted when needed. Considerations related to what type of technology (eg, personal computer, laptop, tablet, or smartphone) is important because portability of such devices may affect location and confidentiality.

Technology and technological issues
To provide adequate teletherapy services, specific recommendations for the provider and patient include: professional grade and reliable high-quality equipment (ie, cameras, microphones, monitors, computers, and speakers), up-to-date antivirus software, personal firewall, adequate bandwidth, and high-speed Internet.[29,30] It is recommended that providers and patients test their technology before an initial session and equipment limitations (eg, poor camera resolution or inadequate lighting) be addressed immediately because any disruption in technology could distract from treatment or lead to premature termination of sessions. In the rare event of a complete technical failure, a backup plan agreed on at the start of treatment may be helpful for the patient and provider. Such a plan could include the temporary transition to voice-only communication.

Close consideration of a well-suited VC platform is necessary. In the United States, a VC platform needs to be compliant with the Health Insurance Portability and Accountability Act (HIPAA) and therefore is required to be confidential and secure, which includes private connections or encryption. Many popular VC platforms that are not designed specifically for health care services are not HIPAA compliant. Some insurers have an approved list of VC platforms. Typically, platforms have a monthly or annual rate depending on the number of clients or providers using the service and/or access to particular features. It is advised to consider the method in which a teletherapist will coordinate sharing documents (eg, administrative forms, consent forms, or therapy worksheets) with the patient, such as using a HIPAA-compliant file share program through the VC platform. Computer scanners or scanner apps may be required. As in face-to-face therapy, clinicians should have guidelines regarding use of email or text messages in the provision of care.

Clinical Considerations

Therapeutic alliance and patient and therapist satisfaction

Teletherapy seems to be well-accepted and patients are satisfied with this delivery method overall[13,22]; however, more research in this area is needed.[31] Clinicians should remain alert to potential influences of VC treatment on the therapeutic alliance. For example, VC's lack of an in-office structure, potential reduced ability to hear vocal tone, inability to astutely read body language, and risk of technical problems have been identified as possible areas of concern. As a result, some patients may be less likely to establish a therapeutic alliance remotely than others. Furthermore, there may be certain aspects of the therapeutic alliance (eg, trust) that are more difficult to develop with remote therapy delivery, although this is an area needing more investigation.[18] In other areas of telehealth, patients seem to prefer a combination of in-person therapy and online sessions versus online sessions alone.[32] For some, blending treatment in this way might allow for the full development of the therapeutic alliance while receiving the benefits of teletherapy.

Given the expectation that teletherapy will continue to expand within the field, therapists' apprehension with providing remote treatment coupled with potential difficulty developing early therapeutic alliance[22] needs to be addressed. The expressed concerns may be the result of inexperience with VC, discomfort with technology, or a general doubt about the VC delivery method. Additional therapist training may be needed. It has been found that comfort and satisfaction with teletherapy by providers increases throughout the course of treatment.[22] Nevertheless, if the therapeutic alliance between the therapist and patient does not become well established, treatment may suffer because it could affect patient openness, self-disclosure, and outcome. If it is perceived by the patient or therapist that the alliance is suffering because of the remote intervention, a transition to in-person therapy is recommended.

Safety

With teletherapy, the management of high-risk patients may pose a unique challenge to the clinician; however, when prepared with emergency protocols, addressing safety through VC has been shown to be safe and effective.[33,34] Therapists treating EDs need to adhere to general teletherapy guidelines[29] and may require additional, more specific, planning for safety with this population. ED teletherapists are necessarily assessing eating, weight, mood, suicidality, self-harm, substance use, and other dangerous behaviors on a regular basis to follow best practices for safe ED treatment.[1-3] Although a high reliability between in-person and VC assessments, across diagnoses, has been demonstrated,[35] there may be some information that is more difficult to obtain (eg, smell of alcohol or subtle scratches from self-harm). As a result, it is recommended that therapists have a low threshold when asking about such behaviors and that assessments, including standardized measures, continue routinely throughout treatment.[36] Obtaining weights for patients with EDs is often a mandatory component of assessment, treatment, and safety monitoring and requires that a teletherapist develops a unique plan to obtain such information. For example, a therapist may ask patients to weigh themselves while observing the process, ask family members to obtain weights and report them through the platform, or require patients to be weighed at a primary care physician's office or the originating site clinic. For the assessment of suicidality or self-harm in teletherapy, it is recommended that a specific emergency plan be written down and discussed fully before initiating therapy.[36] This plan would include the names and contact numbers of a local support person, medical providers, and available community emergency systems, and the terms under which these supports would be contacted. Some have recommended that the teletherapist have a second clinician available to provide assistance with coordination of the care (eg, talking to police or calling 9-1-1) during a crisis situation.[37] Emergency preparedness also includes a familiarity with federal, state, and local laws regarding commitment requirements and duty to warn/protect.

Given the nutritional and medical complications that are associated with EDs, coordination of care with primary medical providers is also an important aspect of safety planning. There will likely be numerous occasions for coordination with primary care physicians, especially for patients with more severe EDs. For instance, it is not uncommon for ED therapists to monitor vital signs at the time of a therapy session, using nursing assistance, when a concern arises; however, this is not possible in a VC session. Although immediate assessment of vitals is ideal in such circumstances, teletherapists instead may need to contact the patient's primary medical provider and ask the patient to be seen as soon as possible. If an agreed on pretreatment plan related to medical monitoring is in place, this could prevent patient delay in following through with such recommendations.

Unique clinical benefits

The benefits of teletherapy are clear. It is cost effective, convenient, and most importantly, provides the opportunity for empirically supported treatment to those without access.[12] Beyond this, key clinical benefits specific to ED treatment have been detected. For example, family meals, environmental modifications, and various behavioral exposures can be conducted in vivo, with therapist support. With teletherapy, as a therapist observes and facilitates, a patient may discard diet products, modify mirrors, prepare and complete an exposure food item, remove exercise equipment, or post grocery lists/menus in a kitchen, all interventions typically discussed as a part of CBT for EDs. In a family meal intervention, meal preparation may be substantially easier, because there may be greater flexibility with menu options, more family members may be available, and families can practice in their natural environment. Finally, clinicians have observed that teletherapy seems to be especially suited for patients with less severe illness. A stepped-care approach for EDs involving teletherapy has been discussed[38] and seems to occur organically in some situations. For instance, for college-aged patients, teletherapy is much more acceptable to the busy student with mild symptoms who is not convinced about the need for treatment. Similarly, for the student returning to college following significant improvement with treatment, teletherapy may allow care to continue uninterrupted.

Clinical indicators that teletherapy may not be appropriate

Despite the growing literature suggesting that teletherapy is an effective and safe way to deliver mental health treatment,[12,19] there may be situations where it is not appropriate. Considerations include patient and therapist comfort level with the out of office environment (discussed previously), a history of repeated in-therapy crisis or problematic behaviors, severe and/or worsening symptoms, follow through with medical care requirements, therapeutic alliance issues, and the level of engagement required for effective therapy.[30,36]

SUMMARY AND FUTURE DIRECTIONS

For clinicians treating EDs, teletherapy is a new field. Because the current body of evidence is limited in scope and methodology,[39] it is recommended that teletherapy not be used as a substitute for traditional in-person therapy when this format is available. It is, however, strongly recommended in situations where there is a compelling reason for this form of treatment, such as a patient's inability to access evidence-based ED treatments within a manageable traveling distance. Many individuals across North America are in such circumstances and it is the hope that there will be a growing application of teletherapy to accommodate those in need. Specific administrative and clinical applications, discussed in this article, are paramount when considering this mode of treatment. There is much future research to be done, including evaluating evidence-based ED treatments, across diagnoses, in randomized controlled trials comparing in-person therapy, VC psychotherapy, and waitlist controls with follow-up data collection. Additional research is required to reevaluate compliance, therapeutic alliance, and comfort with VC psychotherapy as the culture becomes increasingly habituated to technology use. Also, research examining differing age groups, ED group treatment formats, and whether specific interventions may be more efficacious in a teletherapy format (eg, behavioral interventions may be more effective because of in vivo exposure benefits) is indicated.

REFERENCES

1. National Institute for Health and Care Excellence (NICE). Eating disorders: recognition and treatment. NICE guideline 69. 2017. Available at: http://nice.org.uk/guidance/ng69. Accessed October 29, 2018.
2. Yager J, Devlin MJ, Halmi KA, et al. Guideline watch (August 2012): practice guideline for the treatment of patients with eating disorders. 3rd edition. Arlington (VA): American Psychiatric Association; 2012. Available at: https://psychiatryonline.org/pb/assets/raw/sitewide/practice_guidelines/guidelines/eatingdisorders-watch.pdf. Accessed October 29, 2018.
3. Yager J, Devlin MJ, Halmi KA, et al. Practice guideline for the treatment of patients with eating disorders. 3rd edition. Arlington (VA): American Psychiatric Association; 2006. Available at: http://psychiatryonline.org/pb/assets/raw/sitewide/practice_guidelines/guidelines/eatingdisorders.pdf. Accessed October 29, 2018.
4. Cachelin FM, Rebeck R, Veisel C, et al. Barriers to treatment for eating disorders among ethnically diverse women. Int J Eat Disord 2001;30(3):269–78.
5. Cachelin FM, Striegel-Moore RH. Help seeking and barriers to treatment in a community sample of Mexican American and European American women with eating disorders. Int J Eat Disord 2006;39(2):154–61.
6. Mond JM, Hay PJ, Rodgers B, et al. Health service utilization for eating disorders: findings from a community-based study. Int J Eat Disord 2007;40(5):399–408.
7. Agras WS, Fitzsimmons-Craft EE, Wilfley DE. Evolution of cognitive-behavioral therapy for eating disorders. Behav Res Ther 2017;88:26–36.
8. Anastasiadou D, Folkvord F, Lupiañez-Villanueva F. A systematic review of mHealth interventions for the support of eating disorders. Eur Eat Disord Rev 2018;26(5):294–416.
9. Fairburn CG, Murphy R. Treating eating disorders using the Internet. Curr Opin Psychiatry 2015;28(6):461–7.
10. Fairburn CG, Rothwell ER. Apps and eating disorders: a systematic clinical appraisal. Int J Eat Disord 2015;48(7):1038–46.

11. Schlegl S, Bürger C, Schmidt L, et al. The potential of technology-based psychological interventions for anorexia and bulimia nervosa: a systematic review and recommendations for future research. J Med Internet Res 2015;17(3):e85.

12. Hilty D, Yellowlees PM, Parrish MB, et al. Telepsychiatry: effective, evidence-based, and at a tipping point in health care delivery? Psychiatr Clin North Am 2015;38(3):559–92.

13. Backhaus A, Agha Z, Maglione ML, et al. Videoconferencing psychotherapy: a systematic review. Psychol Serv 2012;9(2):111–3.

14. Nelson EL, Barnard M, Cain S. Treating childhood depression over videoconferencing. Telemed J E Health 2003;9(1):49–55.

15. Ruskin PE, Silver-Aylaian M, Kling MA, et al. Treatment outcomes in depression: comparison of remote treatment through telepsychiatry to in-person treatment. Am J Psychiatry 2004;161(8):1471–6.

16. Glueckauf RL, Fritz SP, Ecklund-Johnson EP, et al. Videoconferencing-based family counseling for rural teenagers with epilepsy: phase one findings. Rehabil Psychol 2002;47(1):49–72.

17. Morland LA, Greene CJ, Rosen CS, et al. Telemedicine for anger management therapy in a rural population of combat veterans with posttraumatic stress disorder: a randomized noninferiority trial. J Clin Psychiatry 2010;71(7):855–63.

18. Frueh BC, Monnier J, Yim E, et al. A randomized trial of telepsychiatry for posttraumatic stress disorder. J Telemed Telecare 2007;13(3):142–7.

19. Mitchell JE, Crosby RD, Wonderlich SA, et al. A randomized trial comparing the efficacy of cognitive–behavioral therapy for bulimia nervosa delivered via telemedicine versus face-to-face. Behav Res Ther 2008;46(5):581–92.

20. Crow SJ, Mitchell JE, Crosby RD, et al. The cost effectiveness of cognitive behavioral therapy for bulimia nervosa delivered via telemedicine versus face-to-face. Behav Res Ther 2009;47(6):451–3.

21. Marrone S, Mitchell JE, Crosby R, et al. Predictors of response to cognitive behavioral treatment for bulimia nervosa delivered via telemedicine versus face-to-face. Int J Eat Disord 2009;42(3):222–7.

22. Ertelt TW, Crosby RD, Marino JM, et al. Therapeutic factors affecting the cognitive behavioral treatment of bulimia nervosa via telemedicine versus face-to-face delivery. Int J Eat Disord 2011;44(8):687–91.

23. Anderson KE, Byrne CE, Crosby RD, et al. Utilizing telehealth to deliver family-based treatment for adolescent anorexia nervosa. Int J Eat Disord 2017;50(10): 1235–8.

24. Bakke B, Mitchell J, Wonderlich S, et al. Administering cognitive-behavioral therapy for bulimia nervosa via telemedicine in rural settings. Int J Eat Disord 2001; 30(4):454–7.

25. Simpson S, Bell L, Britton P, et al. Does video therapy work? A single case series of bulimic disorders. Eur Eat Disord Rev 2006;14(4):226–41.

26. Simpson S, Knox J, Mitchell D, et al. A multidisciplinary approach to the treatment of eating disorders via videoconferencing in north-east Scotland. J Telemed Telecare 2003;9(Suppl 1):S37–8.

27. Centers for Medicare and Medicaid Services. Telehealth services, Medicare learning network. Baltimore (MD): Dept of Health and Human Services; 2018. Available at: https://www.cms.gov/Outreach-and-Education/Medicare-Learning-Network MLN/MLNProducts/downloads/TelehealthSrvcsfctsht.pdf. Accessed October 29, 2018.

28. Webb C, Orwig J. Expanding our reach: telehealth and licensure implications for psychologists. J Clin Psychol Med Settings 2015;22(4):243–50.

29. Yellowlees P, Shore JH, Roberts L. American Telemedicine Association: practice guidelines for videoconferencing-based telemental health. Telemed J E Health 2010;16(10):1074–89.

30. Joint Task Force for the Development of Telepsychology Guidelines for Psychologists. Guidelines for the practice of telepsychology. Am Psychol 2013;68(9): 791–800.

31. Whitten PS, Mair F. Telemedicine and patient satisfaction: current status and future directions. Telemed J E Health 2000;6(4):417–23.

32. McClay CA, Waters L, McHale C, et al. Online cognitive behavioral therapy for bulimic type disorders, delivered in the community by a nonclinician: qualitative study. J Med Internet Res 2013;15(3):e46.

33. Luxton DD, Sirotin AP, Mishkin MC. Safety of telemental healthcare delivered to clinically unsupervised settings: a systematic review. Telemed J E Health 2010; 16(6):705–11.

34. Luxton DD, June JD, Kinn JT. Technology-based suicide prevention: current applications and future directions. Telemed J E Health 2011;17(1):50–4.

35. Shore J. Telepsychiatry: videoconferencing in the delivery of psychiatric care. Am J Psychiatry 2013;170(3):256–62.

36. Luxton DD, O'Brien K, McCann RA, et al. Home-based telemental healthcare safety planning: what you need to know. Telemed J E Health 2012;18(8):629–33.

37. Gros DF, Yoder M, Tuerk PW, et al. Exposure therapy for PTSD delivered to veterans via telehealth: predictors of treatment completion and outcome and comparison to treatment delivered in person. Behav Ther 2011;42(2):276–83.

38. Myers TC, Swan-Kremeier L, Wonderlich S, et al. The use of alternative delivery systems and new technologies in the treatment of patients with eating disorders. Int J Eat Disord 2004;36(2):123–43.

39. Aardoom JJ, Dingemans AE, Van Furth EF. E-health interventions for eating disorders: emerging findings, issues, and opportunities. Curr Psychiatry Rep 2016;18(42):2–8.

Intensive Care Unit Telemedicine
Innovations and Limitations

William Bender, MD, MPH[a],
Cheryl A. Hiddleson, MSN, RN, CENP, CCRN-E[b],
Timothy G. Buchman, PhD, MD, MCCM[c],*

KEYWORDS

- Innovation - Limitation - Telemedicine - Intensive care unit

KEY POINTS

- Intensive care unit (ICU) telemedicine denotes an established tool that can help alleviate some of the issues faced by the field of critical care while also serving as a springboard for innovative improvements in the future.
- ICU telemedicine programs have proven to be an effective solution for delivering ICU care in resource-limited environments and in the face of intensivist staffing shortfalls.
- The inclusion of advanced practice providers, more formal inclusion in medical education, and concurrent utilization of machine learning technologies represent future areas of expansion for ICU telemedicine.
- The computational infrastructure of ICU telemedicine promises robust globalization of critical care services.

INTRODUCTION

The demands of critical care continue to grow, fueled by the aging population (and the aging population's disproportionate needs related to chronic medical conditions), by the maldistribution of intensive care resources, by the slow supply of appropriately trained new providers, and by retirement and death of aged providers. The growing demand has been identified by critical care providers and their associated professional societies.[1–4] The delivery of critical care requires considerable investment from a resource perspective and a financial one. In a 10-year period from 2000 until

This article originally appeared in *Critical Care Clinics*, Volume 35, Issue 3, July 2019.
Disclosure Statement: The authors have nothing to disclose.
[a] Division of Pulmonary, Allergy, Critical Care and Sleep Medicine, Emory University School of Medicine, 5673 Peachtree Dunwoody Road, Suite 502, Atlanta, GA 30342, USA; [b] Emory eICU Center, Emory Healthcare Incorporated, 5671 Peachtree Dunwoody Road, Suite 275, Atlanta, GA 30342, USA; [c] Emory University School of Medicine, 1440 Clifton Road Northeast, Suite 313, Atlanta, GA 30322, USA
* Corresponding author.
E-mail address: tbuchma@emory.edu

Clinics Collections 10 (2021) 165–177
https://doi.org/10.1016/j.ccol.2020.12.018

2010, the cost for the provision of critical care to Medicare and Medicaid beneficiaries nearly doubled to just over $100 billion, while accounting for nearly 1% of the US gross domestic product.[5] It is not surprising then that critical care has been the target of numerous attempts to optimize efficiency, effectiveness, and quality.

Intensive care unit (ICU) telemedicine, defined as the remote provision of critical care facilitated by audiovisual conferencing technology, represents 1 strategy to improve efficiency and reduce cost.[6] ICU telemedicine implementations have continued to grow, with approximately 20% of adult ICU beds in the United States currently supported. ICU telemedicine has been associated with successful outcomes, including decreased costs and reduced malpractice claims.[7,8] The implementation models fall into 3 general classes:

Centralized telehealth, where care services originate from a centralized hub and are then delivered out to remote facilities

Decentralized telehealth, which represents more of a process given that there is no established monitoring facility or staff but rather a connected collection of computers and mobile devices often established at sites of convenience

Redisplay/support systems, which allow for collection and analysis of varying types of patient-generated clinical data[9–13]

Leveraging telecommunications technology for the delivery of critical care has not only allowed for novel solutions to issues faced by the field, but also has set the stage for a number of potential innovative enhancements in the future.

RECENT INNOVATIONS IN INTENSIVE CARE UNIT TELEMEDICINE
Critical Care Provider Shortage

The alarm around critical care provider staffing shortages was raised in 2000 in a study commissioned and reported by the Committee on Manpower for Pulmonary and Critical Care Societies, which represented a combined effort from members of the American Thoracic Society, the American College of Chest Physicians, and the Society of Critical Care Medicine. The report foresaw an unrelenting increase in demand for care coupled with a stagnant supply of intensivists, resulting in projections of intensivist hours meeting only 22% of demand by 2020 and 35% of demand by 2030.[2] That report also served as the impetus for the Framing Options for Critical Care in the United States (FOCCUS) report, which was crafted to address strategies to recruit and sustain an adequate critical care workforce.

There are similar supply and demand challenges forecast for critical care nurses. There is a predicted increase of 26% in demand for acute and critical care nurses in the United States from 2010 to 2024. The demand will not be met. Although the shortfall is partially attributable to the care requirements of an aging population and the retirement of large numbers of similarly aging nurses, it is compounded by 2 pipeline problems. One problem relates to insufficient numbers of qualified faculty to teach in accredited nursing schools; more than 60,000 otherwise acceptable candidates are turned away annually.[14] The second problem relates to insufficient graduate training slots; many hospitals hire only experienced nurses into critical care units, leaving new graduates with few options for employment.[15]

FOCCUS included discussion about information technology as a tool to combat this issue, and the authors specifically noted that "continuous remote intensivist staffing with video conferencing and computer-based data transmission may reduce ICU and hospital mortality, ICU complications, and ICU and hospital length of stay and costs. If supported by subsequent studies, the combination of informatics and telemedicine could promote more effective use of intensivists and promote quality, particularly in remote regions."[16] Rosenfeld and colleagues had already reported on experience with around-the-clock remote ICU management of patients in an ICU without continuous presence of an (on-site) intensivist. This observational study was conducted with 2 retrospective baseline periods along with a prospective intervention period in a 450-bed academic-affiliated hospital. During the intervention period, the remote intensivist provided 24-hour monitoring of all the ICU patients via video conferencing, along with transmission and near real-time display of patient care data normally available only at the bedside.[17] The telemedicine intervention was associated with a number of significant improvements, including a reduction in severity-adjusted ICU mortality in the hospital mortality. ICU length of stay declined by 34% and 30% (when compared with both baseline periods), and overall ICU costs decreased by 33% and 36%; additionally, there was a concomitant decrease in the incidence of complications.[17]

Subsequent investigations have continued to suggest that ICU telemedicine is an effective strategy for handling increased ICU staffing needs with associated improvements in quality. Reports emerged from various care environments including that of rural and urban hospitals, as well as community and academic medical centers. Given that over one-third of all US hospitals are rural, Zawada and colleagues examined the effects of the implementation of an ICU telemedicine system across the upper Midwest in the United States.[18–20] This program consisted of around-the-clock staffing of a remote care center by 1 critical care nurse and clerical support person along with 20 hours per day staffing by a critical care physician. The remote teams supported 1 tertiary referral hospital (with a 2- bed mixed medical and surgical ICU without dedicated intensivist staffing), 3 rural regional hospitals (with 10, 6, and 10 ICU beds, respectively), 2 community hospitals (with <100 beds total), and 9 critical access hospitals (<25 beds total). This program was associated with significant reductions in ICU mortality, ICU length of stay, hospital mortality, and hospital length of stay.[19,20] In addition, satisfaction and acceptance of the program were high across all of the participating sites.[19]

Lilly and colleagues examined the association of a telemedicine ICU intervention with hospital mortality, length of stay, and the presence of preventable complications in an academic medical center. This prospective, unblinded, stepped wedge study reported significant reductions in ICU mortality, ICU length of stay, hospital mortality, and hospital length of stay.[21] Significantly higher rates of best clinical practice adherence were attributed to the tele-ICU intervention, including protocols aimed at the prevention of deep vein thrombosis, stress ulcer prophylaxis, and ventilator-associated pneumonia. Interestingly, improvement for the tele-ICU intervention seemed greater for patients admitted after 8 p.m. During the preintervention period, these overnight admissions were reviewed only by telephone by the attending physician at the discretion of the bedside (either house staff or affiliate provider) team. During the intervention period, these overnight admissions were directly assessed by the tele-ICU team with plans of care then being developed and shared with the bedside providers.[21]

A recent meta-analysis examined the effect of ICU telemedicine implementation on ICU mortality.[22] Associated subgroup differences among ICUs with high and low baseline observed-to-predicted mortality ratios were also studied. Implementation was associated with an overall reduction in ICU mortality. In addition, for ICUs with high observed-to-predicted mortality ratios (>1), the introduction of ICU telemedicine was also significantly associated with a reduction in mortality. This relationship did not exist in ICUs with low (<1) baseline observed-to-predicted mortality ratios.[22]

Emory Healthcare gained similar improvements with the initiation of telemedicine ICU coverage. This health care system consists of several tertiary hospitals, each with a variety of subspecialty critical care capabilities, spread across the metropolitan Atlanta area. Emory's eICU Center provides support to 5 hospitals, including 158 ICU beds and mobile carts or in-room systems that allow for ICU without walls support to emergency departments. One of the hospitals served is a rural hospital that is not part of Emory Healthcare. The eICU Center uses an interprofessional and collaborative model of care that emphasizes a pivotal safety officer role for critical care nurses behind the camera who identify and assess threats and then assign tasks either to the eICU physician or to the bedside staff.[1] The Emory critical care model emphasizes advanced practice providers (APPs) at the bedside. The introduction of remote expert nurses and physicians to support APPs in a suburban tertiary hospital making the transition from community- to academic-centered practice resulted in marked and sustained improvements in ICU mortality and hospital length of stay (**Fig. 1**). The authors' local experience suggests that ICU telemedicine roles may be attractive to seasoned critical care physicians and nurses on the cusp of retirement. The physical demands and emotional stresses are perceived to be diminished compared with those experienced at the bedside.

Developing Countries and Resource-Limited Situations

Although ICU telemedicine has continued with increased growth and acceptance within the United States and in the Middle East and Japan, it has also recently begun to gain traction in more resource-limited areas.[23,24] The developing world, natural disasters, and combat environments are increasingly being explored as avenues by which telemedicine can be further utilized. Given that these settings tend to have higher associated levels of morbidity and mortality and also lack the presence of sustained, effective infrastructure along with consistent, appropriate skill sets, it is understandable why they are attractive targets for the specific implementation of ICU telemedicine services.

Critinext represents Asia's first tele-ICU system, and it currently provides coverage to 350 ICU beds in 10 different cities in India.[25,26] Implementation has helped guide the initiation of renal replacement therapy in critically ill patients and has also been associated with improved mortality along with decreased frequency of catheter-associated bloodstream infections.[27,28] In addition, in a retrospective observational study, ICU

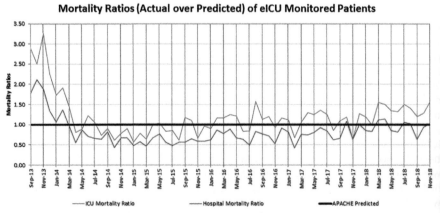

Fig. 1. Mortality rations of eICU monitored patients.

telemedicine services were deployed in Dehradun, India, as part of an attempt to improve cardiac critical care capabilities and specifically, the acute management of patients presenting with acute coronary syndrome. The implementation of an around-the-clock centralized tele-ICU program resulted in significant improvement in 30-day mortality rates (16.4% to 4.8%) along with improved time from door to needle/thrombolytic therapy for patients with ST-elevation myocardial infarctions.[29]

The US military has explored the utilization of ICU telemedicine capabilities as part of its deployments. This has been particularly explored for special forces operators who are often functioning in environments where their medics on the ground represent the most advanced medical provider available, and evacuation of critically ill patients to a more robust care environment may not be possible for a variety of reasons.[30] The Virtual Critical Care (VC3) Consult Service allows for on-demand virtual consultation with experienced critical care physicians. The service is accessed via a single phone line directly to an intensivist, and an email distribution list is used to pass information, including images, flowsheet data, and video clips.[30] Although not as efficient as some of the current civilian technology, particularly from a video or data transfer perspective, cellular telephone-based communication with e-mail supplementation is preferred because of its low bandwidth, minimal equipment requirements, and near-universal familiarity (particularly the act of speaking into a phone).[30] This system was made operational in 2015 with predominant usage with Special Operations Command Africa and Special Operations Command Central. Cases addressed via this system have included penetrating abdominal trauma and complex wound closure. Reported outcomes have been good, and operators have expressed satisfaction with the system.[30,31]

The conflict in Syria has also recently served as an environment for the implementation of an ICU telemedicine system. Because of ongoing fighting, the Syrian Republic's modern medical facilities have been destroyed, and thousands of the country's physicians have been killed or fled the region as refugees.[32] Intact ICUs have been maintained at low capacity because of a lack of staffing also.[32,33] Moughrabieh and Weinert described the implementation of a tele-ICU program that was started in 2012 to help manage the ICU care of patients throughout different parts of the country.[33] It currently has expanded to a network of approximately 20 intensivists providing clinical support 24 hours a day, 365 days a year. This construct has several unique elements to it, particularly when compared with tele-ICU models in the United States. Implementation is rapid (2 months). Care is offered in areas without formal bureaucratic structure, minimizing accreditation and credentialing issues.[33,34] The total operating costs for this construct were noted to be much lower than traditional tele-ICU models due to clinicians donating their time and the use of a virtual network along with commercially available communication applications like WhatsApp.[33,34]

OPPORTUNITIES FOR INTENSIVE CARE UNIT TELEMEDICINE INNOVATION
A Role for the Advanced Practice Provider

ICU telemedicine is now established as a viable solution for delivering ICU care in resource-limited environments and in the face of intensivist staffing shortfalls. There are other opportunities that could be explored to enhance delivery and effectiveness further. One such area is the integration of APPs in the ICU telemedicine environment, serving a clinical role behind the camera.

APPs have been integrated into ICUs as alternative physician trainees (permanent house staff) to offer direct yet supervised management of critically ill patients.[35] This integration improves adherence to coordination of care while not harming specific subgroups of patients.[36,37] It is cost-effective while maintaining or even improving the length of stay and mortality.[35,38,39] Coupling APPs with an ICU telemedicine program has also been associated with significant cost savings.[40]

A centralized continuous care model is a common ICU telemedicine delivery structure.[41,42] This is realized with a remote physical site (the hub) colocating physicians, nurses, and clerical staff who are connected (the spokes) to distant ICUs[41] Within this model, which tends to operate in 24/7/365 fashion, nurses are responsible for providing intense monitoring of between 35 and 45 patients, enabling a collaborating physician to serve up to 250 geographically dispersed patients.[42] As a program grows to include patients with greater and lesser needs, a valuable role for an experienced, critical care advanced practice provider can evolve. Low-acuity issues and routine activities (eg, correcting common electrolyte abnormalities) that otherwise absorb a physician's time could be handled quickly and efficiently by the APP, similar to the division of labor now common in a brick-and-mortar ICU construct. This would be particularly beneficial for ICUs that do not have surrogate providers immediately available at the bedside. Experienced APPs can take on progressive responsibilities, especially in times that an attending tele-intensivist is addressing crises, which are common when covering multiple ICUs. Lags in plans of care (both their creation and approval) would diminish – and coordination with bedside teams will likely accelerate –with the addition of an APP in this role and thus further enhance the capabilities and effectiveness of the centralized continuous care model.

Advanced Machine Learning and Alerting

ICU telemedicine delivers a significant benefit via real-time assessment of physiology and sophisticated trend-based and Boolean alerts.[7] Although bedside teams are structured to be aware of and to respond to bedside alarms, it is not uncommon for alarms to be missed, often because of ongoing alarm fatigue. The consequences of missed alerts are important; ICUs with reported response times to physiologic alerts of less than 3 minutes have significantly shorter ICU length of stays compared with those reporting longer response times.[43] ICU telemedicine support has an effect here as well, as without it, bedside nursing response to 90% of alarms for physiologic instability within 3 minutes of their onset occurs in only 45% of ICUs. Once implemented, ICU telemedicine support that incorporates these more advanced alerting tools has enabled 71% of ICUs to reach the 3 minutes or fewer goal.[44] The authors hasten to add that remote evaluation and adjudication of alerts cannot and will not replace essential bedside responses and responders to immediate life threats such as ventricular tachycardia alarms.

Clinical decision support tools are increasingly being utilized to help forecast a variety of conditions.[45,46] Many use static measurements harvested from the electronic medical record. Dynamic data, such as blood pressure and heart rate collected in real time, can augment predictive power.[47] Recent evidence has demonstrated that a prediction model derived from a combination of EMR data and high-frequency physiologic data (blood pressure and heart rate) can be utilized to predict the onset of sepsis up to 4 hours in advance of its presentation.[45]

These aspects of machine learning, combined with the architectures of ICU telemedicine systems built for robust and consistent response to physiologic alerts, offer a unique opportunity to further enhance and streamline critical care. Running a clinical decision support tool within the background of an ICU telemedicine system that is already equipped to gather real-time physiologic data as well as recognize and prompt the adherence (or lack thereof) to best practices offers enormous potential.[21,48] In the case of sepsis, earlier identification about its pending development can be detected by the telemedicine ICU team and its framework of clinical decision support tools and then relayed to the bedside team prompting further evaluation and early, appropriate management such as volume resuscitation, antibiotic administration, and prompt source control. The authors hasten to add that all predictive tools, including advanced machine learning tools, depend on the reliable flow of high-quality data. Data interruption, confusion, and contamination erode automated analyses, and the authors strongly argue for the use of experienced alert adjudicators (the tele-critical care staff) as essential components in such decision support models.

Medical Education

Concern has been raised that the presence of ICU telemedicine and imagined micromanagement might infringe upon the autonomy with which house-staff operate while within supervised academic environments.[8] This has not been borne out in the literature, and surveys of house-staff have indicated a positive experience with the technology and the education it has provided.[49,50] As attending intensivist staffing patterns remained strained and ACGME duty hours restrictions reduce trainee presence, critical care bedside education can be necessary at off hours. ICU telemedicine offers an extraordinary opportunity to advance the education of not only house-staff but also APP trainees. Utilizing the variety of real-time physiologic data and support systems that it has at hand, the ICU telemedicine intensivist can offer real-time feedback to resident and fellow trainees about a posited intervention while also reinforcing the importance of the implementation of best practices via real-time updates about missed opportunities.[8] Additional skill sets like ultrasound imaging attainment and interpretation can be delivered also.[51]

Bringing trainees into the ICU telemedicine hub and giving them time behind the camera represents another opportunity for innovative medical education. Exposure to the technology and its associated clinical decision support systems offers several opportunities for stimulating further exploration, including research questions and quality improvement projects. At the same time, it offers an opportunity for one-on-one education and discussion directly with an intensivist attending, which can often be difficult to attain within a busy yet dispersed brick and mortar ICU. Insight into operations, plans of care, and patient populations in ICUs in which regular on-the-ground rotations are not available can be beneficial and informative, as can providing care into more remote/community-based ICUs. Large numbers of patients enable assignment of disease-based cohorts to trainees. For example, it is simple to assign 24 patients with sepsis, or a similar number with atrial fibrillation, or a similar number with acute respiratory disease syndrome (ARDS), to a trainee on a given shift. At the authors' institution, elective rotations in the eICU with pulmonary/critical care fellows, anesthesia fellows, and surgical critical care fellows have been well received by faculty and trainees, and discussions are underway to formalize a standing rotation.

Turning Night into Day

Burnout syndromes are common in health care as a whole, and in critical care in particular.[52] Stressful situations, long hours, and night shift work all contribute to burnout. Sustained sleep deprivation can have enormous health consequences.[53] ICU telemedicine, often tasked with providing critical care coverage during the night hours, has the potential to relieve these stresses at the bedside and paradoxically be heavily affected. Indeed, few staff—whether assigned to the bedside or to the telehealth center—are excited about night shift work.

Because telecare is by definition "at a distance," it is up to the operators to determine just how distant the hub and staff should be located. Emory's eICU center has located part of its operations on the other side of the world, where the Georgia night-time corresponds to antipodal daytime. The authors recently completed a 6-month, proof-of-principle study with Macquarie University, where 4 critical care physicians and 3 critical care nurses serially rotated to Sydney, Australia. They delivered critical care during the day back to the Emory Healthcare System in Atlanta, where it was nighttime (**Fig. 2**). The program was well received, with reported improved levels of concentration, efficiency, and job satisfaction. More recently, the authors launched a second phase hosted by Royal Perth Hospital in Perth, Western Australia, which is a full 12- to 13-hour time difference (seasonal variation) from Atlanta, favoring optimal wake-work-sleep patterns.[54]

This element of globalization seeks to leverage the technology of ICU telemedicine and offers the continued provision of efficient and effective care while simultaneously combating direct hindrances to job satisfaction and the development of burnout. Given the ongoing worldwide spread of ICU telemedicine, it is possible that this endeavor represents the beginnings of a global critical care network providing collaborative coverage and serving as a springboard for future investigations.[8,25,26,33]

LIMITATIONS

ICU telemedicine has several limitations to its implementation. These are practically grouped into financial, organizational and behavioral, and technical issues, although there are overlaps among the groupings.

Financial Element

For most ICU telemedicine systems, a significant amount of capital is required for initiation, and this is often cited as a major barrier to its use.[55] Recent analyses have estimated the cost to initiate an ICU telemedicine program for 1 year to be between $50,000 and $123,000 (in 2011 US dollars) per each monitored ICU bed and with total

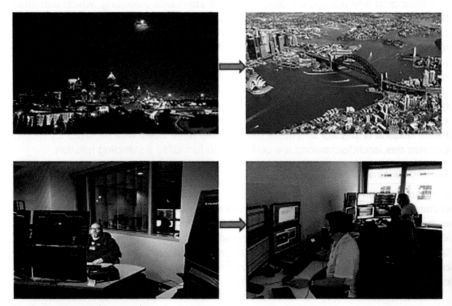

Fig. 2. Turning night into day.

operating costs extending up to $3 million annually.[56–58] The financial return on invest-ment associated with ICU telemedicine has not been well defined in the literature.[59,60] Recent work by Lilly and colleagues, however, found that implementation of ICU tele-medicine led to financial benefits that exceeded program capital and operating costs through increased case volume, higher case revenue relative to direct costs, and shorter length of stay.[59,60]

Another financial component that serves as a significant barrier is the reimburse-ment of services provided. In most cases, reimbursement is limited. In rare cases, reimbursement is provided at the standard rate of brick and mortar ICU care, despite the increased cost associated with the delivery of ICU telemedicine.[40] Category 3 (data collection) codes for ICU telemedicine services exist, but these costs are not currently reimbursed by the Centers for Medicare and Medicaid Services (CMS). At the same time, Medicare beneficiaries are eligible for telehealth services only if they are received at a site located in a rural Health Professional Shortage Area or in a county outside of a Metropolitan Statistical Area.[8]

Organizational and Behavioral Element

The acceptance of ICU telemedicine into an existing medical system relies on a shift of attitudes and the establishment of trust among all care providers. It is not uncommon for clinical providers at the bedside to feel threatened and scrutinized by telemedicine providers.[61] At the same time, the definitive role telemedicine providers are to play in a patient's care can be unclear at various points, and this can lead to disengagement. These difficulties can be particularly pointed in situations where the telemedicine team is providing care and support to a location very distant to its own. Several frequently cited elements that also contribute to this fractured construct include misunderstanding and faulty assumptions regarding onsite resources, equipment, and medication availability; unrealistic expectations about local staff education and abilities; lack of trust; and physician conflicts.[62]

It is not surprising then that robust communication between telemedicine providers and local clinicians can help address and eliminate these issues. Providing familiarity with both parties' workflows can allow a degree of trust and familiarity to develop.[63] At the same time, it needs to be recognized that many of the interactions that permeate ICU telemedicine need to be centered upon the simple tenets that serve as a hallmark for good customer service, notably respect, understanding, listening, responding, and serving. Being able to hold to these principles while concurrently discussing the man-agement of a critically ill patient and navigating advanced technology is a skill set that not every provider will have, nor can they necessarily be taught to produce it repeat-edly. It is key, then, to make sure that staff members are carefully vetted and chosen then adequately trained and educated prior to their deployment in an attempt to address this issue.

Technical Element

Not surprisingly, there is a significant technical limitation to ICU telemedicine also. In general, a substantial amount of manpower must be deployed to get an ICU telemed-icine system installed, and more often than not, a large amount of sophisticated hard-ware must be fitted and set up.[61] Once installed, there are numerous upgrades and updates to software, and ensuring sustained interoperability between these elements and the electronic medical record system is important, time-consuming, and an often cited reason for choosing not to participate with ICU telemedicine.[57]

Maintenance and upkeep of specialized in-room equipment can require separate staffing and skill sets. Such skills must be gained on-site. Ensuring operability across multiple hospitals with appropriate data transfer is complex despite efforts to increase interoperability.[41] With increasing variability in product choices, it is necessary to have a robust understanding of both current and future needs, particularly in light of emerging technologies. This, again, requires advanced expertise and skill set different from that used by providers who use telemedicine systems on a daily basis to help deliver care.[41]

The globalization of critical care, particularly in ultra-long distance construct such as Emory's Night Into Day program, has created new challenges. Contemporary tele-critical care software and hardware use communication protocols within client-server architectures to transmit large quantities of data with each mouse click. So long as the clients are located near servers (ie, within a few hundred miles), the latencies associated with transmission and verification of the accuracy of each data packet prior to transmission of the next packet are imperceptible to clinicians. Once those distances extend to thousands of miles, however, those additional milliseconds add up to perceptible slowness. New software architectures will likely need to take advantage of cloud computing and virtual machines in order to fully globalize such remote care.

SUMMARY

ICU telemedicine represents a well-validated tool to help combat much of the demand that has been placed upon the field of critical care in recent years. Its capabilities to help alleviate heterogeneous intensivist staffing patterns in both the developed and developing world have served as a springboard for further innovations. There appears to be a growing role for APPs in ICU telemedicine along with a role for educating trainees both at the bedside and behind the computer screen. The integration of machine learning into daily ICU telemedicine practice offers new opportunities for the timely evaluation and management of complex conditions like sepsis. The computational infrastructure of ICU telemedicine promises robust globalization of critical care services.

REFERENCES

1. Buchman TG, Coopersmith CM, Meissen HW, et al. Innovative interdisciplinary strategies to address the intensivist shortage. Crit Care Med 2017;45:298–304.
2. Angus DC, Kelley MA, Schmitz RJ, et al, Committee on Manpower for Pulmonary and Critical Care Societies (COMPACCS). Caring for the critically ill patient. Current and projected workforce requirements for care of the critically ill and patients with pulmonary disease: can we meet the requirements of an aging population? JAMA 2000;284:2762–70.
3. Ewart GW, Marcus L, Gaba MM, et al. The critical care medicine crisis: a call for federal action: a white paper from the critical care professional societies. Chest 2004;125:1518–21.
4. Health resources and services administration report to Congress: the critical care workforce: a study of the supply and demand for critical care physicians. 2006. Available at: http://bhpr.hrsa.gov/healthworkforce/reports/studycriticalcarephys.pdf. Accessed November 22, 2018.
5. Halpern NA, Goldman DA, Tan KS, et al. Trends in critical care beds and use among population groups and Medicare and Medicaid beneficiaries in the United States: 2000–2010. Crit Care Med 2016;44:1490–9.
6. Kahn JM. ICU telemedicine: from theory to practice. Crit Care Med 2014;42:2457–8.

7. Fuhrman SA, Lilly CM. ICU telemedicine solutions. Clin Chest Med 2015;36(3): 401–7.
8. Lilly CM, Zubrow MT, Kempner KM, et al. Society of critical care medicine tele-ICU Committee. Critical care telemedicine: evolution and state of the art. Crit Care Med 2014;42(11):2429–36.
9. Reynolds HN, Bander JJ. Options for tele-intensive care unit design: centralized versus decentralized and other considerations: it is not just a "another black sedan." Crit Care Clin 2015;31(2):335–50.
10. Phillips eICU program. Available at: https://www.usa.philips.com/healthcare/product/HC865325ICU/eicu-program-telehealth-for-the-intensive-care-unit. Accessed January 8, 2019.
11. InTouch Health. Available at: https://intouchhealth.com/virtual-care-platform/intouch-os/. Accessed January 8, 2019.
12. PeraHealth. Available at: https://www.perahealth.com/. Accessed January 8, 2019.
13. BedMasterEx. Available at: https://www.bedmaster.net/en/products/bedmasterex. Accessed January 8, 2019.
14. Cox P, Willis K, Coustasse A. (2014, March). The American epidemic: The U.S. nursing shortage and turnover problem. Paper presented at BHAA 2014, Chicago, IL, March 26, 2014.
15. American Association of Colleges of Nursing. Nursing faculty shortage Fact Sheet 2017. 2018. Available at: https://www.aacnnursing.org/News-Information/Fact-Sheets/Nursing-Faculty-Shortage. Accessed January 2, 2019.
16. Kelley MA, Angus D, Chalfin DB, et al. The critical care crisis in the United States: a report from the profession. Chest 2004;125:1514–7.
17. Rosenfeld BA, Dorman T, Breslow MJ, et al. Intensive care unit telemedicine: alternate paradigm for providing continuous intensivist care. Crit Care Med 2000;28:3925–31.
18. American Heart Association. Fast facts on US hospitals 2018. Available at: https://www.aha.org/statistics/fast-facts-us-hospitals. Accessed November 1, 2018.
19. Zawada ET Jr, Herr P, Larson D, et al. Impact of an intensive care unit telemedicine program on a rural health care system. Postgrad Med 2009;121(3):160–70.
20. Zawada ET Jr, Kapaska D, Herr P, et al. Prognostic outcomes after the initiation of an electronic telemedicine intensive care unit (EICU) in a rural health system. S D Med 2006;59(9):391–3.
21. Lilly CM, Cody S, Zhao H, et al. Hospital mortality, length of stay, and preventable complications among critically ill patients before and after tele-ICU reengineering of critical care processes. JAMA 2011;305(21):2175–83.
22. Fusaro MV, Becker C, Scurlock C. Evaluating tele-ICU implementation based on observed and predicted ICU mortality: a systematic review and meta-analysis. Crit Care Med 2019;47(4):501–7.
23. Sturman C. Phillips launches a tele-intensive care eICU programme in Japan. 2018. Available at: https://www.healthcareglobal.com/public-health/philips-launches-tele-intensive-care-eicu-programme-japan. Accessed November 20, 2018.
24. Philips delivers the Middle East's first TeleICU program in collaboration with UAE Ministry of Health. Available at: https://www.albawaba.com/business/pr/philips-delivers-middle-east%E2%80%99s-first-teleicu-program-collaboration-uae-ministry-health-8. Accessed November 20, 2018.

25. GE Healthcare, Fortis pioneer Asia's first eICU. 2012. Available at: https://www.biospectrumasia.com/news/27/3769/ge-healthcare-fortis-pioneer-asias-first-eicu.html. Accessed November 22, 2018.
26. Fortis healthcare EICU. 2018. Available at: https://www.fortishealthcare.com/eicu. Accessed November, 22, 2018.
27. Gupta S, Kaushal A, Dewan S, et al. Can an electronic ICU support timely renal replacement therapy in resource-limited areas of the developing world. Crit Care 2015;19(Suppl 1):P504.
28. Kaushal A, Gupta S, Dewan S, et al. India's first tele-ICU: critinext. Crit Care Med 2013;41(12):A147.
29. Gupta S, Dewan S, Kaushal A, et al. eICU reduces mortality in STEMI patients in resource-limited areas. Glob Heart 2014;9:425–7.
30. Powell D, McLeroy RD, Riesberg J, et al. Telemedicine to reduce medical risk in austere medical environments: the virtual critical care consultation (VC3) service. J Spec Oper Med 2016;16(4):102–9.
31. DellaVolpe J, Lantry J, Powell D, et al. The role of virtual critical care consultation in supporting military combat operations. Crit Care Med 2016;44(12):468.
32. Ahsan S. In Syria, doctors beware. New York Times 2013. Available at: http://www.nytimes.com/2013/10/04/opinion/in-syria-doctors-beware.html. Accessed November 22, 2018.
33. Moughrabieh A, Weinert C. Rapid deployment of international tele–intensive care unit services in War-Torn Syria. Ann Am Thorac Soc 2016;13(2):165–72.
34. Moughrabieh M, Weinert C, Zaza T. Rapid deployment of international tele-ICU services during conflict in Syria. Am J Respir Crit Care Med 2014;189:A3630.
35. Gershengorn HB, Johnson MP, Factor P. The use of nonphysician providers in adult intensive care units. Am J Respir Crit Care Med 2012;185(6):600–5.
36. Hoffman LA, Tasota FJ, Scharfenberg C, et al. Management of patients in the intensive care unit: comparison via work sampling analysis of an acute care nurse practitioner and physicians in training. Am J Crit Care 2003;12:436–43.
37. Hoffman LA, Miller TH, Zullo TG, et al. Comparison of 2 models for managing tracheotomized patients in a subacute medical intensive care unit. Respir Care 2006;51:1230–6.
38. Fry M. Literature review of the impact of nurse practitioners in critical care services. Nurs Crit Care 2011;16(2):58–66.
39. Kleinpell RM, Ely W, Grabenkort R. Nurse practitioners and physician assistants in the intensive care unit: an evidence-based review. Crit Care Med 2008;36(10):2888–97.
40. Trombley MJ, Hassol A, Lloyd JT, et al. The impact of enhanced critical care training and 24/7 (Tele-ICU) support on medicare spending and postdischarge utilization patterns. Health Serv Res 2018;53:2099–117.
41. Reynolds HN, Rogove H, Joseph Bander J, et al. A working lexicon for the tele-intensive care unit: we need to define tele-intensive care unit to grow and understand it. Telemed J E Health 2011;17(10):773–83.
42. Davis TM, Barden C, Dean S, et al. American telemedicine association guidelines for TeleICU operations. Telemed J E Health 2016;22(12):971–80.
43. Lilly CM, McLaughlin JM, Zhao H, et al. A multicenter study of ICU telemedicine reengineering of adult critical care. Chest 2014;145:500–7.
44. Lilly CM, Fisher KA, Ries M, et al. A national ICU telemedicine survey: validation and results. Chest 2012;142:40–7.
45. Nemati S, Holder A, Razmi F, et al. An interpretable machine learning model for accurate prediction of sepsis in the ICU. Crit Care Med 2018;46(4):547–53.

46. Koyner JL, Carey KA, Edelson DP, et al. The development of a machine learning inpatient acute kidney injury prediction model. Crit Care Med 2018;46(7):1070–7.

47. Mayaud L, Lai PS, Clifford GD, et al. Dynamic data during hypotensive episode improves mortality predictions among patients with sepsis and hypotension. Crit Care Med 2013;41:954–62.

48. Kahn JM, Gunn SR, Lorenz HL, et al. Impact of nurse-led remote screening and prompting for evidence-based practices in the ICU. Crit Care Med 2014;42: 896–904.

49. Coletti C, Elliott DJ, Zubrow MT. Resident perceptions of a teleintensive care unit implementation. Telemed J E Health 2010;16:894–7.

50. Mora A, Faiz SA, Kelly T, et al. Resident perception of the educational and patient care value from remote telemonitoring in a medical intensive care unit. Chest 2007;132:443A.

51. Levine AR, McCurdy MT, Zubrow MT, et al. Tele-intensivists can instruct non-physicians to acquire high-quality ultrasound images. J Crit Care 2015;30(5): 871–5.

52. Moss M, Good VS, Gozal D, et al. An official critical care societies collaborative statement: burnout syndrome in critical care healthcare professionals a call for action. Crit Care Med 2016;44(7):1414–21.

53. Haus EL, Smolensky MH. Shift work and cancer risk: potential mechanistic roles of circadian disruption, light at night, and sleep deprivation. Sleep Med Rev 2013; 17:273–84.

54. Emory cares for ICU patients remotely, turning 'night into day' from Australia. Available at: http://news.emory.edu/stories/2018/05/buchman-hiddleson_eicu_perth_australia//. Accessed November 1, 2018.

55. Berenson RA, Grossman JM, November EA. Does telemonitoring of patients–the eICU–improve intensive care? Health Aff 2009;28:w937–47.

56. Kumar G, Falk DM, Bonello RS, et al. The costs of critical care telemedicine programs: a systematic review and analysis. Chest 2013;143:19–29.

57. Lilly CM, Motzkus C, Rincon T, et al, UMass Memorial Critical Care Operations Group. ICU telemedicine program financial outcomes. Chest 2017;151:286–97.

58. Coustasse A, Deslich S, Bailey D, et al. A business case for tele-intensive care units. Perm J 2014;18:76–84.

59. Lilly CM, Motzkus CA. ICU telemedicine: financial analyses of a complex intervention. Crit Care Med 2017;45:1558–61.

60. Vranas KC, Slatore CG, Kerlin MP. Telemedicine coverage of intensive care units: a narrative review. Ann Am Thorac Soc 2018;15(11):1256–64.

61. Avdalovic MV, Marcin JP. When will telemedicine appear in the ICU? J Intensive Care Med 2018;34(4):271–6.

62. Wilkes MS, Marcin JP, Ritter LA, et al. Organizational and teamwork factors of tele-intensive care units. Am J Crit Care 2016;25(5):431–9.

63. Moeckli J, Cram P, Cunningham C, et al. Staff acceptance of a telemedicine intensive care unit program: a qualitative study. J Crit Care 2013;28(6):890–901.

Quality Improvement and Telemedicine Intensive Care Unit

A Perfect Match

Devang K. Sanghavi, MBBS, MD[a], Pramod K. Guru, MBBS, MD[a],
Pablo Moreno Franco, MD[b],*

KEYWORDS

• Critical care • Quality improvement • Tele-ICU • Communication

KEY POINTS

• Telemedicine intensive care can potentially participate in the care of critically ill patients by covering hospital in a multitude of ways.

• The eventual care and overall improvement in the quality of care provided by the telemedicine intensive care team depends on the teams' composition and its relationship with the local practice.

• We describe the synergistic role that quality improvement methodology plays to assist with both implementation science and to facilitate a successful collaboration between the local intensive care practice and the telemedicine team.

INTRODUCTION

There are approximately 5980 intensive care units (ICUs) in the United States caring for about 55,000 patients a day. Based on the results of a survey published by Angus and colleagues,[1] only 4% of the ICU had dedicated attending daytime coverage and any evening physician coverage. Fifty percent of the ICUs had no intensivist coverage, 20% had weekday coverage, 12% had weeknight coverage, and 10% had weekend day coverage, presenting a substantial need for telemedicine intensive care teams (Tele-ICU).

Tele-ICU was first showcased in 1977 as a tool with the potential to enhance care for patients in a smaller private hospital monitored from an academic medical center.[2] Tele-ICU adoption increased from 16 hospitals and 598 beds in 2002 to 213 hospitals and 5799 beds in 2010, based on data from the Centers for Medicare and Medicaid

This article originally appeared in *Critical Care Clinics*, Volume 35, Issue 3, July 2019.
Conflict of Interest: None.
[a] Department of Critical Care Medicine, Mayo Clinic, 4500 San Pablo Road, Jacksonville, FL 32224, USA; [b] Division of Transplant Medicine, Department of Critical Care Medicine, Mayo Clinic, 4500 San Pablo Road, Jacksonville, FL 32224, USA
* Corresponding author.
E-mail address: MorenoFranco.Pablo@mayo.edu

Clinics Collections 10 (2021) 179–190
https://doi.org/10.1016/j.ccol.2020.12.019

Services.[3] Tele-ICU programs support 11% of nonfederal hospital critically ill patients.[4] This number is only going to increase as the quantity of practicing intensivists remain stagnant and demand for around-the-clock specialized intensivist care continues to increase nationwide.[5] The intensivist supply–demand gap seems to be even more marked in rural areas, so the availability of Tele-ICU services guarantees that, in a timely manner, trained specialists are able to assess patients and guide therapy. Without Tele-ICU, patients either have to be transferred to higher levels of care or forgo specialty care; in both of these cases, a margin for error increases and unnecessary delays in care may be introduced.

Beyond increased availability and enhanced timeliness of care, other substantial advantages that Tele-ICU coverage can provide are standardization and continuity of care. The scope of involvement of the Tele-ICU physician can be further classified into comanagement, consultation, and emergent care. The eventual care and the overall improvement in the quality of care provided by the Tele-ICU depend on the composition of the Tele-ICU team, which can potentially include physicians, Advanced Practice Providers (APP), and nurses.[6] The Tele-ICU center can be staffed within the system, wherein the hospital system can manage the Tele-ICU with their clinicians and nurses or outsource it to a vendor that operates a network of ICUs.[2]

There are risks and opportunities that arise as the tele-ICU model is incorporated to an existing local ICU practice, because of the potential differences in policies, procedures, protocols, and process and outcome metrics, along with variations in clinical practice. Potential miscommunication could lead to significant problems in providing appropriate care. That being said, when the tele-ICU implementation process is complete, using quality improvement (QI) methodology, there are many potential advantages. For example, QI has a proven record of closing the gap between evidence-based medicine and clinical practice, bringing the framework and tools that support the implementation of best practices while tracking meaningful outcome indicators and relevant process metrics.

MEDICAL ERRORS IN THE INTENSIVE CARE UNIT AND INCREASING SAFETY IN TELE-INTENSIVE CARE USING QUALITY IMPROVEMENT TOOLS

According to reports from the Agency for Healthcare Research and Quality, roughly 10% of ICU patients develop an adverse effect such as a health care-associated infection, pressure ulcer, preventive all medication-related event, or a fall during hospitalization.[7] Some other potential complications associated with ICU care have frequently been described in the literature and include deep vein thrombosis, pulmonary embolism, gastrointestinal bleeding, catheter-associated urinary tract infection, central line-associated bloodstream infections, ventilator-associated pneumonia, delirium, and acute lung injury.

One of the most critical elements in any industry is QI. The safety level required in each industry determines the extent of the resources needed to achieve it. QI can assist to find a balance between achieving an appropriate level of safety with the correct amount of resources. The spectrum of expected safety could go from ultrasafe industries (eg, commercial aviation; processing industries), which refers to those industries in which safety and the means to achieve it are the absolute priority to ultra-adaptive industries (eg, combat flight, Himalaya mountaineering) that rely heavily on each individuals judgment, adaptability, and resilience, and finally the high-reliability industries (eg, chartered flights), which implies that the teams exhibit characteristics that allow them to operate both in safe conditions and flexibility to respond and manage risk.[8] In medicine, a similar spectrum can be conceived, going from avoiding risk in ultrasafe radiation therapy, managing risk in highly reliable anesthesiology, and mitigating adverse events in ultraadaptive trauma surgery. As in ICUs, clinical providers need to include safety, high reliability, and adaptability moving from ultrasafe conditions to ultraadaptive conditions in emergency situations; therefore, the use of QI in ICUs gains even more relevance to ensure safety.

QUALITY IMPROVEMENT METHODOLOGY EXAMPLES: PLAN–DO–STUDY–ACT CYCLES, DEFINE–MEASURE–ANALYZE–IMPROVE–CONTROL, AND LEAN
Cause and Effect Diagram

Cause and effect diagrams are visual tools designed to group steps and enumerate them in the logical order of the substeps within a process that could breakdown to produce a failure or defect. Very commonly, fishbone diagrams are used to represent causes and effects.

Driver Diagram

Once we understand that each process has steps that are critical to quality and that the visual depiction in a driver diagram helps to identify risks of each stage. Then, attention can be turned to further mitigate the risks based on the primary and secondary drivers. Each one of these drivers could influence performance to a certain degree.

Define–Measure–Analyze–Improve–Control

Define–Measure–Analyze–Improve–Control is one of the most comprehensives tools. It describes the 5 required steps to guide QI projects and teams. Each step is further defined in **Fig. 1**. It is important to mention that all of the requirements in each step are completed before moving to the next stage.

Metrics

To make sure every intervention is leading to a better patient-related outcome, appropriate quality metrics should be defined and tracked. Typically, these metrics can be

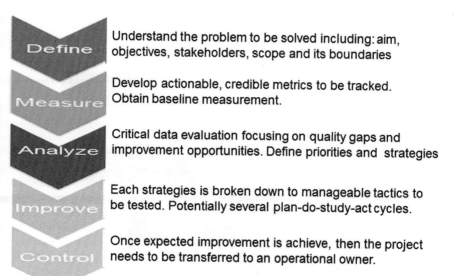

Define — Understand the problem to be solved including: aim, objectives, stakeholders, scope and its boundaries

Measure — Develop actionable, credible metrics to be tracked. Obtain baseline measurement.

Analyze — Critical data evaluation focusing on quality gaps and improvement opportunities. Define priorities and strategies

Improve — Each strategies is broken down to manageable tactics to be tested. Potentially several plan-do-study-act cycles.

Control — Once expected improvement is achieve, then the project needs to be transferred to an operational owner.

Fig. 1. Define–measure–analyze–improve–control: the 5 phases of the methodology.

divided into 2 groups: process and outcome. The health care delivery process ultimately is focused on delivering safety, health maintenance, and patient satisfaction; therefore, outcome metrics should be aligned with patient-related outcomes. When we engineer ICUs, it is recommended that the performance of each critical-to-quality step is tracked as a process metric, which could be done using tele-ICU resources.

Failure Modes and Effects Analysis

Failure modes and effects analysis is one of the most powerful improvement tools, in which all the identified different potential failure modes are stratified in terms of their risk priority index. The frequency, severity, and potential safety mechanisms are accounted for to determine relative importance.

Flowchart

A flowchart is a schematic representation of the different inputs and processes required to deliver high quality to the patient or customers.

Plan–Do–Study–Act Cycles

A plan–do–study–act cycles is a structured approach that uses repeated attempts to modify a process to optimize the performance. Application of consecutive plan–do–study–act cycles in ICU care is essential to improve quality of care (**Fig. 2**).

TELE-INTENSIVE CARE AND ITS ROLE IN ENHANCING INTENSIVE CARE UNIT QUALITY OF CARE

Some of the landmark studies supporting the use of Tele-ICU have been closely linked to specific QI activities. Using QI in Tele-ICU in one study led to an improvement in evidence-based practices adherence and prevention of ICU adverse events.[9]

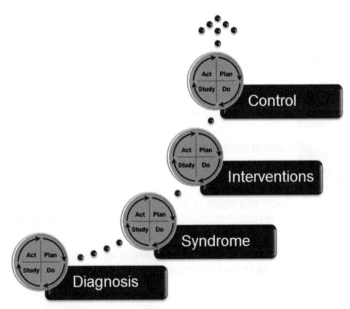

Fig. 2. Plan–do–study–act cycles: a common framework to both critical care and QI.

Providing intensive care requires a fast pace to move from escalation of care to procedures, adaptation, prevention, deescalation, and recovery, which can create tremendous variation in ICU care depending on resources including provider availabilities, ICU census, and patient acuity, among others.

Because of Tele-ICUs advantages in timeliness along with standardization and continuity in care, having a well-organized Tele-ICU team supervising the operation can enhance the safety, patient and provider experience, and quality outcomes. In a systematic review, both centralized monitoring and virtual consultant models have shown improvement in clinical practice adherence.[10]

Length of Stay

Two systematic reviews have been performed to assess the impact of Tele-ICU on patient outcomes, including length of stay. The first by Young and colleagues[11] included 13 eligible studies in 35 ICUs, all of which used a before and after design. The results of this review did not show Tele-ICU coverage to decrease the ICU length of stay (mean difference, −0.64 days; 95% confidence interval [CI], −1.52 to 0.25; P = .16).[11] The second study included 11 articles and reported statistically significant differences in ICU and hospital length of stay (weighted mean difference [telemedicine control], −0.62 days [95% CI −1.21 to −0.04] and −1.26 days [95% CI, −2.49 to −0.03], respectively).[12]

Mortality Impact: Intensive Care Unit and Inpatient

Young and colleagues[11] showed an association between Tele-ICU monitoring and a decrease in ICU mortality (pooled odds ratio [OR], 0.80; 95% CI, 0.66–0.97; P = .02), but not in-hospital mortality for patients admitted to an ICU (pooled OR, 0.82; 95% CI, 0.65–1.03; P = .08). Wilcox and Adhikari[12] Also reported Tele-ICU, compared with standard of care, is associated with a lower ICU (risk ratio, 0.79; 95% CI, 0.65–0.96; 9 studies; n = 23,526 participants) and hospital mortality (risk ratio, 0.83; 95% CI, 0.73–0.94; 9 studies; n = 47,943 participants).

Another systematic review, including only randomized controlled trials and quasiexperimental studies, questioned the methodologic quality of most studies investigating Tele-ICU. This systematic review only included 2 studies meeting the eligibility criteria of appropriate methodology. The first, a nonrandomized, stepped-wedge design in 7 ICUs, showed a decrease in hospital mortality from 13.6% (95% CI, 11.9%–15.4%) to 11.8% (95% CI, 10.9%–12.8%) during the intervention period, with an adjusted OR of 0.40 (95% CI, 0.31–0.52; P = .005).[9] The second study, an unblinded, nonrandomized, preassessment/postassessment of Tele-ICU in 56 adult ICUs, reported a reduction in hospital mortality from 11% to 10% (adjusted hazard ratio, 0.84; 95% CI, 0.78–0.89; P<.001).[13] Both studies confirm a decrease in hospital mortality in patients receiving Tele-ICU care, and they assert that more multisite, randomized, controlled trials or quasiexperimental studies are needed to determine the implementation cost and effectiveness of the intervention.[14]

Intensive Care Unit Emergencies

A significant advantage of Tele-ICU is the ability for alerts and alarms to be initiated by off-site personnel in addition to the standard in-house bedside staff. In a study performed by the University of Massachusetts, most of the day interventions were initiated by the Tele-ICU group.[9] During the Tele-ICU period, there were 6.80 alerts (95% CI, 6.50–7.10) for physiologic instability per patient per day, and from those, 1.75 alerts (95% CI, 1.69–1.81) were managed with a Tele-ICU intervention.[9] The human factor approach and the impact of such alerts in alarm fatigue and staff burnout should be better characterized in future studies.

CONTINUOUS QUALITY IMPROVEMENT BY TELE-INTENSIVE CARE

The concept that every system is perfectly designed to achieve the results has become fashionable in the health care improvement industry. But taking these concepts a little further, one could conceptualize designing a health care system in which every safety event is used as a learning opportunity. Subsequently, QI methodology could be applied to prevent similar events in the future. Then, a continuously learning health care delivery system is born. We propose here that the collaboration between Tele-ICU and local ICU to examine safety events, generate improvement projects, and track metrics will enhance patient outcomes.

LEVERAGING CURRENT AND FUTURE KNOWLEDGE TO ENHANCE INTENSIVE CARE UNIT METRICS BY TELE-INTENSIVE CARE

Many of the diagnostic criteria or risk stratification scoring systems available in the ICU have been the product of traditional research, mainly using logistic regression modeling. One of the limitations of such traditionally derived tools is that only a relatively small number of patients and data points were used to drive them. With the promise of big data, machine learning, and artificial intelligence, one could conceptualize a new future in which Tele-ICU monitoring will also serve as an avenue to capture data, identify variations in care, and follow trends. The data being captured could, in turn, be used to apply machine learning algorithms that can improve the performance of risk stratification models and artificial intelligence–derived decision support tools.

RESOURCE USE AND PROJECT PRIORITIZATION

As the need for appropriate QI projects continues to grow, it is important to identify projects with higher priorities that have more impact and need fewer resources to achieve their goals. Project prioritization is a very simple but very powerful approach that could potentially be used in all ICUs as well as during or after the deployment of a Tele-ICU service. The process steps are as follows.

1. Establish the degree of impact that each QI project will have in the spoke of hub ICU.
2. Define the effort level that will be required, which in part depends on the size of each project.
3. Along with other stakeholders, create an impact–effort prioritization grid or priority matrix.[15]

A frequent question that arises when trying to define the effort that will be required to complete a project is how to determine the scope of the project in a way that could be compared with other projects. **Table 1** proposes a number of elements that could be considered to determine projects scope. **Table 2** demonstrate the calculation of priority score and risk priority matrix. **Table 2** shows how to calculate the impact score by the impact of the project to improve access throughput or clinical outcomes, increase patient safety, enhance public image, improve patient experience and compliance with regulatory requirements, and effects on other stakeholders. **Table 2b** describes the calculation of the estimated effort required for each project. The variables that are taken into account include project scope, extent of time to completion,

Table 1
Plan-do-study-act cycles: a common framework to both critical care and QI

Characteristics	Small and Just Do It	Medium	Large	Extra-Large
Scope example	Single ICU	2 ICUs	2–5 ICUs	>5 ICUs
Speed to mobilize	Rapid	Rapid	Slow	Very Slow
QI expert	From the local practice	From the practice or Tele-ICU	From other areas of the hospital	From outside company
Duration	Days to weeks	Days to <3 mo	3–6 mo	6–24 mo
Cost	Teeny	Small	Big	Bigger
Control	Pulled in	Pulled in–pushed down	Pulled in–pushed down	Pushed down
Sustainability	Easy	Easy-ok	Hard	Very hard
Diffusion of best practices	Usually not required But easily done	Sometimes required Needs some work	Hard	Very hard, usually not needed
Decision drivers	Close to the process/patients	Close to the process/patients	Removed from patient/process	Very removed from patient/process
Patient/voice of the costumer involvement	Easy	Easy-ok	Hard	Very hard
Change management required	Barely any/crowd sourcing	Some but limited to those areas no time required	Moderate to large, usually no time required	Moderate to large, may require some time
Data required	Available within Tele-ICU or IT	Requires IT or extra resources from Tele-ICU to pull	Requires IT, Tele-ICU and EHR vendor	Requires IT, Tele-ICU, EHR vendor and outside agency
Impact	Small	Moderate	Large	Huge
Risk	Minimal	Moderate	Large	Huge
RPN (15 areas)	<50	50–75	75–120	>120

Abbreviations: EHR, electronic health records; IT, information technology; RPN, risk priority number.

Table 2
Impact effort grid for tele-ICU QI projects prioritization

A. Impact scoring

Access to Increase	Outcomes to Improve	Safety to Improve	Public Image to Impact	Patient and Person Experience to Improve	Regulatory Requirement Driven	System/Structure Already in Place	Risk Priority Number
0 N/A	0 N/A	0 N/A	0 N/A	0 N/A	0 Low	0—yes, good	
3 small	3 soft	3 mild	3 mild	3 some	3 Some $	3—borderline	
5 medium	5 medium	5 moderate	5 moderate	5 moderate	5 Moderate $$	5—weak	
10 Strong	10 Important	10 Significant	10 Strong	10 Important	10 High $$$	10—no	

B. Effort scoring

Scope	Speed	Data Required	Resources Required	Change Management Required	Cost	Structure Already in Place?	Similar Project Successfully Completed before?	Risk Priority Number
0 small	0 fast	0 none	0 none	0 none	0 low	0—yes, strong	0—yes, strong	
3 M	3 mid	3 some	3 some	3 some	3 some $	3—moderate	3—moderate	
5 L	5 slow	5 a lot	5 a lot	5 a lot	5 moderate $$	5—weak	5—weak	
10 XL	10 extra slow	10 huge	10 huge	10 huge	10 high $$$	10—no	10—no	

C. Example of a risk priority matrix

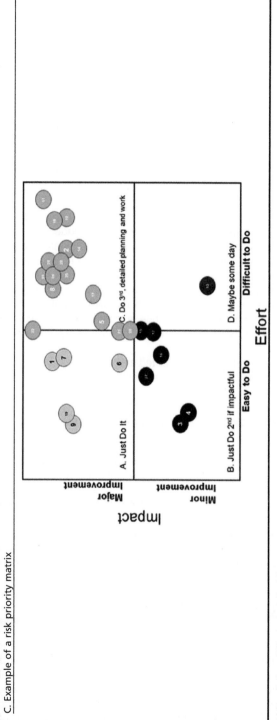

Abbreviation: N/A, not applicable.

amount of data needs to be tracked, the data sources including whether or not the data already exists or needs to be generated, estimation of the required change management efforts, potential cost, availability of infrastructure and historical assessment regarding similar projects that may have been completed before.

Once the impact and effort scoring of all proposed projects are calculated, an impact–effort risk priority matrix can be built to guide resource use (**Table 2**c).

DIFFUSION OF BEST PRACTICES ACROSS ALL INTENSIVE CARE UNITS

For the success of a health care institution, the adoption and implementation of best practices to the bedside for all patients and consistency in health care delivery across the entire system are necessary. Some of the challenges on the path to success, include identification of appropriate best practices, infrastructure to measure and report data, integration into electronic health record, protected time for providers guiding implementation, competing priorities that could affect the speed of diffusion, and cultural challenges to standardized work.[16]

The Tele-ICU infrastructure provides several potential advantages in both discovery and dissemination on the best practices. These opportunities include compiling playbooks with best practices, establishing internal coherency of practices between different ICUs, and organizing teams. The internal dynamics of each ICU or institution need to be taken into account, especially when trying to identify the best implementation approach. Practice adoption could follow the alpha–beta model, wherein a single site defines best practices with the expectation that others follow or the adopt external practices model, in which best evidence is translated directly from other health care organizations, government, national groups, or professional societies.[16]

The big advantage is that, once Tele-ICUs are accepted and embraced by the local ICU practice, then it can serve as the diffusion channel while minimizing friction and maximizing standardization.

IMPACT OF QUALITY IMPROVEMENT BY TELE-INTENSIVE CARE ON INTERHOSPITAL TRANSFERS

Approximately 5% of all ICU patients in the United States are transferred to higher care level centers for a lack of adequate resources or subspecialty support at the referring hospital.[17] Tele-ICU has the potential for fewer transfers of these critically ill patients with a Tele-ICU intensivist helping to manage these patients locally. There are few publications regarding the impact of Tele-ICU on interhospital transfers; the authors reported that there was an increase in interhospital transfer from a less resourced ICU to the referral center, an academic center.[18,19] More QI studies need to be conducted on the pattern of interhospital transfers in the setting of vendors being contracted to cover a particular ICU without an in-network referral ICU.

CONTINUOUS QUALITY IMPROVEMENT USE IN TELE-INTENSIVE CARE

Improving appropriate response to clinically relevant changes in high-stakes environments like an ICU is at the core of QI; therefore, using well-described techniques like plan–do–study–act cycles can provide the appropriate framework (see **Fig. 2**) for a continuously improving health care system. Creating a partnership between the local ICU practice and Tele-ICU to respond to both internal and external risks/opportunities, aggregating data from both process and outcome metrics, safely balance resources provided by local and Tele-ICU groups, depending on the proactive assessment of

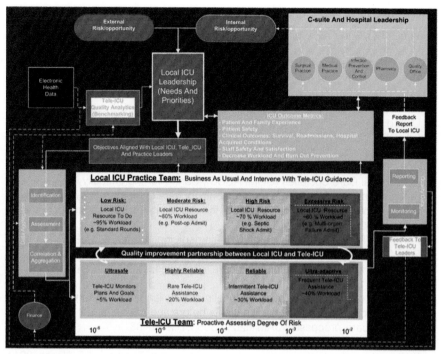

Fig. 3. QI partnership between local ICU and Tele-ICU. C-suite, top senior executives; Tele-ICU, telemedicine intensive care unit.

the degree of risk, and feedback data to hospital leadership pertains important Tele-ICU related potential QI projects (**Fig. 3**). The optimal use of QI tools when establishing, developing, and optimizing partnerships between local and Tele-ICUs can result in improved patient outcomes while making it easier for ICU providers to provide the right care at the right time.

HANDOFF COMMUNICATION

Even after standardized handoff communication projects have been introduced to the ICU, clinicians have reported being unprepared for their shift because of a poor handoff quality in 35 of 343 handoffs events (10.2%), whereas residents using University of Washington Standardized Handoff reported being unprepared in 53 of 740 (7.2%) handoffs (OR, 0.19; 95% CI, 0.03–0.74; P = .03).[20] The presence of Tele-ICU during and after handoff communication might improve clinician preparedness and continuity of care. Tele-ICUs hold standard operating procedures and checklist. As natural language processing technology improves its use during standardized handoff could prepopulate events to be tracked.

SUMMARY

Telemedicine alone does not equate to QI but is merely a tool for QI. The upside is that in the right settings and with the right goals, telemedicine can indeed be used to improve outcomes. Based on the considerations covered here, we recommend that Tele-ICU programs deploy QI methods to monitor process and outcome metrics, and financial impacts closely.

REFERENCES

1. Angus DC, Shorr AF, White A, et al. Critical care delivery in the United States: distribution of services and compliance with Leapfrog recommendations. Crit Care Med 2006;34(4):1016–24.
2. Udeh C, Udeh B, Rahman N, et al. Telemedicine/virtual ICU: where are we and where are we going? Methodist Debakey Cardiovasc J 2018;14(2):126–33.
3. Kahn JM, Cicero BD, Wallace DJ, et al. Adoption of ICU telemedicine in the United States. Crit Care Med 2014;42(2):362–8.
4. Lilly CM, Zubrow MT, Kempner KM, et al. Critical care telemedicine: evolution and state of the art. Crit Care Med 2014;42(11):2429–36.
5. Angus DC, Kelley MA, Schmitz RJ, et al, Committee on Manpower for Pulmonary and Critical Care Societies (COMPACCS). Caring for the critically ill patient. Current and projected workforce requirements for care of the critically ill and patients with pulmonary disease: can we meet the requirements of an aging population? JAMA 2000;284(21):2762–70.
6. Kahn JM. The use and misuse of ICU telemedicine. JAMA 2011;305(21):2227–8.
7. Free from harm. National Patient Safety Foundation.; 2015. p. 59.
8. Vincent C, Amalberti R. Safer healthcare: strategies for the real world. 1st edition. New York: Springer; 2016.
9. Lilly CM, Cody S, Zhao H, et al. Hospital mortality, length of stay, and preventable complications among critically ill patients before and after tele-ICU reengineering of critical care processes. JAMA 2011;305(21):2175–83.
10. Ramnath VR, Ho L, Maggio LA, et al. Centralized monitoring and virtual consultant models of tele-ICU care: a systematic review. Telemed J E Health 2014; 20(10):936–61.
11. Young LB, Chan PS, Lu X, et al. Impact of telemedicine intensive care unit coverage on patient outcomes: a systematic review and meta-analysis. Arch Intern Med 2011;171(6):498–506.
12. Wilcox ME, Adhikari NK. The effect of telemedicine in critically ill patients: systematic review and meta-analysis. Crit Care 2012;16(4):R127.
13. Lilly CM, McLaughlin JM, Zhao H, et al. A multicenter study of ICU telemedicine reengineering of adult critical care. Chest 2014;145(3):500–7.
14. Mackintosh N, Terblanche M, Maharaj R, et al. Telemedicine with clinical decision support for critical care: a systematic review. Syst Rev 2016;5(1):176.
15. Kashani KB, Ramar K, Farmer JC, et al. Quality improvement education incorporated as an integral part of critical care fellows training at the Mayo Clinic. Acad Med 2014;89(10):1362–5.
16. Dilling JA, Swensen SJ, Hoover MR, et al. Accelerating the use of best practices: the Mayo Clinic model of diffusion. Jt Comm J Qual Patient Saf 2013;39(4): 167–76.
17. Iwashyna TJ, Christie JD, Kahn JM, et al. Uncharted paths: hospital networks in critical care. Chest 2009;135(3):827–33.
18. Pannu J, Sanghavi D, Sheley T, et al. Impact of telemedicine monitoring of community ICUs on interhospital transfers. Crit Care Med 2017;45(8):1344–51.
19. Fortis S, Sarrazin MV, Beck BF, et al. ICU telemedicine reduces interhospital ICU transfers in the veterans health administration. Chest 2018;154(1):69–76.
20. Parent B, LaGrone LN, Albirair MT, et al. Effect of standardized handoff curriculum on improved clinician preparedness in the intensive care unit: a stepped-wedge cluster randomized clinical trial. JAMA Surg 2018;153(5):464–70.

Telemedicine and the Management of Insomnia

Caleb Hsieh, MD, MS, Talayeh Rezayat, DO, MPH,
Michelle R. Zeidler, MD, MS*

KEYWORDS

• Insomnia • Telemedicine • Cognitive behavior therapy for insomnia (CBT-i)

KEY POINTS

• Insomnia is a highly prevalent disorder with significant medical and economic consequences best treated with cognitive behavioral therapy for insomnia (CBT-i).
• Behavioral therapies administered through telemedicine are well validated and effective including tele-CBT-i.
• Tele-CBT-i can be delivered through fully directed care with a behavioral therapist or through a self-directed Web or mobile app with varying degrees of therapist interaction.
• Multiple randomized studies as well as meta-analyses show efficacy of both fully directed and self-directed tele-CBT-i.
• Tele-CBT-i increases access for patients with insomnia that are geographically remote.

INTRODUCTION

Insomnia is highly prevalent in the general population with significant economic and social ramifications. Although the exact prevalence of insomnia in the United States is unknown, approximately 30% to 40% of US adults will report insomnia symptoms at some point over a year and approximately 10% will meet criteria for a diagnosis of chronic insomnia. Prevalence of insomnia is increasing, with certain populations, including women and veterans, being more susceptible to developing insomnia.[1] The economic burden due to insomnia is high and includes missed work days and increased rates of occupational and motor vehicle accidents.[2,3] In addition, insomnia is linked to the development of comorbid mental health and medical conditions, including depression, hypertension, diabetes, and heart disease, among others.[3,4]

Treatment options for insomnia include pharmacologic and nonpharmacologic pathways with multiple clinical guidelines recommending utilization of nonpharmacologic approaches, specifically cognitive behavioral therapy (CBT-i), for first-line

This article originally appeared in *Sleep Medicine Clinics*, Volume 15, Issue 3, September 2020.
Pulmonary, Critical Care and Sleep Medicine, David Geffen School of Medicine at UCLA, 10833
Le Conte Avenue, 43-229 CHS, Los Angeles, CA, USA
* Corresponding author.
E-mail address: MZeidler@mednet.ucla.edu

Clinics Collections 10 (2021) 191–202
https://doi.org/10.1016/j.ccol.2020.12.020
2352-7986/21/Published by Elsevier Inc.

treatment of insomnia.[5,6] Although CBT-i is clearly effective and durable for the treatment of insomnia, there are inadequate CBT-i providers to treat the large and rapidly growing insomnia patient population. In addition, most insomnia providers reside within metropolitan areas, which further exacerbates shortages in rural areas. There are currently only 300 CBT-i providers certified by the Society of Behavioral Sleep medicine within the United States.[6] Within the US Department of Veterans Affairs, there were 112 full-time mental health physician and psychologist providers nationwide in 2012 for a population of veterans with diagnosed insomnia estimated to reach a half-million by 2020.[7] Many of these veterans as well as nonveteran patients live in rural areas where the closest provider is often multiple hours away and may be geographically inaccessible during periods of the year.[2] Shortages of CBT-i providers translates to longer appointment wait times, shorter patient visits to accommodate higher volume, and clinician burnout, as well as a need for the primary physician to treat patients with insomnia with pharmacologic therapies rather than referring for CBT-i.

Given the rapid technological advances of recent years, there has been a proliferation of options for the management and treatment of insomnia. Tele-CBT-i, either with a provider or through self-directed CBT-i via the Web or mobile applications, has generated excitement as a bridge to address the barriers to care for a large population of patients.[8] This article reviews and evaluates the evidence for the various telemedicine modalities for the treatment of insomnia.

DEFINITIONS
Insomnia

The International Classification of Sleep Disorders defines insomnia as difficulty with sleep onset, maintenance, duration, or quality, with resulting daytime symptoms in the setting of adequate opportunity and environment for sleep.[9] Insomnia is further categorized as short-term insomnia lasting less than 3 months or chronic insomnia, persisting longer than 3 months.

Cognitive and Behavioral Treatment for Insomnia

Cognitive behavioral therapy for insomnia is considered first-line treatment for insomnia, and has been shown to be more effective and durable than pharmacologic therapy with fewer side effects.[10] Skills and techniques such as stimulus control (behavioral instructions to enhance the bed as stimulus for sleep), sleep restriction (reducing the time in bed to align with sleep time), relaxation, and developing healthy sleep habits help patients address various predisposing, precipitating, and perpetuating causes of chronic insomnia. CBT-i is traditionally completed through face-to-face office visits over a course of 6 to 8 weeks with weekly or every-other-week visits.[7]

Given the time and resource intensity required for CBT-i, brief behavioral therapy for insomnia (BBT-i) was developed as an abridged form of CBT-i accessible to a wider range of clinicians.[11] BBT-i has demonstrated efficacy[12,13] and can reach a larger pool of patients through the training of nonsleep mental health providers to deliver therapy. BBT-i was originally derived from CBT-i and is completed over a shorter duration of 4 weeks (4 sessions) and focuses on sleep restriction and stimulus control[12] (Fig. 1). BBT-i is traditionally done with 2 in-person visits and 2 telephone visits and represents a hybrid of in-office and telemedicine services. Those patients who continue to have residual symptoms following BBT-i can be referred for CBT-i to address components not covered in BBT-i.

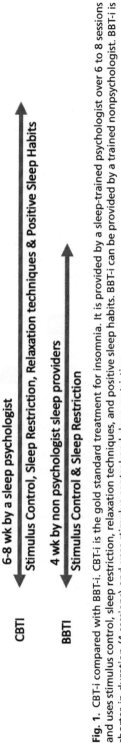

Fig. 1. CBT-i compared with BBT-i. CBT-i is the gold standard treatment for insomnia. It is provided by a sleep-trained psychologist over 6 to 8 sessions and uses stimulus control, sleep restriction, relaxation techniques, and positive sleep habits. BBT-i can be provided by a trained nonpsychologist. BBT-i is shorter in duration (4 sessions) and uses stimulus control and sleep restriction.

Telemedicine

The American Academy of Sleep Medicine separates sleep telemedicine into 2 types: synchronous and asynchronous.[2] In synchronous interactions, patients and providers are separated by distance, but interact in real time via bi-directional telecommunication.[2] The patient may be at a sleep laboratory, a designated clinic, or at their home (provided adequate technical specifications are met) while the provider similarly works from any location with a secure networking connection. Besides the technological intermediary interface, there may be little to distinguish the interaction from an in-person office clinic visit. In asynchronous interactions, patients and providers are separated by both distance and time using "store and forward" technology. Home sleep apnea testing and interpretations, as well as secure e-messaging, are examples already commonly in use. Self-directed care mechanisms are another rapidly growing subset of telemedicine that include mobile phone applications (apps) and Web-based programs that can be enhanced by the use of smart devices or wearable devices. These modalities can be fully self-directed without provider interaction or partially directed, usually through asynchronous interactions. For example, a patient could use a CBT-i app to transmit data on sleep onset and fragmentation through both a sleep diary and from an actigraphy-enabled smart watch. A provider then receives the data and provides counseling on sleep restriction.

TELEMEDICINE FOR INSOMNIA

Although telemedicine has traditionally implied the exchange of health-related services between the clinician and patient via telecommunications, expanding technology enables telemedicine for insomnia to use both synchronous and asynchronous modalities, as well as self-directed care mechanisms using varying levels of clinician support (**Fig. 2**). With synchronous telemedicine, patients with insomnia in varied geographic locations work directly with a CBT-i provider, either in a one-on-one or group setting. Asynchronous telemedicine modalities allow patients to use self-directed insomnia treatments through Web or mobile apps, some of which have access to a provider for support and clarifications.

Telemedicine has significant potential to expand access to nonpharmacologic treatment of insomnia, although with pros and cons depending on the modality used. On one end of the spectrum, completely self-directed therapy is almost universally accessible with relatively low costs compared with using a CBT-i therapist. This may result in a therapy that may be too general and superficial, especially for patients with more severe insomnia or insomnia with comorbid conditions. Conversely, fully directed therapy allows for greater depth of treatment, but as such is much more time and resource intensive (**Table 1**).

Research studies have investigated the efficacy of both synchronous and asynchronous CBT-i in comparison with either an insomnia therapy wait-list or with face-to-face behavioral therapy for insomnia.

Fully Directed Individual Telehealth Cognitive Behavioral Therapy for Insomnia

In recent decades, telemedicine-based psychotherapy has been shown to be effective in the adjunctive treatment of numerous mental health conditions when compared with face-to-face psychotherapy.[14,15] Within the umbrella of fully directed telemedicine-delivered CBT-i, various options exist with varying degrees of clinician interaction, including videoconferencing, telephone visits, and synchronous text chats. For technical and administrative considerations, the reader is referred to the

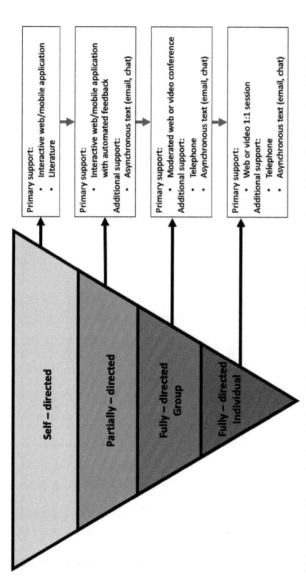

Fig. 2. Modalities of tele-CBT-i with varying levels of provider support. Tele-CBT-i can range from fully self-directed to fully directed with variations in-between. Self-directed CBT-i delivered primarily via the Internet or mobile application is widely available and readily accessible to many patients. Self-directed therapy alone requires few resources but may not be as appropriate for patients with more individualized needs. Varying layers of clinician support can be added to provide better direction for patients from partial to full support.

Table 1
Positive and negative features of tele-CBT-i modalities

Features of tele-CBT-i	Self-Directed Internet/Mobile CBT-i	Partially Directed Internet/Mobile CBT-i	Fully Directed Group Telemedicine CBT-i	Fully Directed Individual Telemedicine CBT-i
Positive	• Least time and resource burden on clinicians • Fewest barriers to accessibility • Allows integration with other wearable devices	• Less time and resource burden on clinicians • Allows for support and feedback that may improve insomnia outcomes • Variable degree of personalization/individualization of treatment depending on site	• Less time and resource burden on clinicians • Allows social support among participants and positive group dynamics	• Most flexibility for treatment individualization/personalization • Most similar to traditional in-person CBT-i
Negative	• Limited personalization/individualization of treatment • Lack of regulation or quality control of Web sites and apps • Increased health-information privacy and security risks • Higher learning curves for less tech-savvy patients • Access to wi-fi or cellular service may be a limiting factor in rural areas	• Lack of regulation or quality control of Web sites and apps • Increased health-information privacy and security risks • Higher learning curves for less tech-savvy patients • Access to wi-fi or cellular service may be a limiting factor in rural areas	• Requires synchronous interactions • Limited by patient social anxieties or negative group dynamics • Less accessible than self-directed therapy	• More time and resource intensive than other tele-modalities • Requires synchronous interactions • Potential adverse effects on the clinician-patient therapeutic relationship as compared with in-person CBT-i

best practices consensus statement published by the American Telehealth Association and the American Psychiatric Association.[16]

Although there have not been large-scale comparisons of face-to-face CBT-i versus telemedicine-delivered CBT-i, preliminary results of 30 patients from a study using the American Academy of Sleep Medicine video telemedicine platform indicate that telemedicine-delivered CBT-i is noninferior to face-to-face delivery.[17] Gieselmann and Pietrowsky[18] randomized individuals with insomnia to a 3-session BBT-i either using face-to-face visit, synchronous text-based chat, or wait-list control. In this novel comparison of 73 patients, the investigators found that chat-based therapy was not only effective based on both objective and subjective measures, but also trended toward outperforming face-to-face therapy. Although the exact cause for the trend is unclear, hypothesized reasons included reduced disruption to patients' daily routines, a more positive patient perception of the process, and the Internet-based treatment setting.

Fully Directed Group Telehealth Cognitive Behavioral Therapy for Insomnia

Although directed individual tele-CBT-i addresses issues of geographic access, it does not address the paucity of providers available to provide CBT-i. Group-directed CBT-i allows clinicians to deliver therapy, training, and education to multiple patients simultaneously, thus reducing costs and time burdens. The efficacy of group-directed therapy is likely similar to both in-person CBT-i and Internet-delivered CBT-i (I-CBT-i).[19] Gehrman and colleagues[20] demonstrated efficacy using this approach to deliver care through the Veterans Health Affairs in Philadelphia. They implemented six 60-minute to 90-minute session protocols and used high-quality video teleconferencing equipment that allowed clinicians to either view a group of 6 to 8 patients in wide-angle format or individual group members close up. In 214 veterans, there were notable improvements in mean insomnia severity index (ISI) (measure of insomnia from 0 to 28 with higher scores indicating worse insomnia), sleep latency, and sleep efficiency that were comparable to published data on group CBT-i. In the preceding format with a teleconference clinician, tele-CBT-i likely suffers from many of the same barriers faced by traditional face-to-face group sessions (eg, patient concerns about group dynamics, limited accessibility, or negative group dynamics).[21]

Holmqvist and colleagues[22] randomized patients with insomnia to either clinical visit telehealth group CBT-i (the patient physically attends their primary care clinic and then undergoes CBT-i via telehealth with a remote provider) or a Web-based CBT-i completed from their home without therapist contact. Both groups completed identical modules. There were significant and similar improvements in insomnia symptoms in both groups, although there was a preference trend for Web-based treatment.

Self-Directed Internet/App Cognitive Behavioral Therapy for Insomnia

The most readily available option for CBT-i is self-directed "on-line" therapy, otherwise known as "Web-based," "Internet-based," "mobile application," or "Internet-delivered" CBT-i (I-CBT-i). I-CBT-i pairs patients with educational material and varying levels of feedback and support directed through either an automated computer program or an insomnia provider. There are more than a dozen different self-directed I-CBT-i options with proprietary solutions and varying efficacy, although many of these programs lack evidence-based data regarding their product. On the whole, randomized studies of self-directed therapy delivered via Internet or mobile devices have demonstrated efficacy for the treatment of insomnia. Use is limited by access to a wireless network or cellular service as well as access to a compatible device to use the program and at least some degree of computer literacy.

Studies as early as 2004 evaluated the use of I-CBT-i for the treatment of insomnia[23] with subsequent multiple randomized studies and 3 meta-analyses being published since then.[24–26] These studies have evaluated the use of I-CBT-i with face-to-face CBT-i visits, placebo, and I-CBT-i with varying levels of support.

Self-Directed Internet/App Cognitive Behavioral Therapy for Insomnia Versus Face-to-Face Cognitive Behavioral Therapy for Insomnia

Blom and colleagues[19] evaluated 48 patients randomized to I-CBT-i or face-to-face group CBT-i for 8 weeks and 6 months of follow-up. I-CBT-i provided asynchronous interaction with an insomnia specialist. Both groups had significant improvement in their ISI scores as well as in their sleep efficiency, latency, and quality. Patient satisfaction with treatment was similar in both groups.

Self-Directed Internet/App Cognitive Behavioral Therapy for Insomnia versus Placebo

A total of 303 adults were randomized to either I-CBT-i for 6 weeks with weekly modules or a Web-based placebo. Follow-up was maintained to 1 year. Individuals randomized to I-CBT-i had significant improvement in their ISI scores as well as sleep latency, which were maintained for a year after treatment.[27]

Meta-Analyses of Self-Directed Internet/App Cognitive Behavioral Therapy for Insomnia

A 2016 meta-analysis by Ye and colleagues[25] evaluated 15 randomized controlled studies comparing more than 1000 patients using I-CBT-i with 591 wait-list controls. Evaluation over 5 to 9 weeks found that I-CBT-i significantly decreased sleep-onset latency by 18.4 minutes, increased total sleep time by 22.3 minutes, increased sleep efficiency by 9.58%, and decreased the ISI by 5.88 points. A similar 2016 meta-analysis of 15 trials by Seyffert and colleagues[24] reached similar conclusions with the addition that Internet-delivered therapy performance was statistically no different from in-person therapy.

Tele-Cognitive Behavioral Therapy for Insomnia and Wearable Devices

As wearable devices such as smart watches and movement trackers become more commonplace, there is also significant potential to further track efficacy of and adherence to CBT-i. In 2017, Kang and colleagues[28] conducted a pilot study evaluating the efficacy of a wearable device in conjunction with use of a mobile application CBT-i program in 19 patients. Using the mobile app, patients in the study demonstrated improved sleep efficiency as measured both by sleep diaries and the wearable device, as well as improvement in ISI scores. No significant differences were noted between the individuals who did or not use the wearable devices.

Stepped-up Care Tele-Cognitive Behavioral Therapy for Insomnia

In light of the inherent advantages and disadvantages of the aforementioned approaches to tele-CBT-i, use of a "stepped care" framework in which patients begin with self-directed therapy and are "stepped-up" to fully directed therapy if nonresponsive, has been proposed to maximize efficacy and minimize costs.[29,30] Mohr and colleagues[30] examined this principle in a randomized noninferiority trial for depression by comparing Internet-based self-directed therapy stepped-up to telephone-administered fully directed therapy (tCBT) versus tCBT alone. Although the stepped-up model was more cost-effective and no less effective than tCBT, patient satisfaction was significantly lower in the stepped model. A recent study in young working adults in Japan comparted tailored I-BBT-i (performed by a computer algorithm) versus I-BBT-i, self-monitoring, and wait-list.[31] The tailored I-BBT-i was comparable with the I-BBT-i in reducing ISI scores, although the improvements in the tailored approaches were noted earlier. Drop-out rates were similar between the 2 groups. Of note, participants in this trial had mild insomnia, were young, and were employed. This population has been shown to do well with I CBT-i. Additional trials of "step-up" therapy targeting individuals with more severe insomnia and additional comorbidities are necessary.

Cognitive Behavioral Therapy for Insomnia and Pharmacologic Discontinuation

Although cognitive and behavioral-based therapies for insomnia are recommended as first-line therapy, there is a large segment of the population still using pharmacologic agents for the treatment of insomnia. Patients on pharmacologic therapy can take advantage of telehealth for insomnia to undergo CBT-i/BBT-i while at the same time titrating medications with the goal to discontinue pharmacotherapy. The current Big Bird trial is randomizing patients on benzodiazepines and z-drugs to either usual care or a blended model with access to a self-directed Internet module that provides education on their sleeping medication as well as cognitive behavioral techniques to assist the patient with deprescription.[32] A different and potential benefit of telemedicine, where CBT-i/BBT-i is not available, is the ability to assess efficacy, side effects, and appropriate use of pharmacologic therapy for insomnia. To date, not many studies are available in the field of insomnia pharmacotherapy discontinuation and use of telemedicine.

Telemedicine and Clinical Visit Telehealth-Insomnia: Pitfalls and Unanswered Questions

Despite a rapidly growing body of literature pointing to the importance and efficacy of I-CBT-i, the proliferation of unregulated applications leads to a number of limitations. Yu and colleagues[4] found that most currently available mobile applications for insomnia do not fully adhere to evidence-based CBT-i principles. Patients with severe insomnia tend to be underrepresented in these studies and thus efficacy in this important demographic may be underevaluated.[24] Many studies in the preceding meta-analyses also still incorporated regular face-to-face sessions, suggesting that self-directed therapy may best be a part of a blended or step care model. In a video-based self-directed study of 242 patients with breast cancer and insomnia, Savard and colleagues[33,34] found that although self-directed video-based treatment was effective, there was considerably more relapse insomnia in patients who did not receive individualized therapy. Leigh and colleagues[35] also raised additional concerns with regard to the regulation (or lack thereof) of I-CBT-i quality, efficacy, and protection of privacy. It is clear that more research is needed to better optimize and ensure quality delivery of self-directed CBT-i.

Although there has been a proliferation of data on the efficacy and utility of tele-CBT-I, many questions still need to be answered, among them are the following:

- What is the ideal level of therapist interaction for a specific patient to allow for optimal treatment results?
- What is the ideal modality for a specific patient to allow for optimal treatment results?
- Most studies predominantly include middle-aged, healthy, white women. What are the optimal treatment modalities for alternate patient populations, including those of different ethnicities and those with additional comorbidities?

- Can specialized programs be developed for individuals with varying levels of computer literacy?
- What unintended or adverse effects can occur with each modality outcomes?

CONCLUSION AND NEXT STEPS

There has been enormous progress in the evolution of tele-CBT-i with development of a variety of options from fully directed therapy with a provider to completely self-directed Internet or app-based CBT-i. Additional work is needed to personalize care based on patient characteristics, preference, and response to therapy.

DISCLOSURE

The authors have nothing to disclose.

REFERENCES

1. Dopheide JA. Insomnia overview: epidemiology, pathophysiology, diagnosis and monitoring, and nonpharmacologic therapy. Am J Manag Care 2020;26(4 Suppl): S76–84.
2. Singh J, Badr MS, Diebert W, et al. American Academy of Sleep Medicine (AASM) position paper for the use of telemedicine for the diagnosis and treatment of sleep disorders. J Clin Sleep Med 2015;11(10):1187–98.
3. Sateia MJ, Buysse DJ, Krystal AD, et al. Clinical practice guideline for the pharmacologic treatment of chronic insomnia in adults: an American Academy of Sleep Medicine Clinical Practice Guideline. J Clin Sleep Med 2017;13(2):307–49.
4. Yu JS, Kuhn E, Miller KE, et al. Smartphone apps for insomnia: examining existing apps' usability and adherence to evidence-based principles for insomnia management. Transl Behav Med 2019;9(1):110–9.
5. Qaseem A, Kansagara D, Forciea MA, et al. Management of chronic insomnia disorder in adults: a clinical practice guideline from the American College of Physicians. Ann Intern Med 2016;165(2):125–33.
6. Management of insomnia disorder in adults: current state of the evidence | Effective Health Care Program. Available at: https://effectivehealthcare.ahrq.gov/products/insomnia/clinician. Accessed April 20, 2020.
7. Koffel E, Bramoweth AD, Ulmer CS. Increasing access to and utilization of cognitive behavioral therapy for insomnia (CBT-I): a narrative review. J Gen Intern Med 2018;33(6):955–62.
8. Ruskin PE, Silver-Aylaian M, Kling MA, et al. Treatment outcomes in depression: comparison of remote treatment through telepsychiatry to in-person treatment. Am J Psychiatry 2004;161(8):1471–6.
9. International Classification of Sleep Disorders. Third edition. Darien: American Academy of Sleep Medicine; 2014.
10. Mitchell MD, Gehrman P, Perlis M, et al. Comparative effectiveness of cognitive behavioral therapy for insomnia: a systematic review. BMC Fam Pract 2012; 13:40.
11. (AASM) AAoSM. Brief behavioral treatment for insomnia. Available at: https://j2vjt3dnbra3ps7ll1clb4q2-wpengine.netdna-ssl.com/wp-content/uploads/2019/03/ProviderFS_BBTI_18.pdf. Accessed January 15, 2020.
12. Troxel WM, Germain A, Buysse DJ. Clinical management of insomnia with brief behavioral treatment (BBTI). Behav Sleep Med 2012;10(4):266–79.

13. Gunn HE, Tutek J, Buysse DJ. Brief behavioral treatment of insomnia. Sleep Med Clin 2019;14(2):235–43.

14. Chakrabarti S. Usefulness of telepsychiatry: a critical evaluation of videoconferencing-based approaches. World J Psychiatry 2015;5(3):286–304.

15. Hilty DM, Ferrer DC, Parish MB, et al. The effectiveness of telemental health: a 2013 review. Telemed J E Health 2013;19(6):444–54.

16. Shore JH, Yellowlees P, Caudill R, et al. Best practices in videoconferencing-based telemental health April 2018. Telemed J E Health 2018;24(11):827–32.

17. Arnedt JT, Conroy D, Mooney A, et al. 0363 efficacy of cognitive behavioral therapy delivered via telemedicine vs. face-to-face: preliminary results from a randomized controlled non-inferiority trial. Sleep 2019;42:A148.

18. Gieselmann A, Pietrowsky R. The effects of brief chat-based and face-to-face psychotherapy for insomnia: a randomized waiting list controlled trial. Sleep Med 2019;61:63–72.

19. Blom K, Tarkian Tillgren H, Wiklund T, et al. Internet- vs. group-delivered cognitive behavior therapy for insomnia: a randomized controlled non-inferiority trial. Behav Res Ther 2015;70:47–55.

20. Gehrman P, Shah MT, Miles A, et al. Feasibility of group cognitive-behavioral treatment of insomnia delivered by clinical video telehealth. Telemed J E Health 2016;22(12):1041–6.

21. Dilgul M, McNamee P, Orfanos S, et al. Why do psychiatric patients attend or not attend treatment groups in the community: a qualitative study. PLoS One 2018; 13(12):e0208448.

22. Holmqvist M, Vincent N, Walsh K. Web- vs. telehealth-based delivery of cognitive behavioral therapy for insomnia: a randomized controlled trial. Sleep Med 2014; 15(2):187–95.

23. Strom L, Pettersson R, Andersson G. Internet-based treatment for insomnia: a controlled evaluation. J Consult Clin Psychol 2004;72(1):113–20.

24. Seyffert M, Lagisetty P, Landgraf J, et al. Internet-delivered cognitive behavioral therapy to treat insomnia: a systematic review and meta-analysis. PLoS One 2016;11(2):e0149139.

25. Ye YY, Chen NK, Chen J, et al. Internet-based cognitive-behavioural therapy for insomnia (ICBT-i): a meta-analysis of randomised controlled trials. BMJ Open 2016;6(11):e010707.

26. Zachariae R, Lyby MS, Ritterband LM, et al. Efficacy of internet-delivered cognitive-behavioral therapy for insomnia - a systematic review and meta-analysis of randomized controlled trials. Sleep Med Rev 2016;30:1–10.

27. Ritterband LM, Thorndike FP, Ingersoll KS, et al. Effect of a web-based cognitive behavior therapy for insomnia intervention with 1-year follow-up: a randomized clinical trial. JAMA Psychiatry 2017;74(1):68–75.

28. Kang SG, Kang JM, Cho SJ, et al. Cognitive behavioral therapy using a mobile application synchronizable with wearable devices for insomnia treatment: a pilot study. J Clin Sleep Med 2017;13(4):633–40.

29. Espie CA. "Stepped care": a health technology solution for delivering cognitive behavioral therapy as a first line insomnia treatment. Sleep 2009;32(12):1549–58.

30. Mohr DC, Lattie EG, Tomasino KN, et al. A randomized noninferiority trial evaluating remotely-delivered stepped care for depression using internet cognitive behavioral therapy (CBT) and telephone CBT. Behav Res Ther 2019;123:103485.

31. Okajima I, Akitomi J, Kajiyama I, et al. Effects of a tailored brief behavioral therapy application on insomnia severity and social disabilities among workers with

insomnia in Japan: a randomized clinical trial. JAMA Netw Open 2020;3(4): e202775.

32. Coteur K, Van Nuland M, Vanmeerbeek M, et al. Effectiveness of a blended care programme for the discontinuation of benzodiazepine use for sleeping problems in primary care: study protocol of a cluster randomised trial, the Big Bird trial. BMJ Open 2020;10(2):e033688.

33. Savard J, Ivers H, Savard MH, et al. Is a video-based cognitive behavioral therapy for insomnia as efficacious as a professionally administered treatment in breast cancer? Results of a randomized controlled trial. Sleep 2014;37(8): 1305–14.

34. Savard J, Ivers H, Savard MH, et al. Long-term effects of two formats of cognitive behavioral therapy for insomnia comorbid with breast cancer. Sleep 2016;39(4): 813–23.

35. Leigh S, Ouyang J, Mimnagh C. Effective? Engaging? Secure? Applying the ORCHA-24 framework to evaluate apps for chronic insomnia disorder. Evid Based Ment Health 2017;20(4):e20.

Telehealth, Telemedicine, and Obstructive Sleep Apnea

Sharon Schutte-Rodin, MD, DABSM, CBSM

KEYWORDS

- Telehealth • Telemedicine • Telemonitoring • Remote patient monitoring (RPM)
- Obstructive sleep apnea (OSA) • Electronic health record (EHR)
- Patient-reported outcomes (PROs) • e-consult

KEY POINTS

- Obstructive sleep apnea (OSA) telehealth options may be used to replace or supplement none, some, or all steps in the evaluation, testing, treatments, and management of OSA. All telehealth steps must adhere to best-practice and quality-measure OSA guidelines.
- OSA telehealth pathways may be adapted for continuous positive airway pressure (CPAP) and non-CPAP treatments.
- Not all patients may be appropriate for 1 common OSA telemanagement pathway. If considering 1 standardized OSA telehealth path, prior evaluation for other sleep breathing, sleep, and medical disorders and comorbidities is needed because these patients may require different telepathways.
- OSA telemanagement may improve communications, workflows, outcomes, patient satisfaction, costs, and e-data collection. E-data collection enhances uses for individual and group analytics, phenotyping, testing and treatment selections, high-risk identification and targeted support, and comparative and multispecialty therapy studies.
- Clinical and consumer sleep and medical technology advancements, deep learning and artificial intelligence algorithms, and the roles of insurers, pharmacies, and Web services will continue to change the evolving landscape of OSA telemanagement.

DEFINITIONS: TELEHEALTH, TELEMEDICINE, AND UNCOMPLICATED OBSTRUCTIVE SLEEP APNEA

There is no 1 definition for either telehealth or telemedicine. There also are a variety of teleservices and e-services. Simply stated, adding tele to the front of a word indicates distant and adding e in front of a word indicates electronic.[1] A broader construct, telehealth, is not a specific service. Telehealth "is a collection of means or methods for enhancing health care, public health, and health education delivery and support using telecommunication technologies."[2] Using the definitions of telehealth and telemedicine similarly, the American Telemedicine Association (ATA) defines telemedicine as

This article originally appeared in *Sleep Medicine Clinics*, Volume 15, Issue 3, September 2020.
Penn Sleep Center, 3624 Market Street, 2nd Floor, Philadelphia, PA 19104, USA
E-mail address: Sharon.Schutte-Rodin@pennmedicine.upenn.edu

Clinics Collections 10 (2021) 203–225
https://doi.org/10.1016/j.ccol.2020.12.021

"the remote delivery of health care services and clinical information using telecommunications technology."[3] Having the most narrow telehealth definition but with impact of the economic feasibility of incorporating OSA telehealth into clinical practice workflows, the definition by the Centers for Medicare and Medicaid Services (CMS) relates to payment to providers for specific telehealth clinical services.[4] These telehealth applications include live (synchronous) videoconferencing, store-and-forward (asynchronous) videoconferencing, remote patient monitoring, and mobile health (mHealth).[5] As the definition associated with payment by CMS and some private insurers, this may be the definition affecting providers when choosing e-technology in practice workflows. In the context of the management of obstructive sleep apnea (OSA), revisiting definitions of telehealth and telemedicine assists OSA clinicians in choosing teleapplications that may be most useful to their practice workflows and available resources.

This article focuses on the broader, more inclusive, telehealth definitions for the evaluation, diagnosis, treatment, and chronic management of OSA (**Fig. 1**). Further, although the evaluation of OSA includes the ability to recognize central sleep apnea and other respiratory breathing and sleep disorders, this article addresses the uses of telehealth specifically for uncomplicated OSA. When considering standard OSA telehealth pathways and options for a patient, it is of critical importance to screen and evaluate for other sleep breathing disorders and related comorbidities because these would require different telehealth management. Ideally, clinicians use unique telehealth pathways using validated preselection algorithms for different patient OSA

Definitions: Telehealth, Telemedicine, Uncomplicated Obstructive Sleep Apnea

OSA Telehealth Implementation: Standardized e-Care Within OSA Best Practice and Quality Measures

OSA Evaluation and Telehealth
Baseline Tele-evaluation Options
Hub-and-spoke Model and E-consults

OSA Diagnosis and Telehealth
OSA Tele-testing
E-Communications of Test Results, OSA Severity, and Treatments
Data Analytics for Testing and Treatment Paths

OSA Treatments and Telehealth

CPAP Tele-management
CPAP: Remote Education and Set-up
CPAP Telemonitoring
Reviewing Remote CPAP Data
Long-term Remote CPAP Data Monitoring

Non-CPAP Device Tele-management
Other Non-CPAP Remote Device Monitoring

Other Telehealth Chronic OSA Management (All treatments)

Discussion

Fig. 1. Article outline.

phenotypes and comorbidities. An interim simplified strategy to identity uncomplicated OSA for standard OSA telehealth care may be similar to the evaluation used when choosing attended polysomnography (PSG) versus unattended home sleep apnea testing (HSAT) for uncomplicated adult OSA.[6–9]

Many sleep medicine clinicians worldwide have been practicing forms of OSA telehealth for decades (such as remote online study interpretations, e-communications, and remote continuous positive airway pressure [CPAP] data monitoring). Likewise, many patients with OSA have been participating in e-care and self-education (eg, online interactive CPAP applications such as MyAir or DreamMapper), with their positive airway pressure (PAP) home medical equipment (HME) companies (using calls, texts, emails, PAP unit messaging), and with providers through EHR message portals.[10–13]

Because the landscape for provider payment of teleservices is rapidly changing and varies from state to state and country to country, OSA providers should be aware of local payments for teleservices.[4,5,14,15] In addition to enhancing and expanding OSA care, providers may find that the integration and implementation of teleservices into daily OSA workflows may realize valuable indirect workflow savings and patient satisfaction benefits.[11,16–21] Recognizing the importance of using sleep telemedicine tools, the American Academy of Sleep Medicine (AASM) launched the SleepTM Web site and provided additional resources (Singh 2015, Implementation Guide, AASM Web site) to assist clinicians with the integration and implementation of telemedicine into sleep practices.[14,22,23]

OBSTRUCTIVE SLEEP APNEA TELEHEALTH: IMPLEMENTATION OF STANDARDIZED E-CARE WITHIN OBSTRUCTIVE SLEEP APNEA BEST-PRACTICE GUIDELINES AND AMERICAN ACADEMY OF SLEEP MEDICINE QUALITY MEASURES

Whether delivered in person or using telehealth technologies, the evaluation, diagnosis, treatment, and chronic management of OSA must be delivered at the same best-practice level using accepted standards of care, quality measures, and guidelines.[6–9,22,24–34] Although clinical care standards for telemedicine should mirror those of in-person visits, OSA telecare and e-care also open opportunities to expand new ways to deliver improved OSA care access, between-visit care, communications, education, cost savings, individual and big data access, and monitoring quality-measure outcomes data.[11,16,17,19–22,35–51] Moreover, in addition to providing a structure for traditional OSA care, the guidelines allow for customized variations in telehealth care implementation using available local practice (technical, staff, financial) resources, regional insurance coverages, and societal best-practice guidelines. This strength provides flexibility for using e-care in none, some, or many of the steps in OSA evaluation, diagnosis, and management. This framework and associated teleopportunities and e-opportunities for OSA care are described in more detail later.

A traditional OSA workflow may include the clinical evaluation, testing, communication of the diagnosis and treatment options with the patient, initial treatment care, and chronic care management. While keeping within OSA best-practice and quality-measure guidelines and the OSA provider's current workflow and resources, there are numerous opportunities for teleservices and e-services to replace, supplement, provide additional interim care and education, or improve practice workflows and costs for each of the OSA treatments (**Fig. 2**). Although many telehealth studies focus on CPAP treatment and outcomes, telehealth applications for other OSA treatments, chronic management strategies, and big-data deep learning applications may be realized.

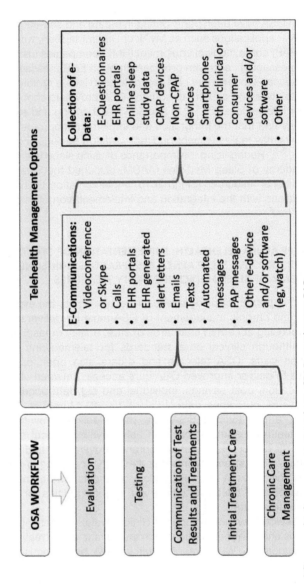

Fig. 2. OSA workflows and telemanagement options. CPAP, continuous PAP.

OBSTRUCTIVE SLEEP APNEA EVALUATION AND TELEHEALTH
Baseline Tele-evaluation Options

Patients with OSA enter sleep-center workflows through varied pathways. Before testing and diagnosis, patients initially may be evaluated by the primary care physician (PCP), by sleep medicine or other specialists, or by self-referral.[22,25,52,53] Thus, identification of possible comorbid apnea conditions and risks during the evaluation and before testing is important in the selection of any OSA workflow path, test type selection, treatment choice, and follow-up care.[6–8,54] Telehealth e-tools and e-consults offer added opportunities to document screening and evaluation for appropriate OSA telehealth uses and management.[22,23,35]

For OSA, whether done at a face-to-face visit or using telehealth options, baseline and follow-up OSA symptoms, sleepiness, quality of life (QoL), weight, blood pressure, comorbid disorders, and motor vehicle accident assessment are documented.[22,24,26,29,55] Evaluation e-tool examples include patient-reported outcomes (PROs), quality measures, and sleep symptom questionnaires that may be completed by patients through EHR patient portals, sleep middleware or other medical or consumer OSA risk assessment software, or by phone.[56,57] Cukor and colleagues[57] used phone call OSA educational dialogue to show improved likelihood of scheduling an OSA evaluation in a black community sample. Moreover, consumer sleep technologies and digital health tools continue to advance from entertainment to validated sleep and physiologic collection devices.[58–60] Alerted by feedback about sleep questionnaire completion, snoring, heart rate variations, and/or sleep disruption, consumers may collect increasingly valuable apnea-related symptom data to share in the apnea evaluation process either as an individual self-referral or through computer algorithm risk identification and device alerts.[61,62] Likewise, whether done at a face-to-face visit or using telehealth options (such as video or blood pressure/weight tele-collection), baseline and follow-up blood pressure and weight assessments with appropriate counseling are performed.[26,30,58,63–66]

Hub-and-Spoke Model and E-consults

Sarmiento and colleagues[42] provide a concise summary of the Veterans' Affairs (VA) TeleSleep hub-and-spoke model of (synchronous) video teleconferencing and Remote Veteran Apnea Management Platform (REVAMP), a VA web-application which allows veterans to complete PRO questionnaires, communicate with providers, use online self-help tutorials, and view CPAP data. REVAMP providers either review the PRO and electronic health record (EHR) information during the televisit or provide an (asynchronous) e-consult determination to proceed directly to HSAT testing (without the televisit). Later, test results, CPAP prescriptions, and modem data are incorporated in the EHR for further telemanagement. E-consults also are gaining use outside of the VA system, particularly when providers are practicing within 1 EHR.[67,68] Although e-consults improve access, costs, and time to diagnosis and treatment, there are reported concerns about increased PCP workload, unpaid time for provider and practice support services, ownership of follow-up services, potential liability issues, and unanticipated consequences such as missed comorbidities.[18,53,67–70]

OBSTRUCTIVE SLEEP APNEA DIAGNOSIS AND TELEHEATH
Obstructive Sleep Apnea Teletesting Options

PSG and HSAT provide accepted pathways for the diagnosis of OSA.[6–9,28,31,71] Both PSG and HSAT commonly use forms of (asynchronous store-and-forward) remote data review.[22] Of note, HSAT and consumer device technologies continue to evolve and undergo direct gold standard and/or outcomes-based OSA validation testing to further expand telehealth testing options.[50,72–77] Several wearables with pulse oximetry SpO$_2$, heart rate variability, actigraphy, and deep learning algorithms are currently under US Food and Drug Administration (FDA) evaluation as HSAT-type devices.[78] Further, ongoing HSAT validation studies for specific subgroups of at-risk patients continue to expand possible HSAT telehealth services. Saletu and colleagues[76] described the use of HSAT OSA diagnosis for inpatient rehabilitation of cerebrovascular accident, Kauta and colleagues[79] described the use of inpatient HSAT and PAP therapy reducing 30-day readmission rates, and Choi and colleagues[80] reported the use of Watch-PAT for adolescent OSA diagnosis. Although the use of autoCPAP for high-risk patients with OSA without formal testing has been proposed, the exclusion of comorbidities (such as obesity hypoventilation), lack of OSA severity assessment, validated preselection algorithms for patient phenotypes and comorbidity exclusions, and inconclusive correlation with low autoCPAP pressures currently preclude treatment of patients without any OSA testing and severity assessment.[6,24,27,30,81,82]

E-communications of Test Results, Obstructive Sleep Apnea Severity, and Treatment Options

In keeping with OSA best-practice and quality-measure guidelines, the communications of the test results, OSA severity, and treatment options with patients may be done at face-to-face visits or using e-communications such as videoconferencing, phone, EHR portal messaging, Skype, or other e-communications.[21,35,42,44,45,50] Education of OSA risks, test results, treatment options, sleepiness and driving, and weight and blood pressure monitoring may be supplemented with video links, Web sites, and other e-communication formats.[8,22,24,35,44] With respect to the e-communication of test results on OSA telehealth outcomes, there is considerable variation in who provides the test results to patients in many telehealth studies. Test results may be e-communicated to patients by sleep medicine or other physicians, nurses, nurse practitioners, physician assistants, laboratory technicians, respiratory therapists, home equipment therapists, or other trained staff.[20–22,39,42,44–46,49,52,83] Teasing out the use of only e-communication of test results on treatment outcomes is further confounded by OSA telehealth studies using different telecommunication forms as well as different timing for the e-evaluation, PAP adherence monitoring, and PAP e-support combined with the e-communication of the test results.[84] Nevertheless, many OSA telehealth studies and reviews include combinations of e-visits for e-communication of test results, some type of adherence telemonitoring, and CPAP support e-communications, which are discussed later.[11,19–22,35–38,40–51,85,86]

Data Analytics for Testing and Treatment Paths

In addition to clinical guidelines for OSA test type and promising OSA testing technologies, deep learning and artificial intelligence models using phenotyping, EHR data, and/or other consumer or medical sensor devices and applications may provide insights for OSA risk assessment and test prioritization, choosing the optimum test type, or selection of personalized treatment paths.[87–96] Stretch and colleagues[87] proposed a machine learning model to predict patients having nondiagnostic HSATs and requiring PSG, whereas Mencar and colleagues[97] and Huang and colleagues[92,93] suggested models to predict OSA severity risk for testing prioritization. Using HL-7 integration of software or internal EHR portals, PRO and sleep questionnaire data within EHRs may allow the interface of comorbid and other clinical EHR big data to further enhance identification of OSA risk, phenotypes, optimum test type, and outcomes.[56,98]

OBSTRUCTIVE SLEEP APNEA TREATMENTS AND TELEHEALTH

Current recommended OSA treatment options include PAP, positional apnea devices, oral appliances, and upper airway surgeries.[8,24,26–28,30,31,99,100] Adjunct OSA management includes, but is not limited to, weight loss; HME and PAP device patient engagement technologies; cognitive behavior therapy for insomnia (CBT-I) with comorbid insomnia; and the use of supportive education, coaching, monitoring, and management e-communications.[22,30,44–47,86,101]

CONTINUOUS POSITIVE AIRWAY PRESSURE TELEMANAGEMENT
Continuous Positive Airway Pressure: Remote Education and Setup

For patients who receive CPAP as initial therapy, a PAP Rx often is sent from the provider (EHR) to an HME for either face-to-face, group class, Skype, or videoconference remote CPAP setup and education.[35,36,42,45,47,49,50,85] For appropriate patients, the use of autoCPAP allows the Rx to be in either fixed or auto-Rx modes and also permits flexibility in resetting the Rx remotely through online pressure adjustments as clinically needed.[27,30] Initial education and mask choice by sleep technicians or HME therapists is thought to influence early compliance but is recognized to be labor intensive, particularly if done in person in the patient's home. When adhering to AASM telemedicine standards, both remote education and video CPAP setups may offer decreased labor time while maintaining equivalent or improved CPAP compliance and satisfaction.[22] Close relationships and monitoring of HMEs by providers are key in minimizing setup errors and ensuring telemonitoring protocols.[102] Mask fitting facial recognition software, use of mask sizers (during video or Skype setups), mask fit packs (containing several cushion sizes), and deep learning analysis of mask fitting selection phenotypes may expand remote CPAP mask selection and setup options.[103–105]

Using e-questionnaires, insurance and clinical EHR data, and phenotyping models, patients at high risk for nonadherence might receive added or targeted tele-educational and support protocols such as adjunct CBT-I with comorbid insomnia.[86,96,101,104,106,107] Although early educational interventions before CPAP initiation are strongly recommended and behavioral and troubleshooting interventions are suggested, specific standard or tele-education formats are not mandated.[30] This noted, the effect of tele-education alone on compliance overall does not seem robust,[45] which may be because of confounding factors such as the variability of the initial and following tele-education deliveries, as well as easy availability of Internet sites and industry-sponsored Web OSA and CPAP educational resources for patients with OSA. Kuna and colleagues,[108] Malhotra and colleagues,[109] Hostler and colleagues,[12] Hardy and colleagues,[10] Lynch and colleagues,[110] and Shaughnessy and colleagues[111] found improved compliance for patients given Web access to their data and companion educational resources. Isetta and colleagues[85,112] and Fields and colleagues[21] reported improved compliance and satisfaction with videoconference training. Parikh and colleagues[20] showed similar compliance and patient satisfaction with videoconferencing compared with standard visit care. Hwang and colleagues[45] explored the use of telemedicine OSA education (teled) and automated compliance messaging and found that teled alone did not increase adherence, but teled did improve clinic attendance and further increased compliance in the automated messaging group. For patients identified as being at risk for poor CPAP compliance, Guralnick and colleagues[113] noted that educational videos did not improve compliance or clinic show rates.

Continuous Positive Airway Pressure Telemonitoring

Numerous studies have shown similar or increased CPAP compliance with various forms of CPAP data telemonitoring, which may include automated message data alerts, coaching and reinforcement emails/texts/calls/EHR messages/online educational and motivational support, and Skype or videoconferencing.[11,37–39,41,43–46,48,114,115] Turino and colleagues[38] showed similar compliance with telemonitoring but improved patient satisfaction and cost savings. Murase and colleagues[51] proposed that telemedicine may assist adherence even with users for more than 3 months. Nilius and colleagues[116] and Kotzian and colleagues[117] showed improved compliance of patients with strokes with proactive telemonitoring. Further, telemonitoring of CPAP data may enable early identification of central sleep apnea/Cheyne-Stokes and congestive heart failure/cardiac disease occurrence or progression.[46,118] Tung and colleagues[118] followed 2912 patients over 5 years and found central sleep apnea and Cheyne-Stokes to be a predictor of incident atrial fibrillation.

As noted earlier, many patients are empowered to improve adherence with Web access to CPAP use, leak, and residual apnea-hypopnea index (AHI) data as well as access to online support tools.[12,13,43,44,88,108,109,111] Self-monitoring of blood pressure and weight is gaining interest. Although limited to a 4-month trial, Mendelson and colleagues[119] showed the feasibility of patient entry of blood pressure, CPAP use, sleepiness, and QoL data into smartphones for clinician review. McManus and colleagues[58] reported that patient self-monitoring of blood pressure, with or without telemonitoring, decreased blood pressure after 12 months. Personal patient cost savings have been shown to improve medication adherence, suggesting that telecare without copays also may improve adherence.[120] Likewise, HMEs are using CPAP vendor telemonitoring software such as ResMed's U-Sleep and Philips Patient Adherence Monitoring Service to improve initial CPAP compliance.[121,122]

Reviewing Remote Continuous Positive Airway Pressure Data

Sleep providers are familiar with CPAP remote data monitoring, which often focuses on initial CPAP adherence. However, the presence of significant air leak may confound the interpretation of CPAP use time, residual AHI data, and minimum/maximum/average autoCPAP pressure data. Remote data interpretation and clinical caution are indicated if an acceptable air seal is not first confirmed. Note that leak data are not included in adherence reporting in many studies. The choice of the date range also affects interpretation of remote data monitoring. For example, normal data for the past averaged 3 or 6 or 12 months may not represent recent normal or abnormal data over the past weeks. In addition, definitions and algorithms for leak, AHI, and use times may vary between CPAP unit brands.[123,124] Spo_2 monitoring is available to add separately or directly into some home CPAP unit brands, but typically Spo_2 monitoring is not part of standard OSA CPAP data monitoring. For patients empirically set up with autoCPAP, Koivumaki and colleagues[125] suggested oximetry as part of CPAP initiation of patients with baseline Spo_2 less than 92% or body mass index greater than 30 kg/m^2. Further, users may overlook that CPAP unit residual AHI is based on recording time and may include snoring and vibration in the total residual event calculations (ie, CPAP AHI is not equal to PSG AHI).[126,127] Nonetheless, CPAP remote data monitoring improves CPAP adherence and outcomes and is standard care for CPAP management.[30,33]

Long-Term Remote Continuous Positive Airway Pressure Data Monitoring

After the initial 90 days, some HMEs may decrease remote data monitoring of CPAP adherence. In a review, Murphie and colleagues[36] found variability in the frequency of long-term PAP visit or call follow-up. Telehealth offers increased care access options. However, office staff telemonitoring of voluminous nightly data from entire practices of patients is daunting and generally not reimbursable. Ideally, patients are, and continue to be, engaged in self-monitoring of Web-based data and are instructed to notify providers with changes in leak, residual AHI, use times, or clinical problems. The use of vendor software notice applications, EHR applications, middleware algorithms, and automated data alert messaging may provide a feasible solution for practices attempting to manage huge amounts of nightly CPAP data for PAP patients over years.[44,88] Using Health Level 7 (HL7) integrated PAP data within the EHR, Tan and colleagues[128] showed how an EHR could be used as the workhorse to identify real-time, abnormal PAP data on a quarterly or scheduled basis, and then send EHR-generated alert e-messages (to seek follow-up) to a large practice of clinic patients with OSA with abnormal PAP data.

OBSTRUCTIVE SLEEP APNEA TELEMANAGEMENT OF NON–CONTINUOUS POSITIVE AIRWAY PRESSURE TREATMENTS
Other Non–continuous Positive Airway Pressure Remote Device Monitoring

Although not as commercially available to patients as online CPAP data access, data alerts, and education, telemonitoring of other OSA therapy data seems to be forthcoming. Positional OSA (POSA) devices are an OSA treatment option that has more recent telemonitoring capabilities.[129–133] Although there remain discussions on definitions, subclassifications, and associated use guidelines for POSA, new technologies are allowing sleep position and compliance e-monitoring capabilities.[129–131,134–136] The addition of remote POSA adherence data to PRO and EHR data allows clearer outcomes analytics and also the valuable dimension of comparative therapy studies.[134,136,137] Similar to CPAP teleapplications, some POSA devices are FDA cleared; may be combined with other therapies; and offer online educational resources, data access, and downloadable reports to share with sleep clinicians.[132,133]

Abilities to telemonitor oral appliance (OA) compliance data are evolving. Although not yet as common as online CPAP and some POSA device data access, the use of temperature-sensing data chips embedded in the OA have provided objective OA adherence data in studies.[136–141] Commercially available SomnoDent OA uses patented software, temperature sensor, and triple axis accelerometer technologies that allow patients to upload OA use times and supine/nonsupine data for Web report access.[140] The use of OA compliance data with PRO, EHR, and AHI study data allows comparative treatment studies, quality-measure and outcomes analysis, and prediction models.[136,137,140] Expansion of online software for OA therapy data access seems the next logical step toward OA telemanagement. In addition, like POSA and other non-CPAP therapies, such OA adherence telemonitoring would require supplemental, periodic OSA reassessment long term and as clinically indicated.[32,138,142] The American Academy of Dental Medicine recommends at least annual OA therapy follow-up.[143]

Using an implantable pulse generator and stimulation and sensing leads, hypoglossal nerve stimulation (HGNS) offers the promise of expanded future telemanagement applications. Remembering how CPAP data were originally downloaded using cards to software, HGNS compliance data currently are available using cloud-based reports after USB upload.[144] Marrying HGNS data with PRO, EHR, and AHI study data opens possibilities for comparative studies and for phenotyping, patient selection, outcomes, cost analysis, and prediction models.[145–149] Looking toward the future, although wireless transmission is not yet available, such telemonitoring software and workflows could be a next step in HGNS remote data telemanagement. Cardiologists are familiar with remote pacemaker data monitoring, including event documentation.[150–152] In the IN-TIME study, Husser and colleagues[150] described an analysis of pacemaker workflow for remote data collection and alert messages sent to clinics that then phone patients for clinical correlation. In addition, pacemaker technologies continue to advance. According to a January 2020 press release by Medtronic, the FDA recently approved the first leadless pacemaker for atrioventricular synchrony using accelerometer-based atrial sensing and a patented algorithm.[153]

Other Telehealth Chronic Obstructive Sleep Apnea Management (All Treatments)

Although the same telehealth evaluation, testing, diagnosis, and educational options are available for other OSA treatments, fewer studies have explored the use of telehealth for non-CPAP treatments. However, regardless of the chosen OSA treatment, the same best-practice initial and chronic OSA management are recommended.[8,24,32,99,100] In addition to long-term remote device data monitoring, chronic OSA management for all treatments includes reassessment of sleep and apnea symptoms, sleepiness, QoL, weight, and blood pressure, which may be assessed in person or using telehealth methods used during initial tele-evaluations.[8,24,154] E-communications with patients may help clinicians to standardize blood pressure and weight assessments and counseling.[66,155] Ideally, clinical and PRO data may be collected using scheduled e-questionnaires or device data and used within the EHR for individual and group monitoring, for creation of patient high-risk list follow-up, for comparative treatment studies, and for big data AASM and CMS quality measures.[64,91,97,98] Using PRO, EHR, compliance, and other e-data, benefits and comparisons with CPAP e-data have been explored. Mendelson and colleagues[119] did not find a difference in smartphone-collected blood pressures after 4 months of CPAP use. In separate OA studies, de Vries and colleagues[156,157] reported reductions of systolic and diastolic blood pressures comparable with CPAP and adherence comparable with CPAP. Cillo and colleagues[158] showed long-term QoL improvement and patient satisfaction with maxillomandibular advancement. Analyzing 5-year outcomes of HGNS, Woodson and colleagues[149] reported improvement of sleepiness, QoL, and AHI response.

Because OSA may change with aging, weight, menopause, and some medications, long-term OSA monitoring for all treatments is indicated.[159–161] Although autoCPAPs may adjust with weight changes, aging, menopause, disease progression, and changing medications and comorbidities over time, other treatments may not offer long-term permanent protection or adapting therapy coverage.[162–165] It seems reasonable to use HSAT-type testing for long-term follow-up of ongoing treatment efficacy, but the frequency of follow-up teletesting for non-CPAP therapies does not seem clear. For POSA and OA devices, ongoing remote data monitoring of adherence is needed. Sutherland and Cistulli[138] and Sato and Nakajima[142] discussed the importance of long-term monitoring of OA adherence and for late side effects.[32] In particular, because weight changes over time affect OSA management, long-term weight monitoring remains important. Wang and colleagues[166] showed a correlation between weight loss, reduction of tongue fat, and improved AHI following weight loss interventions. This correlation noted, weight gain has been observed years after weight loss surgeries, with some patients requiring surgical revisions for further weight reduction.[165,167] Thus, even with apparent initial successful resolution of OSA, such as with airway or weight loss surgeries, long-term monitoring for OSA reoccurrence or progression is warranted.[161–164]

Like the initial e-evaluation and e-testing, scheduled telehealth e-questionnaires, weight and comorbidity monitoring, and home screening or testing devices may offer an option for long-term tele–follow-up of non-CPAP OSA treatment. Moreover, with ongoing validation studies, some consumer sleep technologies are transitioning to reliably track snoring, sleep, oximetry, heart rate variability, and OSA screening. As well, deep learning algorithms and software to collect individual and group analysis of weight, blood pressure, sleepiness, and other quality-measure data for prediction models are advancing. For example, Cistulli and Sutherland[89] proposed the use of analytics of phenotype and other tools to help guide personalized OSA therapy approaches.

DISCUSSION

The execution of OSA clinical guidelines and practice standards is possible using traditional, hybrid, and telehealth OSA workflows. Face-to-face visits or telehealth applications may be inserted in 1 or more of the workflow steps for (1) evaluation pathways, (2) diagnosis pathways, (3) CPAP and non-CPAP treatments, and (4) long-term follow-up. Telehealth e-applications may be used for communications, education, and support in any or all of these steps. OSA telehealth offers the opportunities to increase patient access, between-visit care, consultant-provider-HME-patient communications and education, cost savings, testing and treatment type selections, and patient satisfaction.[21,35,42,47,49,50] In addition, e-data collection using telehealth expands possibilities for individual and group data analysis for AASM and CMS quality measures, phenotyping, outcomes, comparative studies, and deep learning predictive models for OSA evaluation, testing, treatment selection, and best-practice workflows.[45,46,90] Farré and colleagues pose[168] the question of whether all patients with OSA or particular phenotypes are better served for different aspects of telehealth options. Incorporation of OSA-related data and other EHR discrete data opens dimensions to better understand the relationships of OSA with OSA-related comorbidities, multispecialty therapies, and outcomes-driven practices.

However, the promise of expanded OSA telehealth applications is accompanied with cautious considerations. Practical implementation into clinical OSA workflows requires an understanding of local payment for teleservices as well as assessment of available investment, staff, EHR, and information technology resources. In addition, clear OSA telehealth algorithms to screen and identify appropriate patients are essential. Separate telehealth pathways need to be clarified for special populations or patients with combination breathing, sleep, medical, or comorbid disorders.

Telehealth offers flexibility in who delivers and takes ownership of initial and chronic OSA care and workflows. As previously described, telehealth applications may be used in none, some, or all of the OSA workflow steps. However, this workflow assumes that a boarded clinician is the OSA workflow supervisor and monitor. On its chronic disease HealthHUB Web site, a national pharmacy chain advertises that its HealthHUB providers may perform an OSA risk assessment, order home testing, review results and options, and prescribe CPAP and supplies.[169] Another pharmacy chain advertises sleep links and live provider video calls for sleep and chronic disease evaluation.[170] In these proposed care models, tele and electronic data sharing with clinicians seem vital in long-term OSA follow-up and management, particularly if these patients include those with unscreened comorbidities, requiring therapy changes, or requiring OSA problem solving. It also is unclear whether and how mergers of insurers, pharmacies, and retail chains will affect standard and telehealth OSA care and delivery.[171] How to best incorporate these and other new entities into best-practice standard, hybrid, and telehealth OSA workflows currently seems a moving environment.

The volumes of available OSA e-data also present questions on how best to monitor and use these huge datasets in daily practices as well as how to use them in deep learning predictive models.[91,95,172–174] Assuming the feasibility of automated machine alerts of abnormal OSA clinical or device data or high-risk groups, how frequently should e-alerts be advised and how will such alerts be handled in an expanded tele-workflow? While monitoring practice support resources as ample, Tan and colleagues[128] found that quarterly clinic EHR-generated alerts of abnormal PAP and other OSA therapy data provided adequate time for the correction of PAP issues and then time to generate new PAP (postintervention) data. Education and scheduled engagement of patients in self-monitoring of abnormal PRO, sleep, weight, blood pressure, and PAP e-data through e-communications with providers may be an option for some practices.[50,119] Moreover, evolving validation of clinical and consumer sleep-related technologies, sensors, devices/applications, and deep learning/artificial intelligence algorithms affect telehealth options and explosively increase available big datasets.[44,59,91,172,175–185] How telehealth will play a role in EHR information exchange with insurers and with Apple and Web service consumer e-data is developing.[186–189] For example, Apple's Healthkit offers wireless blood pressure cuffs for home blood pressure and heart rate data to interface with the EHR for clinician review. In addition, refill and health tips may be e-sent to the patient Apple Watch.[186] Other large health and sleep e-dataset resources available for OSA prediction models and telehealth applications include access to the National Institutes of Health Big Data to Knowledge and National Sleep Research Resource.[91,190] Although AASM has dedicated task forces for telemedicine, EHR, clinical and consumer sleep technologies, and artificial intelligence, the fast rate of technology development and e-datasets seems to continue to outpace clinical studies on how to best incorporate new OSA technologies, telehealth, and voluminous clinical and consumer daily data into clinical practice guidelines.

Revisiting the telehealth construct of "a collection of means or methods for enhancing health care, public health, and health education delivery and support using telecommunication technologies,"[2] it is clear that increasing applications of telehealth into the OSA workflow will continue to enhance and expand OSA care. Although there are potential future challenges in standard, hybrid, and telehealth OSA care options, AASM and other specialty groups have provided a framework and clear standards on best-practice clinical guidelines for OSA evaluation, diagnosis, treatment, and follow-up.[6–9,22,24–34] The use of telehealth in any of the OSA care steps requires the same level of attention to accepted standards of OSA care, quality measures, and clinical guidelines. With the ongoing development and validation of clinical and consumer sleep technologies, remote data monitoring, expansion of e-communications, and data analytics, the role of OSA telehealth applications and management will continue to evolve and expand. While maintaining best-practice standards, telehealth offers new dimensions and strengths in flexibility and enhancement of standard OSA workflows, and the promise for improved OSA care.

DISCLOSURE

The author has nothing to disclose.

REFERENCES

1. California telemedicine and eHealth center: a glossary of telemedicine and eHealth. Available at: http://www.caltrc.org/wp-content/uploads/2013/10/ctec_glossary_final.pdf. Accessed November 6, 2019.
2. Center for Connected Health Policy (The National Telehealth Policy Resource Center): What is Telehealth?. Available at: https://www.cchpca.org/about/about-telehealth. Accessed January 26, 2020.
3. American Telemedicine Association: What is Telemedicine?. Available at: http://legacy.americantelemed.org/main/about/about-telemedicine/telemedicine-faqs. Accessed January 26, 2020.
4. Centers for Medicare and Medicaid Services (CMS) Medical Learning Network: Telehealth Service. Available at: https://www.cms.gov/Outreach-and-Education/Medicare-Learning-Network-MLN/MLNProducts/downloads/TelehealthSrvcsfctsht.pdf. Accessed November 26, 2019.
5. HealthIT.gov (Official website of the Office of the National Coordinator for Health Information Technology- ONC): ONC): Telemedicine and Telehealth. Available at: https://www.healthit.gov/topic/health-it-initiatives/telemedicine-and-telehealth. Accessed November 26, 2019.
6. Kapur VK, Auckley DH, Chowdhuri S, et al. Clinical practice guideline for diagnostic testing for adult obstructive sleep apnea: an American Academy of Sleep Medicine Clinical Practice Guideline. J Clin Sleep Med 2017;13:479–504.
7. Rosen IM, Kirsch DB, Carden KA, et al. Clinical use of a home sleep apnea test: an updated American Academy of Sleep Medicine position statement. J Clin Sleep Med 2018;14(12):2075–7.
8. Epstein LJ, Kristo D, Strollo PJ Jr, et al. Clinical guideline for the evaluation, management and long-term care of obstructive sleep apnea in adults. J Clin Sleep Med 2009;5(3):263–76.
9. Collop NA, Anderson WM, Boehlecke B, et al. Clinical guidelines for the use of unattended portable monitors in the diagnosis of obstructive sleep apnea in adult patients. Portable Monitoring Task Force of the American Academy of Sleep Medicine. J Clin Sleep Med 2007;3(7):737–47.
10. Hardy W, Powers J, Jasko JG, et al. DreamMapper white paper: a mobile application and website to engage sleep apnea patients in PAP therapy and improve adherence to treatment. Available at: http://incenter.medical.philips.com/doclib/enc/fetch/2000/4504/577242/577256/588723/588747/sleepmapper-tx-whitepaper.pdf%3fnodeid%3d11228847%26vernum%3d-2.
11. Munafo D, Hevener W, Crocker M, et al. A telehealth program for CPAP adherence reduces labor and yields similar adherence and efficacy when compared to standard of care. Sleep Breath 2016;20(2):777–85.
12. Hostler JM, Sheikh KL, Andrada TF, et al. A mobile, web-based system can improve positive airway pressure adherence. J Sleep Res 2017;26(2):139–46.
13. ResMed My Air. Available at: https://myair.resmed.com/. Accessed April 30, 2020.
14. American Academy of Sleep Medicine Clinical Resources: Telemedicine. Available at: https://aasm.org/clinical-resources/telemedicine/. Accessed January 20, 2020.
15. Telligen, gpTRAC. Telehealth: Start-Up and Resource Guide. Version 1.1. 2014. Available at: https://gptrac.org/wp-content/uploads/2015/01/TelligenTelehealthGuide-Final-2014.pdf.

16. Isetta V, Negrín M, Monasterio C, et al. A Bayesian cost-effectiveness analysis of a telemedicine-based strategy for the management of sleep apnoea: a multicentre randomised controlled trial. Thorax 2015;70(11):1054–61.

17. Russo JE, McCool RR, Davies LVA. Telemedicine: an analysis of cost and time savings. Telemed J E Health 2016;22(3):209–15.

18. Thaker DA, Monypenny R, Olver I, et al. Cost savings from a telemedicine model of care in northern Queensland, Australia. Med J Aust 2013;199:414–7.

19. Dullet NW, Geraghty EM, Kaufman T, et al. Impact of a university-based outpatient telemedicine program on time savings, travel costs, and environmental pollutants. Value Health 2017;2:542–6.

20. Parikh R, Touvelle MN, Wang H, et al. Sleep telemedicine: patient satisfaction and treatment adherence. Telemed J E Health 2011;17:609–14.

21. Fields BG, Behari PP, McCloskey S, et al. Remote ambulatory management of veterans with obstructive sleep apnea. Sleep 2016;39(3):501–9.

22. Singh J, Badr MS, Diebert W, et al. American Academy of Sleep Medicine (AASM) position paper for the use of telemedicine for the diagnosis and treatment of sleep disorders. J Clin Sleep Med 2015;11(10):1187–98.

23. Singh J, Badr MS, Epstein L, et al. Sleep telemedicine implementation guide. American Academy of Sleep Medicine; 2015. Available at: https://aasm.org/clinical-resources/telemedicine/. Accessed November 22, 2019.

24. Aurora RN, Collop NA, Jacobowitz O, et al. Quality measures for the care of adult patients with obstructive sleep apnea. J Clin Sleep Med 2015;11(3):357–83.

25. Aurora RN, Quan SF. Quality measure for screening for adult obstructive sleep apnea by primary care physicians. J Clin Sleep Med 2016;12(8):1185–7.

26. Morgenthaler TI, Aronsky AJ, Carden KA, et al. Measurement of quality to improve care in sleep medicine. J Clin Sleep Med 2015;11(3):279–91.

27. Morgenthaler TI, Aurora RN, Brown T, et al. Practice parameters for the use of autotitrating continuous positive airway pressure devices for titrating pressures and treating adult patients with obstructive sleep apnea syndrome: an update for 2007. An American Academy of Sleep Medicine report. Sleep 2008;31(1):141–7.

28. Fleetham J, Ayas N, Bradley D, et al. Canadian Thoracic Society 2011 guideline update: diagnosis and treatment of sleep disordered breathing. Can Respir J 2011;18(1):24–47.

29. Gamaldo C, Buenaver L, Chernyshev O, et al, OSA Assessment Tools Task Force of the American Academy of Sleep Medicine. Evaluation of clinical tools to screen and assess for obstructive sleep apnea. J Clin Sleep Med 2018;14(7):1239–44.

30. Patil SP, Ayappa IA, Caples SM, et al. Treatment of adult obstructive sleep apnea with positive airway pressure: an American Academy of Sleep Medicine clinical practice guideline. J Clin Sleep Med 2019;15(2):335–43.

31. Qaseem A, Holty J, Owens D, et al. Management of obstructive sleep apnea in adults: a clinical practice guideline from the American College of Physicians. Ann Intern Med 2013;159(7):471–83.

32. Ramar K, Dort LC, Katz SG, et al. Clinical practice guideline for the treatment of obstructive sleep apnea and snoring with oral appliance therapy: an update for 2015. J Clin Sleep Med 2015;11(7):773–827.

33. Schwab RJ, Badr SM, Epstein LJ, et al. An official American Thoracic Society statement: continuous positive airway pressure adherence tracking systems.

The optimal monitoring strategies and outcome measures in adults. Am J Respir Crit Care Med 2013;188:613–20.

34. Kushida CA, Littner MR, Morgenthaler T, et al. Practice parameters for the indications for polysomnography and related procedures: an update for 2005. Sleep 2005;28:499–521.

35. Bruyneel M. Telemedicine in the diagnosis and treatment of sleep apnoea. Eur Respir Rev 2019;28:180093.

36. Murphie P, Little S, Paton R, et al. Defining the core components of a clinical review of people using continuous positive airway pressure therapy to treat obstructive sleep apnea: an international e-Delphi study. J Clin Sleep Med 2018;14(10):1679–87.

37. Hoet F, Libert W, Sanida C, et al. Telemonitoring in continuous positive airway pressure-treated patients improves delay to first intervention and early compliance: a randomized trial. Sleep Med 2017;39:77–83, 26(2):139-146.

38. Turino C, de Batlle J, Woehrle H, et al. Management of continuous positive airway pressure treatment compliance using telemonitoring in obstructive sleep apnoea. Eur Respir J 2017;49:1601128.

39. Smith CE, Dauz ER, Clements F, et al. Telehealth services to improve nonadherence: a placebo-controlled study. Telemed J E Health 2006;12:289–96.

40. Smith I, Nadig V, Lasserson TJ. Educational, supportive and behavioural interventions to improve usage of continuous positive airway pressure machines for adults with obstructive sleep apnoea. Cochrane Database Syst Rev 2009;(2):CD007736.

41. Sparrow D, Aloia M, Demolles DA, et al. A telemedicine intervention to improve adherence to continuous positive airway pressure: a randomised controlled trial. Thorax 2010;65:1061–6.

42. Sarmiento KF, Folmer RL, Stepnowsky CJ, et al. National expansion of sleep telemedicine for veterans: the telesleep program. J Clin Sleep Med 2019; 15(9):1355–64.

43. Schoch OD, Baty F, Boesch M, et al. Telemedicine for continuous positive airway pressure in sleep apnea. A randomized, controlled study. Ann Am Thorac Soc 2019;16(12):1550–7.

44. Hwang D. Monitoring progress and adherence with positive airway pressure therapy for obstructive sleep apnea: the roles of telemedicine and mobile health applications. Sleep Med Clin 2016;11:161–71.

45. Hwang D, Chang JW, Benjafield AV, et al. Effect of telemedicine education and telemonitoring on continuous positive airway pressure adherence. The Tele-OSA randomized trial. Am J Respir Crit Care Med 2018;197(1):117–26.

46. Pepin JL, Tamisier R, Hwang D, et al. Does remote monitoring change OSA management and CPAP adherence? Respirology 2017;22(8):1508–17.

47. Suarez-Giron M, Bonsignore MR, Montserrat JM. New organisation for follow-up and assessment of treatment efficacy in sleep apnoea. Eur Respir Rev 2019;28: 190059.

48. Fox N, Hirsch-Allen A, Goodfellow E, et al. The impact of a telemedicine monitoring system on positive airway pressure adherence in patients with obstructive sleep apnea: a randomized controlled trial. Sleep 2012;35(4):477–81.

49. Lugo VM, Garmendia O, Suarez-Girón M, et al. Comprehensive management of obstructive sleep apnea by telemedicine: clinical improvement and cost-effectiveness of a Virtual Sleep Unit. A randomized controlled trial. PLoS One 2019;14(10):e0224069.

50. Villanueva JA, Suarez MC, Garmendia O, et al. The role of telemedicine and mobile health in the monitoring of sleep-breathing disorders: improving patient outcomes. Smart Homecare Technology TeleHealth 2017;4:1–11.

51. Murase K, Tanizawa K, Minami T, et al. A randomized controlled trial of telemedicine for long-term sleep apnea CPAP management. Ann Am Thorac Soc 2019. https://doi.org/10.1513/AnnalsATS.201907-494OC.

52. Chai-Coetzer CL, Antic NA, Rowland LS, et al. Primary care vs specialist sleep center management of obstructive sleep apnea and daytime sleepiness and quality of life: a randomized trial. JAMA 2013;309(10):997–1004.

53. Osman MA, Schick-Makaroff K, Thompson S, et al. Barriers and facilitators for implementation of electronic consultations (eConsult) to enhance access to specialist care: a scoping review. BMJ Glob Health 2019;4(5):e001629.

54. Mokhlesi B, Masa JF, Brozek JL, et al. Evaluation and management of obesity hypoventilation syndrome. An official American Thoracic Society Clinical Practice Guideline. Am J Respir Crit Care Med 2019;200(3):e6–24.

55. Ibáñez V, Silva J, Cauli O. A survey on sleep assessment methods. PeerJ 2018; 6:e4849.

56. Chang Y, Staley B, Simonsen S, et al. Transitioning from paper to electronic health record collection of Epworth sleepiness scale (ESS) for quality measures. Sleep 2018;41(1):404.

57. Cukor D, Pencille M, Ver Halen N, et al. An RCT comparing remotely delivered adherence promotion for sleep apnea assessment against an information control in a black community sample. Sleep Health 2018;4(4):369–76.

58. McManus RJ, Mant J, Franssen M, et al. Efficacy of self-monitored blood pressure, with or without telemonitoring, for titration of antihypertensive medication (TASMINH4): an unmasked randomised controlled trial. Lancet 2018; 391(10124):949–59.

59. Consumer Technology Association and Heart Rhythm Society. Guidance for wearable health solutions white paper. 2020. Available at: https://shop.cta. tech/products/guidance-for-wearable-health-solutions. Accessed January 26, 2020.

60. Dias D, Paulo Silva Cunha J. Wearable health devices—vital sign monitoring, systems and technologies. Sensors 2018;18(8):2414.

61. Katyayan A, Yadav V, Mishra P, et al. Computer algorithms in assessment of obstructive sleep apnoea syndrome and its application in estimating prevalence of sleep related disorders in population. Indian J Otolaryngol Head Neck Surg 2019;71(3):352–9.

62. Turakhia M, Perez M, Desai M, et al. Results of a large-scale, app-based study to identify atrial fibrillation using a smartwatch: the Apple Heart Study. Presented at the 68th American College of Cardiology Scientific Session, New Orleans, Louisiana; March 16–18, 2019. Abstract 19-LB-20253.

63. Rifkin DE, Abdelmalek JA, Miraclev CM, et al. Linking clinic and home: a randomized, controlled clinical effectiveness trial of real-time, wireless blood pressure monitoring for older patients with kidney disease and hypertension. Blood Press Monit 2013;18(1):8–15.

64. Margolis KL, Asche SE, Dehmer SP, et al. Long-term outcomes of the effects of home blood pressure telemonitoring and pharmacist management on blood pressure among adults with uncontrolled hypertension: follow-up of a cluster randomized clinical trial. JAMA Netw Open 2018;1(5):e181617.

65. Houser SH, Joseph R, Puro N, et al. Use of technology in the management of obesity: a literature review. Perspect Health Inf Manag 2019;16(Fall):1c.

66. Casey DE, Thomas RJ, Bhalla V, et al. 2019 AHA/ACC clinical performance and quality measures for adults with high blood pressure: a report of the American College of Cardiology/American Heart Association Task Force on Performance Measures. Circ Cardiovasc Qual Outcomes 2019;12:e000057.
67. Deeds SA, Dowdell KJ, Chew LD, et al. Implementing an Opt-in eConsult program at seven academic medical centers: a qualitative analysis of primary care provider experiences. J Gen Intern Med 2019;34(8):1427–33.
68. Kent J. How eConsults could transform care coordination and access. In: mHealth Intelligence. 2019. Available at: https://mhealthintelligence.com/news/how-econsults-could-transform-care-coordination-and-access. Accessed November 18, 2019.
69. Lee MS, Ray KN, Mehrotra A, et al. Primary care practitioners' perceptions of electronic consult systems: a qualitative analysis. JAMA Intern Med 2018; 178(6):782–9.
70. Vimalananda VG, Gupte G, Seraj SM, et al. Electronic consultations (e-consults) to improve access to specialty care: a systematic review and narrative synthesis. J Telemed Telecare 2015;21(6):323–30.
71. Kuna ST, Gurubhagavatula I, Maislin G, et al. Noninferiority of functional outcome in ambulatory management of obstructive sleep apnea. Am J Respir Crit Care Med 2011;183(9):1238–44.
72. Sands SA, Owens RL, Malhotra A. New approaches to diagnosing sleep-disordered breathing. Sleep Med Clin 2016;11(2):143–52.
73. Yalamanchali S, Farajian V, Hamilton C, et al. Diagnosis of obstructive sleep apnea by peripheral arterial tonometry: meta-analysis. JAMA Otolaryngol Head Neck Surg 2013;139(12):1343–50.
74. Watson NF, Lawlor C, Raymann RJ. Will consumer sleep technologies change the way we practice sleep medicine? J Clin Sleep Med 2019;15(1):159–61.
75. Khosla S, Deak MC, Gault D, et al. Consumer sleep technology: an American Academy of Sleep Medicine position statement. J Clin Sleep Med 2018;14(5): 877–80.
76. Saletu MT, Kotzian ST, Schwarzinger A, et al. Home sleep apnea testing is a feasible and accurate method to diagnose obstructive sleep apnea in stroke patients during in-hospital rehabilitation. J Clin Sleep Med 2018;14(9):1495–501.
77. Penzel T, Schöbel C, Fietze I. New technology to assess sleep apnea: wearables, smartphones, and accessories [version 1; peer review: 2 approved]. F1000Res 2018;7(F1000 Faculty Rev):413.
78. American Academy of sleep medicine clinical resources for #SleepTechnology. Available at: https://aasm.org/consumer-clinical-sleep-technology/. Accessed January 20, 2020.
79. Kauta SR, Keenan BT, Goldberg L, et al. Diagnosis and treatment of sleep disordered breathing in hospitalized cardiac patients: a reduction in 30-day hospital readmission rates. J Clin Sleep Med 2014;10(10):1051–9.
80. Choi JH, Lee B, Lee JY, et al. Validating the Watch-PAT for diagnosing obstructive sleep apnea in adolescents. J Clin Sleep Med 2018;14(10):1741–7.
81. Nigro CA, Borsini E, Dibur E, et al. Indication of CPAP without a sleep study in patients with high pretest probability of Obstructive Sleep Apnea. Sleep Breath 2019. https://doi.org/10.1007/s11325-019-01949-6.
82. Drummond F, Doelken P, Ahmed QA, et al. Empiric auto-titrating CPAP in people with suspected obstructive sleep apnea. J Clin Sleep Med 2010;6(2):140–5.
83. Parthasarathy S, Subramanian S, Quan SF. A multicenter prospective comparative effectiveness study of the effect of physician certification and center

accreditation on patient-centered outcomes in obstructive sleep apnea. J Clin Sleep Med 2014;10:243–9.

84. Pamidi S, Knutson KL, Ghods F, et al. The impact of sleep consultation prior to a diagnostic polysomnogram on continuous positive airway pressure adherence. Chest 2012;141:51–7.

85. Isetta V, Negrín MA, Monasterio C, et al. A Bayesian cost-effectiveness analysis of a telemedicine-based strategy for the management of sleep apnoea: a multi-centre randomised controlled trial. Thorax 2015;70(11):1054–61.

86. Wozniak DR, Lasserson TJ, Smith I. Educational, supportive and behavioural interventions to improve usage of continuous positive airway pressure machines in adults with obstructive sleep apnoea. Cochrane Database Syst Rev 2014;(1):CD007736.

87. Stretch R, Ryden A, Fung CH, et al. Predicting nondiagnostic home sleep apnea tests using machine learning. J Clin Sleep Med 2019;15(11):1599–608.

88. Cistulli PA, Armistead J, Pepin JL, et al. Short-term CPAP adherence in obstructive sleep apnea: a big data analysis using real world data. Sleep Med 2019;59:114–6.

89. Cistulli PA, Sutherland K. Phenotyping obstructive sleep apnoea- bringing precision oral appliance therapy. J Oral Rehabil 2019;46:1185–91.

90. Mostafa SS, Mendonça F, Ravelo-García AG, et al. A systematic review of detecting sleep apnea using deep learning. Sensors (Basel) 2019;19(22). https://doi.org/10.3390/s19224934.

91. Budhiraja R, Thomas R, Kim M, et al. The role of big data in the management of sleep-disordered breathing. Sleep Med Clin 2016;11:241–55.

92. Huang W, Lee P, Liu Y, et al. 0495 prediction of obstructive sleep apnea using machine learning technique. Sleep 2018;41(S1):A186.

93. Huang W-C, Lee P-L, Liu Y, et al. Support vector machine prediction of obstructive sleep apnea in a large-scale Chinese clinical sample. Sleep 2020;zsz295. https://doi.org/10.1093/sleep/zsz295.

94. Bates DW, Saria S, Ohno-Machado L, et al. Big data in health care: using analytics to identify and manage high-risk and high-cost patients. Health Aff 2014;33(7):1123–31.

95. Liu Y, Chen PC, Krause J, et al. How to read articles that use machine learning: users' guides to the medical literature. JAMA 2019;322(18):1806–16.

96. Sunwoo BY, Light M, Malhotra A. Strategies to augment adherence in the management of sleep-disordered breathing. Respirology 2020;25:363–71.

97. Mencar C, Gallo C, Mantero, et al. Application of machine learning to predict obstructive sleep apnea syndrome (OSAS) severity. Health Inform J 2019. https://doi.org/10.1177/1460458218824725.

98. Staley B, Keenan BT, Simonsen S, et al. Using an Electronic Health Record (EHR) to collect and use quality-of-life data for AASM process and outcomes quality measures. Sleep 2018;41(1):402.

99. Aurora RN, Casey KR, Kristo D, et al. Practice parameters for the surgical modifications of the upper airway for obstructive sleep apnea in adults. Sleep 2010;33(10):1408–13.

100. Morgenthaler TI, Kapen S, Lee-Chiong T, et al. Practice parameters for the medical therapy of obstructive sleep apnea. Sleep 2006;29(8):1031–5.

101. Sweetman A, Lack L, Catcheside PG, et al. Cognitive and behavioral therapy for insomnia increases the use of continuous positive airway pressure therapy in obstructive sleep apnea participants with comorbid insomnia: a randomized clinical trial. Sleep 2019;42(12) [pii:zsz178].

102. Orbea CP, Dupuy-McCaulry KL, Morgentahler T. Prevalence and sources of errors in positive airway pressure therapy provisioning. J Clin Sleep Med 2019; 15(5):697–704.
103. Mehrtash M, Bakker JP, Ayas N. Predictors of continuous positive airway pressure adherence in patients with obstructive sleep apnea. Lung 2019;197: 115–21.
104. Sawyer AM, Gooneratne NS, Marcus CL, et al. A systematic review of CPAP adherence across age groups: clinical and empiric insights for developing CPAP adherence interventions. Sleep Med Rev 2011;15:343–56.
105. Rowland S, Aiyappan V, Hennessy C, et al. Comparing the efficacy, mask leak, patient adherence, and patient preference of three different CPAP interfaces to treat moderate-severe obstructive sleep apnea. J Clin Sleep Med 2018;14(1): 101–8.
106. Shapiro GK, Shapiro CM. Sleep breath. Factors that influence CPAP adherence. Sleep Breath 2010;14(4):323–35.
107. Mastromatto N, Killough N, Keenan BT, et al. CPAP adherence varies with type of patient insurance. Sleep 2018;41(1):402–3.
108. Kuna ST, Shuttleworth D, Chi L, et al. Web-based access to positive airway pressure usage with or without an initial financial incentive improves treatment use in patients with obstructive sleep apnea. Sleep 2015;38(8):1229–36.
109. Malhotra A, Crocker ME, Willes L, et al. Patient engagement using new technology to improve adherence to positive airway pressure therapy: a retrospective analysis. Chest 2018;153:843–50.
110. Lynch S, Blasé A, Erikli L, et al. Retrospective descriptive study of CPAP adherence associated with use of the ResMed myAir application. In: ResMed. 2015. Available at: https://pdfs.semanticscholar.org/bc8e/2341489e89cf76eeae0e 76aaccb82a091c92.pdf. Accessed November 14, 2019.
111. Shaughnessy GF, Morgenthaler TI. The effect of patient-facing applications on positive airway pressure therapy adherence: a systematic review. J Clin Sleep Med 2019;15(5):769–77.
112. Isetta V, Leon C, Torres M, et al. Telemedicine-based approach for obstructive sleep apnea management: building evidence. Interact J Med Res 2014;3(1):e6.
113. Guralnick AS, Balachandran JS, Szutenbach S, et al. Educational video to improve CPAP use in patients with obstructive sleep apnoea at risk for poor adherence: a randomised controlled trial. Thorax 2017;72(12):1132–9.
114. Stepnowsky CJ, Palau JJ, Marler MR, et al. Pilot randomized trial of the effect of wireless telemonitoring on compliance and treatment efficacy in obstructive sleep apnea. J Med Internet Res 2007;9(2):e14. Available at: http://www.jmir. org/2007/2/e14/.
115. Sedkaoui K, et al. Efficiency of a phone coaching program on adherence to continuous positive airway pressure in sleep apnea hypopnea syndrome: a randomized trial. BMC Pulm Med 2015;15:102.
116. Nilius G, Schroeder M, Domanski U, et al. Telemedicine improves continuous positive airway pressure adherence in stroke patients with obstructive sleep apnea in a randomized trial. Respiration 2019;98:410–20.
117. Kotzian ST, Saletu MT, Schwarzinger A, et al. Proactive telemedicine monitoring of sleep apnea treatment improves adherence in people with stroke- a randomized controlled trial (HOPES study). Sleep Med 2019;64:48–55.
118. Tung P, Levitzky YS, Wang R, et al. Obstructive and central sleep apnea and the risk of incident atrial fibrillation in a community cohort of men and women. J Am Heart Assoc 2017;6:e004500.

119. Mendelson M, Vivodtzev I, Tamisier R, et al. CPAP treatment supported by telemedicine does not improve blood pressure in high cardiovascular risk OSA patients: a randomized, controlled trial. Sleep 2014;37:1863–70.

120. Persaud N, Bedard M, Boozary AS, et al. Effect on treatment adherence of distributing essential medicines at no charge: the CLEAN meds randomized clinical trial. JAMA Intern Med 2020;180(1):27–34.

121. Crotti N. ResMed and Philips Respironics use new tools to boost sleep apnea mask adherence. MedCity News; 2016. Available at: https://medcitynews.com/2016/10/resmed/. Accessed January 26, 2020.

122. Woehrle H, Arzt M, Graml A, et al. Effect of a patient engagement tool on positive airway pressure adherence: analysis of a German healthcare provider database. Sleep Med 2018;41:20–6.

123. Isetta V, Navajas D, Montserrat JM, et al. Comparative assessment of several automatic CPAP devices' responses: a bench test study. ERJ Open Res 2015; 1(1). 00031-2015.

124. Farré R, Navajas D, Montserrat JM. Technology for noninvasive mechanical ventilation: looking into the black box. ERJ Open Res 2016;2(1). 00004-2016.

125. Koivumaki V, Maasilta P, Bachour A. Oximetry monitoring recommended during PAP initiation for sleep apnea in patients with obesity or nocturnal hypoxemia. J Clin Sleep Med 2018;14(11):1859–63.

126. Stepnowsky C, Zamora T, Barker R, et al. Accuracy of positive airway pressure device-measured apneas and hypopneas: role in treatment followup. Sleep Disord 2013;2013:314589.

127. Rotty MC, Mallet JP, Suehs CM, et al. Is the 2013 American Thoracic Society CPAP-tracking system algorithm useful for managing non-adherence in long-term CPAP-treated patients? Respir Res 2019;20(1):209.

128. Tan M, Keenan B, Staley B, et al. Using an Electronic Health Record (EHR) to identify chronic CPAP users with abnormal HL7 CPAP data. Sleep 2018; 41(1):402.

129. Omobomi O, Quan SF. Positional therapy in the management of positional obstructive sleep apnea-a review of the current literature. Sleep Breath 2018; 22:297–304. Available at: https://doi-org.proxy.library.upenn.edu/10.1007/s11325-017-1561-y.

130. Ravesloot MJ, White D, Heinzer R, et al. Efficacy of the new generation of devices for positional therapy for patients with positional obstructive sleep apnea: a systematic review of the literature and meta-analysis. J Clin Sleep Med 2017; 13(6):813–24.

131. Bignold JJ, Mercer JD, Antic NA, et al. Accurate position monitoring and improved supine-dependent obstructive sleep apnea with a new position recording and supine avoidance device. J Clin Sleep Med 2011;7(4):376–83.

132. Philips sleep position therapy: NightBalance. Available at: https://www.usa.philips.com/c-e/hs/sleep-solutions/nightbalance.html. Accessed January 26, 2020.

133. Advanced Brain monitoring: NightShift. Available at: https://www.advancedbrainmonitoring.com/night-shift/. Accessed January 26, 2020.

134. Berry RB, Uhles ML, Abaluck BK, et al. NightBalance sleep position treatment device versus auto-adjusting positive airway pressure for treatment of positional obstructive sleep apnea. J Clin Sleep Med 2019;15(7):947–56.

135. Levendowski DJ, Seagraves S, Popovic D, et al. Assessment of a neck-based treatment and monitoring device for positional obstructive sleep apnea. J Clin Sleep Med 2014;10(8):863–71.

136. De Ruiter M, Benoist L, de Vries N, et al. Durability of treatment effects of sleep position trainer versus oral appliance therapy in positional OSA: 12-month follow-up of a randomized controlled trial. Sleep Breath 2018;22:441–50.
137. Benoist L, de Ruiter M, de Lange J, et al. A randomized, controlled trial of positional therapy versus oral appliance therapy for position-dependent sleep apnea. Sleep Med 2017;34:109–17.
138. Sutherland K, Cistulli P. Oral appliance therapy for obstructive sleep apnoea: state of the art. J Clin Med 2019;8:2121.
139. Gjerde K, Lehmann S, Naterstad IF, et al. Reliability of an adherence monitoring sensor embedded in an oral appliance used for treatment of obstructive sleep apnoea. J Oral Rehabil 2018;45(2):110–5.
140. Dieltjens M, Vanderveken OM. Oral appliances in obstructive sleep apnea. Healthcare (Basel) 2019;7(4) [pii:E141].
141. SomnoDent with compliance recorder. Available at: https://somnomed.com/en/physicians/compliance-recording/. Accessed January 26, 2020.
142. Sato K, Nakajima T. Review of systematic reviews on mandibular advancement oral appliance for obstructive sleep apnea: the importance of long-term follow-up. Jpn Dent Sci Rev 2020;56(1):32–7.
143. American Academy of Dental Sleep Medicine: oral appliance therapy. Available at: https://aadsm.org/oral_appliance_therapy.php. Accessed January 20, 2020.
144. Inspire sleep apnea innovation: table of contents. Available at: https://professionals.inspiresleep.com/bibliography/. Accessed January 20, 2020.
145. Thaler E, Schwab R, Maurer J, et al. Results of ADHERE upper airway stimulation and predictors of therapy efficacy. Laryngoscope 2019. https://doi.org/10.1002/lary.28286.
146. Dedhia RC, Woodson BT. Standardized reporting for hypoglossal nerve stimulation outcomes. J Clin Sleep Med 2018;14(11):1835–6.
147. Vandervekem OM, Beyers J, Op de Beek S, et al. Development of a clinical pathway and technical aspects of upper airway stimulation therapy for obstructive sleep apnea. Front Neurosci 2017;11:523.
148. Pietzsch JB, Richter AK, Randerath W, et al. Clinical and economic benefits of upper airway stimulation for obstructive sleep apnea in a european setting. Respiration 2019;98:38–47.
149. Woodson BT, Strohl KP, Soose RJ, et al. Upper airway stimulation for obstructive sleep apnea: 5-year outcome. Otolaryngol Head Neck Surg 2018;159(1): 194–202.
150. Husser D, Christoph Geller J, Taborsky M, et al. Remote monitoring and clinical outcomes: details on information flow and workflow in the IN-TIME study. Eur Heart J Qual Care Clin Outcomes 2019;5(2):136–44.
151. Parahuleva MS, Soydan N, Divchev D, et al. Home monitoring after ambulatory implanted primary cardiac implantable electronic devices: the home ambulance pilot study. Clin Cardiol 2017;40(11):1068–75.
152. Burri H, Senouf D. Remote monitoring and follow-up of pacemakers and implantable cardioverter defibrillators. Europace 2009;11(6):701–9 [published correction appears in Europace. 2009 Nov;11(11):1569].
153. Chinitz L. Leadless pacemaker for patients with atrioventricular block nets FDA approval. 2020. Available at: https://www.healio.com/cardiology/arrhythmia-disorders/news/online/%7Baf7e44bf-d1b2-4f10-8ffe-5fdad7e3927b%7D/leadless-pacemaker-for-patients-with-atrioventricular-block-nets-fda-approval. Accessed January 26, 2020.

154. American Academy of sleep medicine clinical resources for clinical guidelines and guidelines in development. Available at: https://aasm.org/clinical-resources/practice-standards/practice-guidelines/. Accessed January 26, 2020.

155. Fitzpatrick AL, Wischenka D, Appelhans BM, et al. An evidence-based guide for obesity treatment in primary care. Am J Med 2016;129:115.e1-7.

156. de Vries GE, Hoekema A, Claessen JQPJ, et al. Long-term objective adherence to mandibular advancement device therapy versus continuous positive airway pressure in patients with moderate obstructive sleep apnea. J Clin Sleep Med 2019;15(11):1655–63.

157. de Vries GE, Wijkstra PJ, Houwerzijl EJ, et al. Cardiovascular effects of oral appliance therapy in obstructive sleep apnea: a systematic review and meta-analysis. Sleep Med Rev 2018;40:55–68.

158. Cillo JE, Robertson N, Dattilo DJ. Maxillomandibular advancement for obstructive sleep apnea is associated with very long-term overall sleep-related quality-of-life improvement. J Oral Maxillofac Surg 2020;78:109–17.

159. Benca RM, Teodorescu M. Sleep physiology and disorders in aging and dementia. Handb Clin Neurol 2019;167:477–93.

160. Zolfaghari S, Yao C, Thompson C, et al. Effects of menopause on sleep quality and sleep disorders: Canadian Longitudinal Study on Aging. Menopause 2020; 27(3):295–304.

161. Cowan DC, Livingston E. Obstructive sleep apnoea syndrome and weight loss: review. Sleep Disord 2012;163296:11.

162. Friberg D, Carlsson-Nordlander B, Larsson H, et al. UPPP for habitual snoring: a 5-year follow-up with respiratory sleep recordings. Laryngoscope 1995;105(5 Pt 1):519–22.

163. Boot H, van Wegen R, Poublon RM, et al. Long-term results of uvulopalatopharyngoplasty for obstructive sleep apnea syndrome. Laryngoscope 2000;110(3 Pt 1):469–75.

164. Levin BC, Becker GD. Uvulopalatopharyngoplasty for snoring: long-term results. Laryngoscope 1994;104(9):1150–2.

165. Neagoe R, Muresan M, Timofte D, et al. Long-term outcomes of laparoscopic sleeve gastrectomy - a single-center prospective observational study. Wideochir Inne Tech Maloinwazyjne 2019;14(2):242–8.

166. Wang SH, Keenan BT, Wiemken A, et al. Effect of weight loss on upper airway anatomy and the apnea hypopnea index: the importance of tongue fat. Am J Respir Crit Care Med 2020. https://doi.org/10.1164/rccm.201903-0692OC.

167. Callahan ZM, Su B, Kuchta K, et al. Five-year results of endoscopic gastrojejunostomy revision (transoral outlet reduction) for weight gain after gastric bypass. Surg Endosc 2019. https://doi.org/10.1007/s00464-019-07003-6.

168. Farré R, Navajas D, Montserrat JM. Is telemedicine a key tool for improving continuous positive airway pressure adherence in patients with sleep apnea? Am J Respir Crit Care Med 2018;197:12–4.

169. CVS HealthHub: a new approach to healthcare. Available at: https://www.cvs.com/content/health-hub/sleep-apnea. Accessed June 17, 2020.

170. Walgreens: a new way to find care. Available at: https://www.walgreens.com/findcare/services. Accessed January 26, 2020.

171. Definitive healthcare: the top 3 most important pharmacy mergers and acquisitions of 2018. 2019. Available at: https://blog.definitivehc.com/top-3-pharmacy-acquisitions-2018. Accessed January 26, 2020.

172. Luo J, Wu M, Gopukumar D, et al. Big data application in biomedical research and health care: a literature review. Biomed Inform Insights 2016;8:1–10.
173. Price WN, Gerke S, Cohen IG. Potential liability for physicians using artificial intelligence. JAMA 2019;322(18):1765–6.
174. Hwang TJ, Kesselheim AS, Vokinger KN. Lifecycle regulation of artificial intelligence– and machine learning–based software devices in medicine. JAMA 2019;322(23):2285–6.
175. Shi H, Zhao H, Liu Y, et al. Systematic analysis of a military wearable device based on a multi-level fusion framework: research directions. Sensors 2019; 19(12):2651.
176. Kamišalić A, Fister I, Turkanović M, et al. Sensors and functionalities of non-invasive wrist-wearable devices: a review. Sensors 2018;18(6):1714.
177. Walch O, Huang Y, Forger D, et al. Sleep stage prediction with raw acceleration and photoplethysmography heart rate data derived from a consumer wearable device. Sleep 2019;20(20):1–19.
178. Auerbach AD. Evaluating digital health tools—prospective, experimental, and real world. JAMA Intern Med 2019;179(6):840–1.
179. Chen CE, Harrington RA, Desai SA, et al. Characteristics of digital health studies registered in ClinicalTrials.gov. JAMA Intern Med 2019;179(6):838–40.
180. Guk K, Han G, Lim J, et al. Evolution of wearable devices with real-time disease monitoring for personalized healthcare. Nanomaterials 2019;9(6):813.
181. Qureshi F, Krishnan S. Wearable hardware design for the internet of medical things (IoMT). Sensors 2018;18(11):3812.
182. Ko PR, Kientz JA, Choe EK, et al. Consumer sleep technologies: a review of the landscape. J Clin Sleep Med 2015;11(12):1455–61.
183. Khosla S, Deak MC, Gault D, et al. Consumer sleep technologies: how to balance the promises of new technology with evidence-based medicine and clinical guidelines. J Clin Sleep Med 2019;15(1):163–5.
184. Sharman JE, O'Brien E, Alpert B, et al. Lancet commission on hypertension group position statement on the global improvement of accuracy standards for devices that measure blood pressure. J Hypertens 2019. https://doi.org/10.1097/HJH.0000000000002246.
185. US Food and Drug Administration. Digital health software precertification (Pre-Cert) program. Available at: https://www.fda.gov/MedicalDevices/DigitalHealth/DigitalHealthPreCertProgram/default.htm. Accessed November 14, 2019.
186. Apple healthcare. 2020. Available at: https://www.apple.com/healthcare/. Accessed January 26, 2020.
187. Gramling, A. How Hospitals are using Apple HealthKit and ResearchKit. In 2020 Healthcare IT Leaders. 2015. Available at: https://www.healthcareitleaders.com/blog/how-hospitals-are-using-apples-healthkit-and-researchkit/. Accessed January 26, 2020.
188. Oschner Health System. Hypertension digital medicine program. Available at: https://www.ochsner.org/hypertension-digital-medicine. Accessed January 26, 2020.
189. Cohen IG, Mello MM. Big data, big tech, and protecting patient privacy. JAMA 2019;322(12):1141–2.
190. National Sleep Research Resources (funded by the National Heart, Lung, and Blood Institute). Available at: https://sleepdata.org/. Accessed January 26, 2020.

Telehealth Use to Promote Quality Outcomes and Reduce Costs in Stroke Care

Kelsey Halbert, MSN, RN, CNL, SCRN, CNRN[a],*,
Cynthia Bautista, PhD, APRN, FNCS[b]

KEYWORDS

• Telehealth • Telestroke • Telemedicine • Stroke • Outcomes • Cost

KEY POINTS

• Use of telestroke can increase access to acute stroke care in neurologically underserved areas to improve stroke care.
• Improving functional outcome in acute stroke patients is one important quality outcome that can occur with the use of telestroke.
• Telestroke practice can be cost-effective, improve continuity of care, shorten hospital stays, and avoid unnecessary stroke patient transfers.

INTRODUCTION

Stroke can cause severe disability and death in the adult population. When an ischemic stroke occurs, there is a need to administer intravenous thrombolytics within a defined treatment window in order to significantly improve patient clinical outcomes. Many stroke patients do not have access to the resources required to provide a timely diagnosis and treatment. Telestroke can provide these ischemic stroke patients the accurate diagnosis and appropriate treatment they require, thus promoting quality outcomes and reducing costs.

STROKE AND USE OF TELESTROKE

Stroke is the fifth most common cause of death and ranks first as the leading cause of disability in the United States.[1] For many years, the gold standard in the treatment of acute ischemic stroke has been thrombolytic therapy with intravenous alteplase.

This article originally appeared in *Critical Care Nursing Clinics*, Volume 31, Issue 2, June 2019.
Disclosure: The authors have nothing to disclose.
[a] Yale New Haven Hospital, New Haven, CT 06510, USA; [b] Egan School of Nursing and Health Studies–Fairfield University, Fairfield, CT 06824, USA
* Corresponding author.
E-mail address: rkelsey.halbert@ynhh.org

Clinics Collections 10 (2021) 227–233
https://doi.org/10.1016/j.ccol.2020.12.022

Functional outcomes have been shown to improve when thrombolytic therapy is administered within 3 hours of symptom onset.[2] Despite this, it is estimated that only 3.7% of eligible patients receive this therapy.[2] One contributing factor is that many of these stroke patients live in rural areas where acute stroke care is not readily available. Approximately 61 million Americans are considered underserved regarding access to specialty medical care.[3] In the United States there are roughly 4.0 neurologists per 100,000 people who provide care for more than 700,000 acute strokes annually.[4] As a growing number of neurologists opt out of call coverage for acute stroke and other neurologic emergencies, the gap between supply and demand widens and a greater number of patients become underserved. State and local regulations that require hospitals to provide emergency call coverage to be recognized as an acute stroke–capable or primary stroke center also contribute to the provider gap. As a result, many patients who present to community hospitals with stroke symptoms have to be transferred to a comprehensive stroke center. Transferring patients is expensive, labor-intense, and time consuming; delays created by such a transfer might preclude thrombolytic and/or endovascular therapies because the patient might arrive outside of the treatment window or irreversible brain damage might have already occurred.[5] The estimated total cost of stroke in the United States in 2009 exceeded $36 billion resulting from health care expenses and lost productivity.[6] Stroke does not affect the nation evenly; rural areas experience a 20% higher stroke-related death rate than urban areas.[6] Telestroke provides an effective solution for providing rural, community, or underresourced hospitals with on-demand access to acute stroke expertise.

Two models of telestroke exist: an off-site stroke specialist uses digital technology to communicate with on-site health care providers who are treating patients at a spoke facility that lacks stroke expertise, assisting with diagnosis and treatment including administration of intravenous alteplase; and a spoke hospital provider receives guidance from a stroke specialist at a hub hospital regarding diagnosis and treatment, but the patient can be transferred to the hub facility if a higher level of care is warranted.[5] In the first model, the teleneurologist is located anywhere in the country, whereas in the second model, the teleneurologist is at a primary or comprehensive stroke center nearest the spoke hospital.

QUALITY OUTCOMES OF TELESTROKE

The teleneurologist can visualize, assess, and converse with the patient as if they were in-person at the bedside, while at the same time review clinical and diagnostic results, developing an individualized treatment plan that takes into account the patient's health history, stroke risk factors, current presentation, and anticipated outcome.[7]

Telemedicine has been recommended by the American Stroke Association and the American Academy of Neurology as a strategy to increase access to acute stroke care and rapid acute stroke evaluation.[8] Spoke hospitals participating in a telestroke network have access to vascular fellowship trained neurologists for an immediate audiovisual consultation; this relationship with an academic hub site fosters ongoing education and formal processes for clinical improvement.[8] Quality outcomes of telestroke utilization (eg, **Box 1**) can occur when this real-time consultation provides timely assessment, accurate diagnosis, and possibly effective treatment.

Rapid recognition and an accurate diagnosis are critical elements of acute stroke care. Because many conditions can mimic the symptoms of acute stroke, the ability to rapidly and accurately differentiate between stroke and stroke mimic is challenging

Box 1
Quality outcomes of telestroke utilization
Timely assessment
Accurate diagnosis
Effective treatment
Improved functional outcomes
Reduced morbidity and mortality

for physicians without neurologic expertise. Delays in diagnosis and failure to diagnose acute stroke limit the use of proven therapies, such as intravenous alteplase. Telestroke provides neurology specialists at a comprehensive stroke center (hub) with the data necessary to assist the bedside physician at a community hospital (spoke) with stroke-related decision-making for patients who initially present to rural or underresourced facilities. Remote image transmission of a neurologic assessment is as valid as a face-to-face examination by a stroke neurologist and has been shown to shorten the time to complete a stroke patient's evaluation when compared with traditional methods of stroke diagnosis.[3]

Ischemic strokes account for approximately 87% of all acute strokes. Selected patients are good candidates for intravenous alteplase, a thrombolytic agent that can help restore blood flow and potentially reverse or prevent disability if administered within the guideline-recommended time window. The more quickly this agent is administered, the greater the chances for recovery with minimal or no neurologic deficits.[9] Studies have shown that clinical outcomes after alteplase therapy are time-dependent.[10] This urgency of treatment, when coupled with the shortage of onsite stroke expertise, contributes to difficulties for rural and underresourced hospitals to deliver alteplase in a timely manner. Telestroke promotes the safe and reliable administration of alteplase at these remote locations, resulting in a significant increase in the rates of alteplase utilization and shorter door-to-needle times before access to telestroke services.[4,8,11]

Telestroke utilization is linked to improved functional outcomes in the treatment of acute ischemic stroke. Patients who receive intravenous alteplase within 90 minutes of symptom onset are more than three times likely to experience favorable outcomes than patients who did not receive alteplase.[9] Additionally, patients treated with intravenous alteplase at a comprehensive stroke center showed no difference in functional outcomes at 90 days or in discharge outcome and treatment complications when compared with patients who received alteplase at community hospitals via telestroke.[5]

In addition to being among the leading causes of death, stroke also leads to physical and cognitive impairments that impact functional abilities and quality of life. Prompt identification, emergency response, and acute treatment and management of early stroke symptoms impact clinical outcomes. Telestroke has emerged as an important resource to ensure timely access to stroke neurology specialists fostering acute stroke diagnosis and treatment recommendations, recognition of stroke cause and risk, and provision of tools for health promotion strategies for stroke prevention.[7]

It is challenging to quantify quality of life, but the quality-adjusted life-year has been used as a measure to assess the value for cost of a health care intervention. A 2013 model to estimate the incremental costs and effectiveness of a telestroke network found that when compared with no network, a telestroke network yielded a discounted cost savings of $1000 to $1900 per patient and an incremental effectiveness of 0.01 to 0.03 quality-adjusted life-years per patient.[12] These results illustrate the health care resource utilization savings and cost-effective benefits from a societal perspective caused by improved clinical outcomes ameliorated by telestroke.

BARRIERS TO USE OF TELESTROKE

Despite the overall benefit of telestroke utilization, many barriers (eg, **Box 2**) exist that may limit stroke hospital participation in a telestroke network. Common challenges related to licensure and liability include infrastructure funding, regulatory changes to promote the development of acute stroke–capable or primary stroke centers, reimbursement for services, physician adoption and participation, licensure and credentialing issues, technology assessment and deployment, medical liability, compliance with privacy laws, and compliance with fraud and abuse statutes.[4] Under the telestroke model, the on-site treating physician and the remote consulting physician need to be licensed to practice medicine in the state where the patient is located, and both providers must be credentialed and privileged at the originating site. For a telestroke hub serving multiple spokes, consulting neurologists must be credentialed at all spoke hospitals in the network. This process is time-consuming and cumbersome, requiring significant administrative resources to ensure that all credentialing requirements are met. This process is more limiting when the spoke hospital is in a different state than the hub. Under the traditional state-based physician licensure system, each state requires that physicians practicing medicine in the state are licensed by that state. Telemedicine advocates are lobbying for relaxing the methods of telemedicine licensure by instituting reciprocity between states or developing a national licensure system.[6]

Widespread use of telemedicine is hindered by limitations in reimbursement; legal issues, such as state licensure laws; the need for multiple-site credentialing; and liability concerns. Insurance coverage for telehealth is fragmented: only 29 states (double the number for 3 years ago) have telehealth parity laws that require private insurers to cover telehealth services to the same extent that they cover in-person care.[7] There exist 48 state Medicaid programs, each with its own restrictions, that cover telehealth services. Medicare only reimburses telemedicine services to clinical facilities in areas where there is a shortage of health professionals.[13] Potential solutions to these limitations include the accelerated implementation of the Interstate Medical Licensure Compact and the Tele-Med Act of 2015, which enable Medicare-participating providers to provide services to any Medicare beneficiary; streamlining the credentialing process at spoke sites by allowing reliance on privileging decisions at hub sites; and providing informed consent to stroke patients regarding telemedicine.[4]

Box 2 Barriers to telestroke utilization
Reimbursement
Licensure and liability laws
Technological
Financial
Compliance

Telestroke reimbursement must also comply with two federal statutes, the Antikickback Statute and the Stark Law, which determine the allowable relationship between hospitals and the sharing of information technology. These statutes prohibit reimbursement for services in exchange for referrals that are payable under programs such as Medicare and Medicaid. This prohibits the hub hospital from providing services or equipment at less than fair market value in exchange for patient referrals to the hub.[4]

The technology necessary for telestroke services poses a challenge to spoke hospitals seeking to engage and sustain membership in a telestroke network. Inadequate training and needlessly complex and sophisticated equipment diminish the efficacy of telemedicine. Technical problems, such as nonconnection, poor broadband access, and malfunctioning devices, are major barriers to successful telestroke programs. The necessity of cloud-based imaging transfer can also cause technological difficulties leading to low levels of satisfaction by hub and spoke. This can delay care, especially in spoke facilities that lack immediate image interpretation by a radiologist. The lack of interoperability between computer systems and between electronic medical records may delay adoption of telestroke because of the rapid obsolescence of technology and potentially wasted capital.[4]

Financial barriers to telestroke utilization exist on the hub and spoke side. Spoke hospitals must invest in the purchase and maintenance of computer hardware and software; they need to maintain a secure way to transmit stroke-related data that is compliant with federal privacy standards. Hub hospitals must recruit and provide round-the-clock access to vascular neurologists while also providing training and support for spoke hospital clinical staff. The lack of adequate reimbursement to physicians and hospitals has played a crucial role in delaying the development of sufficient acute stroke call coverage, which may profoundly affect smaller, nonacademic hospitals.[4] A surprising financial barrier to telestroke is the reimbursement policy for "drip and ship," a term referring to cases in which thrombolytic therapy is initiated at the spoke hospital during a telestroke consultation, and then the patient is transferred to a comprehensive stroke center, typically the hub hospital, for the remainder of treatment. In this drip-and-ship scenario, Medicare does not permit either the spoke or hub hospital to obtain enhanced payment, even if alteplase is still infusing on arrival to the hub hospital; rather, the spoke hospital is only paid on an outpatient basis for the medication, and the receiving hospital is only paid the traditional inpatient payment rate for stroke care of patients not receiving thrombolytic therapy.[5] A final financial barrier is the lack of resources a spoke hospital may experience providing postacute stroke care for patients not transferred to the hub hospital, with or without thrombolytic therapy.[11]

REDUCING COSTS WITH TELESTROKE

Research suggests that telestroke utilization can be cost-effective, can improve continuity of care, can shorten hospital stays, avoid unnecessary transfers, enhance education, and improve research trial enrollment.[4] Although telestroke has an upfront implementation cost, its utilization can lead to reduced health care costs, direct and indirect, by reducing acute care lengths of stay and long-term care needs.[5] It is clear that when considering the overall lifetime costs of managing patients impacted by stroke, reducing or eliminating complications and disability results in health care resource savings.[8] It has been estimated that the use of remote patient monitoring for certain patients with chronic conditions could yield $1.8 billion in savings over 10 years.[10]

Telestroke also contributes to cost reduction by reducing complications and disabilities by initiating timely cost-effective interventions at the point of care, such as intravenous alteplase, or by identifying and facilitating patient transfer to higher levels of care for specific interventions, such as neurointensive care, decompressive hemicraniectomy for life-threatening cerebral infarction with swelling, and emergent surgical or endovascular repair of ruptured aneurysms and mechanical thrombectomy.[4]

The overall lifetime costs of managing stroke is estimated to be $62.7 billion annually in the United States, with a 15% to 30% rate of permanent disability and 20% of stroke victims requiring institutional care 3 months post-stroke.[4] The national increase in intravenous alteplase administration rates because of telestroke has been estimated to avoid direct costs of $13.6 million, reduce acute care days by 4351, reduce residential care days by 43,902, and save $5.2 million in indirect costs annually.[5] Telestroke can provide better access to post-stroke care. Newer applications of telestroke include virtual rehabilitation therapies, offering patients the opportunity to participate in physical and occupational therapist-supervised therapies closer to their homes and support systems, eliminating long transfers and reducing family travel costs.[5]

NURSES ROLE IN TELESTROKE

The stroke delivery model at the spoke hospital is greatly impacted by telestroke utilization. Nurses at the spoke level become coordinators of acute stroke care. Several elements of nursing care include triage in the emergency department, care of the patient including vital signs, intravenous access, blood work, timely computed tomography scan arrival, blood pressure evaluation and management, neurologic assessment using the National Institutes of Health Stroke Scale, documentation of a stroke code, and administration of intravenous alteplase.[14] Depending on the spoke hospital policy, nurses may be responsible for calculating the alteplase dose; mixing the medication; administering a bolus; starting the infusion; and monitoring the patient receiving alteplase for complications, such as angioedema and hemorrhagic transformation.[14] Improving the scope, quality, and speed of stroke treatment requires nurse leaders to create a structure for a spoke hospital's stroke care delivery model.

SUMMARY

Stroke is a leading cause of disability and death in the United States in the adult population. Telestroke can provide increasing access to expert stroke care and treatment that promote quality outcomes and reduce costs in stroke care. It provides an effective solution for providing underresourced hospitals access to acute stroke expertise. With access to stroke experts, stroke disability and death could decrease.

Many quality outcomes are achieved with the use of telestroke. It can increase the access to acute stroke care, thereby providing timely assessment, accurate diagnosis, and effective treatment. Telestroke has been linked to improve functional outcomes in the treatment of acute ischemic strokes.

There are currently several barriers to providing a telestroke service. Common challenges include: licensure and liability, reimbursement, technology, and financial issues. It is important to recognize these barriers and begin to implement strategies to overcome these barriers.

Telestroke engages nurses at the spoke hospital to become coordinators of acute stroke care, which identifies the need and avenues for educational and professional development.

Telestroke utilization can be cost-effective. It can reduce complications and disabilities by initiating timely interventions. The future of telestroke is beginning to provide improved access to post-stroke care.

REFERENCES

1. Centers for Disease Control and Prevention. Stroke. 2018. Available at: https://www.cdc.gov/stroke/index.htm. Accessed December 19, 2018.
2. LaMonte M, Bahouth M, Xiao Y, et al. Outcomes from a comprehensive stroke telemedicine program. Telemed J E Health 2008;4:339–44.
3. Burch S, Gray D, Sharp J. The power and potential of telehealth what health systems should know: proposed legislation in Congress offers the promise that the nation's healthcare policy will support the expansion of telehealth, allowing hospitals and health systems to fully realize the benefits of this important emerging approach to care. Healthc Financ Manage 2017;2:46–50.
4. Dorsey E, Topol E. State of telehealth. N Engl J Med 2016;2:154–61.
5. Kulcsar M, Gilchrist S, George M. Improving stroke outcomes in rural areas through telestroke programs: an examination of barriers, facilitators, and state policies. Telemed J E Health 2014;1:3–10.
6. Bowen P. Early identification, rapid response, and effective treatment of acute stroke: utilizing teleneurology to ensure optimal clinical outcomes. Medsurg Nurs 2016;4:241.
7. Adler-Milstein J, Kvedar J, Bates D. Telehealth among US hospitals: several factors, including state reimbursement and licensure policies, influence adoption. Health Aff 2014;2:207–15.
8. Demaerschalk B, Berg J, Chong B, et al. American Telemedicine Association: telestroke guidelines. Telemed J E Health 2017;5:376–89.
9. Almallouhi E, Holmstedt CA, Harvey J, et al. Long-term functional outcome of telestroke patients treated under drip-and-stay paradigm compared with patients treated in a comprehensive stroke center: a single center experience. Telemed J E Health 2018. https://doi.org/10.1089/tmj.2018.0137.
10. Al Kasab S, Harvey J, Debenham E, et al. Door to needle time over telestroke: a comprehensive stroke center experience. Telemed J E Health 2018;2:111–5.
11. Baratloo A, Rahimpour L, Abushouk A, et al. Effects of telestroke on thrombolysis times and outcomes: a meta-analysis. Prehosp Emerg Care 2018;22(4):472–84.
12. Demaerschalk B, Switzer J, Xie J, et al. Cost utility of hub-and-spoke telestroke networks from societal perspective. Am J Manag Care 2013;12:976–85.
13. Amorim E, Shih M, Koehler S, et al. Impact of telemedicine implementation in thrombolytic use for acute ischemic stroke: the University of Pittsburgh Medical Center telestroke network experience. J Stroke Cerebrovasc Dis 2013;4:527–31.
14. Rafter R, Kelly T. Nursing implementation of a telestroke programme in a community hospital in the US. J Nurs Manag 2011;19:193–200.

Telemedicine in Rehabilitation

Marinella DeFre Galea, MD

KEYWORDS

• Telerehabilitation • Telehealth • Telemedicine

KEY POINTS

• Telemedicine offers the opportunity to deliver rehabilitative services in the patients' home, closing geographic, physical, and motivational gaps.
• The exponential growth of telerehabilitation has yielded the proliferation of studies with varying methodologies.
• Several methods of telerehabilitation delivery alone and in conjunction with traditional rehabilitation methodology have been explored based on available technology, patient literacy and level of function, and caregiver availability.

INTRODUCTION

In the past decade, the use of technology for remote assessment and intervention in rehabilitation has grown exponentially, paving the way for the development of telerehabilitation. The services provided under this term are wide in scope and can include evaluation, assessment, monitoring, prevention, intervention, supervision, education, consultation, and coaching. There is no formal structure for the delivery of telehealth, and the exchange of data may occur in numerous forms. Telephone, messaging and e-mail, or multimodal systems, such as videoconferencing, virtual therapists, and interactive Web-based platforms are some examples. In the field of rehabilitation, the patient-centered team approach has guided the identification of ad hoc solutions to overcome geographic, temporal, social, and financial barriers.[1]

Telerehabilitation has been shown to strengthen the patient-provider connection by (1) enhancing the knowledge of the patients and their contextual factors, (2) providing information exchange and facilitating education, and (3) establishing shared goal setting and action planning.[2] In the inpatient setting, telerehabilitation has been used to shorten hospital stay, facilitate discharge home, and provide patient and caregiver education and support.[3–5] In the outpatient setting, telemedicine supplements or

This article originally appeared in *Physical Medicine and Rehabilitation Clinics*, Volume 30, Issue 2, May 2019.
The author has nothing to disclose.
Department of Spinal Cord Injury and Disorder, Amyotrophic Lateral Sclerosis Program, Multiple Sclerosis Regional Center, The James J Peters VAMC, SCI/D Unit, 130 West Kingsbridge Road, Bronx, NY 10468, USA
E-mail address: Marinella.galea@va.gov

substitutes face-to-face encounters in acute and chronic neurologic, cardiac, and musculoskeletal conditions commonly treated by physiatrists.

As the application of telehealth proliferates, a central concern is how to protect data to preserve patient privacy. The Office of the National Coordination for Health Information Technology reported that health information is at a high risk for breaches, with more than 113 million individuals affected in 2015.[6] Although health care providers routinely receive mandatory training about how to safeguard the privacy and security of health care information during face-to-face encounters, the same is not true for virtual visits. In fact, very few studies have reported on the privacy and security of health care information in the context of telehealth. A systematic review by Peterson and colleague[7] shows that health care providers do not have a clear idea of how to protect health information when using telehealth. The investigators conclude that existing best practices are inconsistent across telehealth services and tools to assist health care providers are needed. To address this gap, the American Telemedicine Association (ATA) has recently developed a document to inform and assist practitioners in providing effective and secure telerehabilitation services, laying the foundation for developing discipline-specific standards, guidelines, and practice requirements.[8]

The development of a user-friendly, cost-effective, integrated telerehabilitation system aligned with existing policies will necessitate a business model that ensures effective, sustainable, and value-based services.[9] A forecast by Goldman Sachs estimates the comprehensive value of the US telerehabilitation market at $32.4 billion, of which 45% derives from remote patient monitoring; 37% from telehealth; and 18% from behavioral modifications.[10] Data from the QYR Pharma & Healthcare Research Center confirm the growth trend of the telerehabilitation market in the United States.[11] Cost-effectiveness has been shown in the application of tele-stroke,[12] cardiac rehabilitation,[13,14] traumatic brain injury,[15] and hip replacement rehabilitation.[4] Although insurance coverage for telerehabilitation services varies, the cost of technology is decreasing, making telerehabilitation modalities more affordable.[9] The 2017 ATA State Telemedicine Gap analysis[16] shows that, of the 37 states analyzed, 13 states do not cover telerehabilitation services for their Medicaid recipients. Although state policies vary in scope and application, 24 states reimburse for telerehabilitative services in their Medicaid plans. Only 12 states reimburse for telerehabilitative services within home health benefits.

This article presents recent applications of this burgeoning field of telerehabilitation by various medical subspecialties. These case studies demonstrate the evidence base for telerehabilitation, highlight potential areas of improvement, and propose potential future directions and applications.

CONTENT
Neurologic Telerehabilitation

The use of telemedicine in acute stroke has validated the proof-of-concept that specialized services can be delivered virtually when they cannot be easily provided face-to-face.[17] Several teleneurology applications have been proposed to manage patients with chronic neurologic diseases where impaired mobility hinders access.[18]

Stroke
Research has shown that more time spent on exercise therapy in the first weeks to months after stroke leads to better functioning.[19] Under the present health care system, transitional care programs are insufficient to address the barriers preventing community stroke survivors from achieving their highest potential, leading to hospital readmission, poorer outcome, and permanent disability.[20] Several randomized

controlled trials have used alternative solutions to provide and/or supplement care in the patient's home after discharge.

Caregiver-delivered rehabilitation services have been evaluated to augment intensity of practice. A Cochrane review[21] showed that caregiver-mediated exercises (CME) administered alone or in combination with standard therapy have no significant effect on basic activities of daily living. However, CME significantly improved patients' standing balance and quality of life with no significant effects on caregiver strain. A more recent review showed that telerehabilitation interventions were associated with significant improvements in recovery from motor deficits, higher cortical dysfunction, and depression in the intervention groups in all studies assessed. Modalities used included tele-supervision, virtual reality, game-based virtual reality, and interactive mobile phone applications.[12]

Ongoing studies promise to provide more definitive evidence on CME and to assess the utility of televisits by the interdisciplinary team using more rigorous methodology.[22,23]

Approximately one-third of all people with stroke suffer from depressive symptoms,[24] using more health care services and increasing costs. In addition, the presence of depression is associated with poor functional outcomes after stroke.[24] Telerehabilitation has been successfully applied to address motor and nonmotor domains measured by the Stroke Impact Scale in a study comparing the effects of home-based robot-assisted rehabilitation coupled with a home exercise program versus home-based exercise alone.[25] The investigators were not able to determine why the quality-of-life and depression outcomes improved. They hypothesized that the positive trend could be attributed to the intervention per se, the resulting modest motor improvement, or the weekly interaction between the participants and the therapists.

Spinal cord injury

Individuals with spinal cord injury (SCI) experience substantial physical, psychological, and social challenges, requiring frequent, specialized, and interdisciplinary care. Several telerehabilitation modalities have been proposed to deliver specialized care and provide education and training. As described in a recent literature review,[26] to date there are a limited number of randomized controlled studies with different patient selection, outcomes, and modalities. The investigators conclude that there is not enough evidence about optimal methods of utilization, policy, and efficacy of telerehabilitation in SCI. Of note is that the reviewed studies showed high patient satisfaction and engagement.

Within the SCI system of care, the Veterans Health Administration (VHA) has developed a robust telehealth structure to address the postacute and chronic consequences of SCI. The Disease Management Protocol consist of semicustomized questions delivered to the patients' home via data messaging devices to evaluate changes in comorbidity severity and health-related quality of life.[27] The system has been shown to be most beneficial to newly injured patients recently discharged from acute rehabilitation that live far from specialty SCI care facilities. In recent years, the VHA has supported the use of Clinical Video Telehealth, a real-time videoconferencing system, to provide health care services. Qualitative analysis has shown that the system is complex and requires coordination and communication among stakeholders.[27,28] Video connect is a new secure provider to patient solution that is used to supplement face-to-face visits; data regarding its efficacy in delivering care and comparability with face-to-face encounters are not yet available. Notably, the VHA has invested in extensive health care provider education and training, constructed a safe and secure telemedicine structure, and marketed to its consumers.

Limited tele-exercise studies have been successfully executed in small cohorts of individuals with SCI.

One pilot study[29] used a platform consisting of a home monitoring system to record physiologic parameters, a hand ergometer to perform a customized home exercise program (HEP), and a tablet to conduct video training. The therapy sessions were led by a telecoach. Results showed 100% adherence to the HEP, that all participants experienced a modest improvement in aerobic capacity (24%), and physical activity and increased satisfaction with life scores. Subjects valued the motivation and disability-related expertise provided by the telecoach, consistent with the theory of Supportive Accountability,[30] which accounts for the complex interaction of a health care professional and consumer when communicating through electronic health technology.

Van Straaten and colleagues[31] studied the effectiveness of a HEP on pain and function. Results showed that after a 12-week intervention consisting of a high-dose scapular stabilizer and rotator cuff strengthening program using telerehabilitation for supervision, shoulder pain was reduced even in individuals with longstanding symptoms. The study was limited by sample size, lack of a control group, and low to moderate levels of pain at baseline.

Video visits have been used in SCI to provide nonurgent specialized consultation in lieu of, or in addition to, face-to-face visits. A recent pilot study[32] using iPads in the SCI population confirmed previous findings[33,34] that videoconferencing is a clinically viable and effective tool. The type of interactions between clinicians and participants varied from generalized hospital follow-up and SCI–primary care to specific questions on medications and coordination with subspecialty clinics. This modality has been well-accepted by patients and caregivers and has reduced rate of hospitalization and overall length of stay.

Multiple sclerosis

Individuals with multiple sclerosis (MS) are at risk for developing long-term disability. Rehabilitation provides treatments and therapies to lessen the impact of disability and improve function; however, access to those services is complicated by limited mobility, fatigue, and related issues. It has been shown that individuals with MS are willing to receive rehabilitative services through telemedicine. However, patients with moderate-to-severe disability may experience technical difficulties due to cognitive and physical impairment.[35]

Charvet and colleagues[36] have used an adaptive online cognitive improvement program to train individuals with MS at home. The patients were randomly assigned to either a conventional adaptive cognitive remediation program or an active control of ordinary computer games. This telerehabilitation modality provided modest improvement in cognitive performance as measured by changes in a composite of neuropsychological tests.

Khan and colleagues[37] conducted a systematic review of the use of telerehabilitation to provide or supplement therapy to individuals with MS. The studies evaluated included multiple delivery modalities, some complex, with more than one rehabilitation component and included physical activity, educational, behavioral, and symptom management programs. With such heterogeneous methodology, it was concluded that there is limited evidence on the efficacy of telerehabilitation in improving functional activities, fatigue, and quality of life in adults with MS. The review also found that evidence supporting telerehabilitation in the longer term for improved function, impairment, quality of life, and psychological outcomes is poor. A very recent randomized trial[38] provides higher-quality evidence that telerehabilitation is technically feasible, desirable, and effective in improving gait and other outcomes in patients with MS.

An ongoing study is evaluating the delivery of complementary and alternative medicine sessions at home to rural and low-income individuals with MS versus the same intervention delivered in the clinic by a therapist.[39]

Traumatic brain injury

It has been shown that many people with traumatic brain injury (TBI) are interested in accessing telerehabilitative services to assist with problems in memory, attention, problem-solving, and activities of daily living.[40] In addition, as their caregivers assume increased responsibility for providing support, they receive limited access to services leading to increased risk of anxiety and depression.[41]

Rietdijk and colleagues[42] conducted a systematic review searching for interventions delivered at distance with the use of technology, involving caregivers of adults and children with TBI. They concluded that telehealth can be used to increase access to services for families in rural areas, to train family members in the skills required to facilitate recovery after TBI, to provide appropriate and timely intervention for problems arising at home, or to create a forum for peer support. Significant outcomes included improved cognitive functioning of the person with TBI as well as psychological well-being, support skills, and burden of caregivers. Several studies demonstrated that participants reported training to be beneficial over the long-term after program completion, and that improvements in outcomes were maintained over time.

A more recent systematic review by Ownsworth and colleagues[15] aimed to determine whether telerehabilitation interventions are effective for improving outcomes relative to usual care, alternative interventions, and baseline functioning. Of the modalities described, telephone interventions focused on managing self-identified concerns through tailored interventions, providing education and strategies for enhancing cognitive skills and physical exercise, and encouraging compliance with prescribed therapy, were most used. Of interest, Web-based platforms were rarely used compared with other neurologic conditions, possibly because of TBI-related impairments and dependence on caregiver assistance. Telephone-based interventions were found to improve global functioning, posttraumatic symptoms, sleep quality, and depressive symptoms for individuals with mild and moderate-to-severe TBI relative to usual care; however, the durability of these effects was either not demonstrated or not examined by these studies.

Cardiac Telerehabilitation

Coronary artery disease

Cardiac rehabilitation has beneficial effects on morbidity and mortality in patients with coronary artery disease (CAD); however, it is underused and short-term improvements are often not sustained. Several randomized controlled trials[13,14] have shown that telerehabilitation provided positive results when compared with conventional hospital rehabilitation. Of interest, these studies use a combination of communication technologies (Internet, video-consultation), on-demand coaching to encourage compliance, and individually tailored coaching on both training intensity and physical activity.[43] Frederix and colleagues[14] have shown that a prolonged (1 year), Internet-based comprehensive telerehabilitation program in addition to conventional cardiac rehabilitation is cost-effective, and can reduce cardiovascular rehospitalization.

Congestive heart failure

In a recent study by Hwang and colleagues,[44] patients with stable congestive heart failure were randomized to 12 weeks of real-time exercise and education intervention using online videoconferencing software versus a traditional hospital-outpatient program. The group-based video telerehabilitation program was noninferior to an outpatient rehabilitation program and promoted greater attendance yielding few adverse effects. These findings confirm previous reports[45,46] that telerehabilitation is a safe care delivery modality. Similarly, Nouryan and colleagues[47] conducted a randomized controlled trial, studying Medicare outpatients with heart failure after discharge from home care for 6 months. Patients were randomized to home telehealth or comprehensive outpatient management. The telehealth intervention consisted of weekly televisits and daily vital signs monitoring. The results showed that the telehealth intervention group improved all causes of emergency department utilization, length of stay, and quality of life. A trend toward cost savings was reported in the telehealth intervention group; however, it did not reach statistical significance.

Musculoskeletal

Orthopedic care provides a fertile ground for the utilization of telerehabilitation in an aging population prone to osteoarthritis. In fact, procedures involving the musculoskeletal system are among the most common in the United States.[48] These interventions are paired with a rehabilitation program aimed at maximizing functional outcome.

A recent systematic review[49] identified several studies in which postsurgical telerehabilitation programs were implemented after total knee arthroplasty,[50] total hip arthroplasty,[4] and upper limb and hand surgeries.[51] Methods of administration included real-time videoconferencing, asynchronous programs, telephone follow-up, and interactive virtual systems. The investigators found strong evidence in favor of telerehabilitation in patients following total knee and hip arthroplasty and limited evidence in the upper limb interventions. Another review by Cottrell and colleagues[52] analyzed evidence exclusively for the use of real-time telerehabilitation for the treatment of musculoskeletal conditions. The investigators concluded that there was strong evidence that the management of musculoskeletal conditions via real-time telerehabilitation is effective in improving physical function, disability, and pain. At least one study has been proposed to study the delivery of a pre-habilitation program in surgical candidates awaiting total hip or knee arthroplasty, to address the reported long wait times before surgery.[53] Results are pending.

Occupational therapists often assess a patient's home for safety before discharge as part of their role in acute care and rehabilitation teams.[54] When the evaluation cannot be completed in a timely manner, delays in discharge and increased length of stay ensue, or the patient is discharged without the assessment, potentially leading to an increased risk of early readmission. The World Federation of Occupational Therapists has published a position statement on the use of telehealth to improve accessibility to occupational therapy. Telehealth has been suggested as an effective and reliable way to access home modification services.[55] Nix and Comans[5] described an initiative to improve the timeliness of occupational therapy home visits for discharge planning by implementing technology solutions while maintaining patient safety. The project demonstrated that on-site home visits can be safely and efficiently performed or augmented using technology. The study also highlighted the positive impact of the project on the occupational therapy department productivity.

Chronic Pain

Chronic pain is a major public health problem, which is expected to increase as the population ages. Physical training has been proven to decrease pain and improve function[56] and therefore plays an important role in current pain rehabilitation programs. Improvements in chronic low back pain seen in physical therapy do not appear to be retained over the long term, providing an opportunity for telerehabilitation services to provide continuity and ensure sustainability.[57]

Patients with chronic pain were favorable to an "intermediate" telerehabilitation program offering feedback and monitoring technology with some face-to-face consulting and exercise location.[58] However, Adamse and colleagues[59] conducted a systematic review of exercise-based telemedicine in patients with chronic pain and found no difference compared with usual care on physical activity, activities of daily living, and quality of life.

Telerehabilitation interventions have proven to be beneficial to retain improvement in low back pain and increase attrition, respectively, via booster sessions delivered through a mobile phone application[57] and videoconferencing.[60]

For patients with chronic knee pain, an Internet-delivered, physiotherapist-prescribed home exercise and pain-coping skills training provided clinically meaningful and sustained improvements in pain and function.[61]

Virtual complementary and integrative health modalities, such as yoga and tai chi sessions, to treat chronic pain are being investigated.

Rheumatology

A recent systematic review[62] shows that telemedicine has been applied to the field of rheumatology in the form of remote consultations, monitoring of treatment strategies, and Web-based self-management programs. Some of the chronic conditions treated include rheumatoid arthritis, systemic sclerosis, fibromyalgia, osteoarthritis, and juvenile idiopathic arthritis. Types of intervention have included remote disease activity assessment, tele-monitoring of treatment strategies, and information communication technology–delivered self-management programs.

In the application of tele-consultation, it was concluded that this modality resulted in high patient satisfaction rates, albeit lacking in diagnostic accuracy. Internet-delivered programs revealed high feasibility and satisfaction rates, although effectiveness data lacked homogeneity. Remote monitoring programs were also well received by patients. Cost-effectiveness needs to be evaluated, as readmission rates were higher in patients on tight control and treat-to-target approaches. Self-directed kinesiotherapy sessions were effective in improving hand function after drug-induced remission.

In a recent study by Pani and colleagues,[63] the patients reported increased motivation and greater engagement of the medical staff in their therapy when using an ad hoc telerehabilitation platform. Although the investigators did not perform a formal cost analysis, they concluded that the proposed solution appeared to be cost-effective compared with face-to-face therapy sessions.

SUMMARY

Studies have provided evidence that telerehabilitation is well received by patients whether applied alone or to supplement conventional therapy; it does not add burden to the caregiver; it is advantageous for patients recovering from motor deficits, higher cortical dysfunction, and depression after stroke; and to recover after hip and knee arthroplasty.

Lack of methodological rigor and variability of approaches used in telerehabilitation studies to date hinder the ability to conclude that telehealth services can and should be deployed more broadly in the delivery of rehabilitation.

Larger, well-powered, longer-term studies are needed to provide definitive evidence and establish the indications and limitations of telerehabilitation utilization in the treatment of acute and chronic conditions.

There is a need for best practices that are consistent across all types of telehealth services for all health care providers. In this rapidly evolving field, existing research may not reflect the most recent developments in practice or technology and best practice may be moving ahead of the research reported in publications.

Strong, evidence-based telerehabilitation methodologies together with best practices will provide the matrix to create effective services that can be both delivered by health care structures and reimbursed by health insurance providers.

REFERENCES

1. Hailey D, Roine R, Ohinmaa A, et al. Evidence of benefit from telerehabilitation in routine care: a systematic review. J Telemed Telecare 2011;17(6):281–7.
2. Wang S, Blazer D, Hoenig H. Can eHealth technology enhance the patient-provider relationship in rehabilitation? Arch Phys Med Rehabil 2016;97(9):1403–6.
3. Tsavourelou A, Stylianides N, Papadopoulos A, et al. Telerehabilitation solution conceptual paper for community-based exercise rehabilitation of patients discharged after critical illness. Int J Telerehabil 2016;8(2):61–70.
4. Nelson M, Bourke M, Crossley K, et al. Telerehabilitation versus traditional care following total hip replacement: a randomized controlled trial protocol. JMIR Res Protoc 2017;6(3):e34.
5. Nix J, Comans T. Home quick–occupational therapy home visits using mHealth, to facilitate discharge from acute admission back to the community. Int J Telerehabil 2017;9(1):47–54.
6. Office of the National Coordinator for Health Information Technology. Breaches of unsecured protected health information. Health IT Quick-Stat #53. 2016. Available at: https://dashboard.healthit.gov/quickstats/pages/breaches-protected-health-informatio.
7. Peterson C, Watzlaf V. Telerehabilitation store and forward applications: a review of applications and privacy considerations in physical and occupational therapy practice. Int J Telerehabil 2015;6(2):75–84.
8. Richmond T, Peterson C, Cason J, et al. American Telemedicine Association's principles for delivering telerehabilitation services. Int J Telerehabil 2017;9(2):63–8.
9. Marzano G, Ochoa-Siguencia L, Pellegrino A. Towards a new wave of telerehabilitation applications. The Open Public Health Journal 2017;1(1):1–9.
10. The digital revolution comes to US Healthcare. 2015. Available at: www.Wur.Nl/Upload_mm/0/f/3/8fe8684c-2a84-4965-9dce-550584aae48c_Internet%20of%20Things%205%20-%20Digital%20Revolution%20Comes%20to%20US%20Healtcare.Pdf.
11. QYR Pharma & Healthcare Research Center. Global and United States telerehabilitation systems market size, status and forecast 2022. 2017.
12. Sarfo FS, Ulasavets U, Opare-Sem OK, et al. Tele-rehabilitation after stroke: an updated systematic review of the literature. J Stroke Cerebrovasc Dis 2018;27(9):2306–18.
13. Frederix I, Solmi F, Piepoli MF, et al. Cardiac telerehabilitation: a novel cost-efficient care delivery strategy that can induce long-term health benefits. Eur J Prev Cardiol 2017;24(16):1708–17.
14. Frederix I, Vandijck D, Hens N, et al. Economic and social impact of increased cardiac rehabilitation uptake and cardiac telerehabilitation in Belgium—a cost-benefit analysis. Acta Cardiolo 2017;73(3):222–9.

15. Ownsworth T, Arnautovska U, Beadle E, et al. Efficacy of telerehabilitation for adults with traumatic brain injury: a systematic review. J Head Trauma Rehabil 2017;33(4):E33–46.
16. Capistrant G, Thomas L. State telemedicine gaps analysis: coverage and reimbursement. American Telehealth Association 2017. Available at: https://utn.org/resources/downloads/50-state-telemedicine-gaps-analysis-physician-practice-standards-licensure.pdf.
17. Schwamm LH, Pancioli A, Acker JE, et al. American Stroke Association's Task force on the development of stroke systems. Recommendations for the establishment of stroke systems of care: recommendations from the American Stroke Association's task force on the development of stroke systems. Circulation 2005; 111(8):1078–91.
18. Wechsler LR, Tsao JW, Levine SR, et al, American Academy of Neurology Telemedicine Work Group. Teleneurology applications: report of the telemedicine work group of the American Academy of Neurology. Neurology 2013;80(7):670–6.
19. English C, Veerbeek J. Is more physiotherapy better after stroke? Int J Stroke 2015;10(4):465–6.
20. Lichtman JH, Leifheit-Limson EC, Jones SB, et al. Preventable readmissions within 30 days of ischemic stroke among Medicare beneficiaries. Stroke 2013; 44(12):3429–35.
21. Vloothuis JDM, Mulder M, Veerbeek JM, et al. Caregiver-mediated exercises for improving outcomes after stroke. Cochrane Database Syst Rev 2016;(12):CD011058.
22. Vloothius J, Mulder M, Nijland RH. Caregiver-mediated exercises with e-health support for early supported discharge after stroke (CARE4STROKE): study protocol for a randomized controlled trial. BMC Neurol 2017;15:193.
23. Jhaveri MM, Benjamin-Garner R, Rianon N, et al. Telemedicine-guided education on secondary stroke and fall prevention following inpatient rehabilitation for Texas patients with stroke and their caregivers: a feasibility pilot study. BMJ Open 2017; 7(9):e017340.
24. Wulsin L, Alwell K, Moomaw CJ, et al. Comparison of two depression measures for predicting stroke outcomes. J Psychosom Res 2012;72(3):175–9.
25. Linder SM, Rosenfeldt AB, Bay RC, et al. Improving quality of life and depression after stroke through telerehabilitation. Am J Occup Ther 2015;69(2). 6902290020p1-10.
26. Irgens I, Rekand T, Arora M, et al. Telehealth for people with spinal cord injury: a narrative review. Spinal Cord 2018;56(7):643–55.
27. Woo C, Seton JM, Washington M, et al. Increasing specialty care access through use of an innovative home telehealth-based spinal cord injury disease management protocol (SCI DMP). J Spinal Cord Med 2016;39(1):3–12.
28. Martinez RN, Hogan TP, Balbale S, et al. Sociotechnical perspective on implementing clinical video telehealth for veterans with spinal cord injuries and disorders. Telemed J E Health 2017;23(7):567–76.
29. Lai B, Rimmer J, Barstow B, et al. Teleexercise for persons with spinal cord injury: a mixed-methods feasibility case series. JMIR Rehabil Assist Technol 2016;3(2):e8.
30. Mohr DC, Cuijpers P, Lehman K. Supportive accountability: a model for providing human support to enhance adherence to eHealth interventions. J Med Internet Res 2011;13(1):e30.
31. Van Straaten MG, Cloud BA, Morrow MM, et al. Effectiveness of home exercise on pain, function, and strength of manual wheelchair users with spinal cord injury: a

high-dose shoulder program with telerehabilitation. Arch Phys Med Rehabil 2014; 95(10):1810–7.e2.

32. Shem K, Sechrist SJ, Loomis E, et al. SCiPad: effective implementation of tele-medicine using iPads with individuals with spinal cord injuries, a case series. Front Med (Lausanne) 2017;4:58.

33. Veerbeek JM, Van Wegen E, Van Peppen R, et al. What is the evidence for phys-ical therapy poststroke? A systematic review and meta-analysis. PLoS One 2014; 9(2):e87987.

34. Phillips VL, Vesmarovich S, Hauber R, et al. Telehealth: reaching out to newly injured spinal cord patients. Public Health Rep 2001;116(Suppl 1):94–102.

35. Remy C, Valet M, Stoquart G. Telecommunication and rehabilitation among pa-tients with multiple sclerosis: access and willingness to use. Ann Phys Rehabil Med 2018;61:e99.

36. Charvet LE, Yang J, Shaw MT, et al. Cognitive function in multiple sclerosis im-proves with telerehabilitation: results from a randomized controlled trial. PLoS One 2017;12(5):e0177177.

37. Khan F, Amatya B, Kesselring J, et al. Telerehabilitation for persons with multiple sclerosis. Cochrane Database Syst Rev 2015;(4):CD010508.

38. Conroy SS, Zhan M, Culpepper WJ, et al. Self directed exercise in multiple scle-rosis: Evaluation of a home automated tele-management system. J Telemed Tele-care 2018;24(6):410–9.

39. Rimmer J, Thirumalai M, Young H, et al. Rationale and design of the tele-exercise and multiple sclerosis (TEAMS) study: a comparative effectiveness trial between a clinic- and home-based telerehabilitation intervention for adults with multiple sclerosis (MS) living in the deep south. Contemp Clin Trials Commun 2018;71: 186–93.

40. Ricker JH, Rosenthal M, Garay E, et al. Telerehabilitation needs: a survey of per-sons with acquired brain injury. J Head Trauma Rehabil 2002;17(3):242–50.

41. Kreutzer JS, Rapport LJ, Marwitz JH, et al. Caregivers' well-being after traumatic brain injury: a multicenter prospective investigation. Arch Phys Med Rehabil 2009;90(6):939–46.

42. Rietdijk R, Togher L, Power E. Supporting family members of people with trau-matic brain injury using telehealth: A systematic review. Journal of Rehabilitation Medicine 2012;44:913–21.

43. Brouwers RWM, Kraal JJ, Traa SCJ, et al. Effects of cardiac telerehabilitation in patients with coronary artery disease using a personalised patient-centred web application: protocol for the SmartCare-CAD randomised controlled trial. BMC Cardiovasc Disord 2017;17(1):46.

44. Hwang R, Bruning J, Morris NR, et al. Home-based telerehabilitation is not inferior to a centre-based program in patients with chronic heart failure: a randomised trial. J Physiother 2017;63(2):101–7.

45. Piotrowicz E, Baranowski R, Bilinska M, et al. A new model of home-based tele-monitored cardiac rehabilitation in patients with heart failure: effectiveness, qual-ity of life, and adherence. Eur J Heart Fail 2010;12(2):164–71.

46. Piotrowicz E, Zieliłski T, Bodalski R, et al. Home-based telemonitored Nordic walking training is well accepted, safe, effective and has high adherence among heart failure patients, including those with cardiovascular implantable electronic devices: a randomised controlled study. Eur J Prev Cardiol 2015;22(11):1368–77.

47. Nouryan C, Morahan S, Pecinka K, et al. Home telemonitoring of community-dwelling heart failure patients after home care discharge. Telemed J E Health 2018. [Epub ahead of print].

48. Fingar KR, Stocks C, Weiss AJ, et al. Most frequent operating room procedures performed in U.S. Hospitals, 2003–2012. HCUP statistical brief #186. Rockville (MD): Agency for Healthcare Research and Quality; 2014.

49. Kairy D, Lehoux P, Vincent C, et al. A systematic review of clinical outcomes, clinical process, healthcare utilization and costs associated with telerehabilitation. Disabil Rehabil 2009;31(6):427–47.

50. Moffet H, Tousignant M, Nadeau S, et al. Patient satisfaction with in-home telerehabilitation after total knee arthroplasty: results from a randomized controlled trial. Telemed J E Health 2017;23(2):80–7.

51. Pastora-Bernal JM, Martín-Valero R, Barón-López FJ, et al. Evidence of benefit of telerehabilitation after orthopedic surgery: a systematic review. J Med Internet Res 2017;19(4):e142.

52. Cottrell MA, Galea OA, O'Leary SP, et al. Real-time telerehabilitation for the treatment of musculoskeletal conditions is effective and comparable to standard practice: a systematic review and meta-analysis. Clin Rehabil 2017;31(5):625–38.

53. Doiron-Cadrin P, Kairy D, Vendittoli PA, et al. Effects of a tele-prehabilitation program or an in-person prehabilitation program in surgical candidates awaiting total hip or knee arthroplasty: protocol of a pilot single blind randomized controlled trial. Contemp Clin Trials Commun 2016;4:192–8.

54. Cumming RG, Thomas M, Szonyi G, et al. Home visits by an occupational therapist for assessment and modification of environmental hazards: a randomized trial of falls prevention. J Am Geriatr Soc 1999;47(12):1397–402.

55. World Federation of Occupational Therapists. World Federation of Occupational Therapists' position statement on telehealth. Int J Telerehabil 2014;6(1):37–9.

56. Van Tulder M, Malmivaara A, Esmail R, et al. Exercise therapy for low back pain: a systematic review within the framework of the Cochrane collaboration back review group. Spine (Phila Pa 1976) 2000;25(21):2784–96.

57. Peterson S. Telerehabilitation booster sessions and remote patient monitoring in the management of chronic low back pain: a case series. Physiother Theory Pract 2018;34(5):393–402.

58. Cranen K, Groothuis-Oudshoorn CGM, Vollenbroek-Hutten MMR, et al. Toward patient-centered telerehabilitation design: understanding chronic pain patients' preferences for web-based exercise telerehabilitation using a discrete choice experiment. J Med Internet Res 2017;19(1):e26.

59. Adamse C, Dekker-Van Weering MG, van Etten-Jamaludin FS, et al. The effectiveness of exercise-based telemedicine on pain, physical activity and quality of life in the treatment of chronic pain: a systematic review. J Telemed Telecare 2018; 24(8):511–26.

60. Herbert MS, Afari N, Liu L, et al. Telehealth versus in-person acceptance and commitment therapy for chronic pain: a randomized noninferiority trial. J Pain 2017;18(2):200–11.

61. Bennell KL, Nelligan R, Dobson F, et al. Effectiveness of an Internet-delivered exercise and pain-coping skills training intervention for persons with chronic knee pain: a randomized trial. Ann Intern Med 2017;166(7):453–62.

62. Piga M, Cangemi I, Mathieu A, et al. Telemedicine for patients with rheumatic diseases: systematic review and proposal for research agenda. Semin Arthritis Rheum 2017. https://doi.org/10.1016/j.semarthrit.2017.03.014.

63. Pani D, Piga M, Barabino G, et al. Home tele-rehabilitation for rheumatic patients: impact and satisfaction of care analysis. J Telemed Telecare 2017; 23(2):292–300.

Safety of Surgical Telehealth in the Outpatient and Inpatient Setting

Shawn Purnell, MD, MS, Feibi Zheng, MD, MBA*

KEYWORDS

• Telehealth • Telemedicine • mHealth • Surgical safety

KEY POINTS

• Telemedicine replacement for routine in-person postoperative care appears to be safe for carefully selected low-risk patients undergoing low-risk procedures.
• High-quality trials studying telehealth interventions to improve patient safety and patient outcomes are ongoing in all surgical subspecialties.
• Telehealth interventions must be designed in an iterative fashion with consideration for local resources, processes, and end-user patient preferences and needs.

INTRODUCTION

The COVID-19 pandemic has accelerated the adoption of telehealth in all phases of surgical care (**Table 1**). Both CMS and commercial payers have loosened guidelines for billing and reimbursement in both the inpatient and the outpatient settings. Medicare has waived originating site requirements, which previously required reimbursed care to be provided to patients in health care shortage or rural areas and for the visits to be conducted with the patient physically present at a remote health care facility. Before the COVID-19 crisis, telemedicine could not be provided across state lines unless the surgeon had a license to practice in the neighboring state. Since April 2020, state licensing requirements have been loosened in order to provide increased flexibility to provide care across state lines. Most states have also implemented telemedicine parity laws, which allow for synchronous video visits to be reimbursed at the same rate as in-person visits for both established and new patient visits. These rapid developments necessitate an examination of the safety of telehealth platforms and interventions that are proliferating globally.

This article originally appeared in Surgical Clinics, Volume 101, Issue 1, February 2021.
Department of Surgery, Houston Methodist Hospital, 6550 Fannin Street, Smith 16, Houston, TX 77030, USA
* Corresponding author.
E-mail address: fzheng@houstonmethodist.org

| Table 1 | |
Key definitions	
Telehealth	Digital health care activities, platforms, services
Telemedicine	Remote diagnosis and treatment of patients by means of telecommunication technology
mHealth	Use of smartphones and tablets for telehealth
Remote patient monitoring	The use of wearable devices, mobile devices, applications for physiologic data transmission, analysis, and monitoring
Tele-ICU	A platform that uses remote patient monitoring technology to augment care of intensive care unit patients

Data from NEJM Catalyst. What is Telehealth? *Massachusetts Medical Society.* 2018. Available at: https://catalyst.nejm.org/doi/full/10.1056/CAT.18.0268.

EVALUATION OF TELEHEALTH FOR PATIENT SAFETY

There is no widely accepted framework for the evaluation of telehealth interventions or platforms. However, most frameworks examine the following outcomes: patient access and acceptability, surgeon and staff satisfaction, efficacy of intervention, safety of intervention, patient-reported outcomes and use of institutional resources to deploy intervention, and cost-effectiveness. Additional domains related to the development of the intervention include stakeholder input, interoperability with existing electronic medical record (EMR) software, and data security and governance.[1]

TELEHEALTH IN THE OUTPATIENT SETTING

Telehealth modalities in the outpatient setting, which have been previously studied, include substitution of in-person visits for routine postoperative care, patient education, medication adherence, and home-based virtual ward recovery programs. Many of these programs have been evaluated for feasibility and safety in carefully selected populations. The authors examine several of these programs across different surgical subspecialties in later discussion.

The Veterans Administration was an early adopter of telemedicine technologies. It was one of the first hospital systems to evaluate the safety of telemedicine for routine postoperative care for low-risk procedures.[2] Eisenberg and colleagues[3] examined 62 patients undergoing laparoscopic inguinal hernia repair. These patients were given a telephone-only postoperative visit. Eighty-nine percent of patients were able to successfully complete the visit; 5% never completed any follow-up visit, and 7% were accidentally scheduled an in-person visit. Of the patients who had a telephone-only postoperative visit, 9% returned for an in-person visit for issues that could not be addressed via the telephone visit. One was found to have an early recurrence, and one was found to have a seroma.

More recently, in a randomized prospective trial, a tertiary care hospital in Spain randomized 200 carefully selected patients to telemedicine follow-up video visits or in-person office follow-up visits. The 3 most commonly performed procedures in this group of patients were laparoscopic cholecystectomy, inguinal hernia repair, and laparoscopic appendectomy. In their primary endpoint of successful completion of the assigned visit type, 90% of the patients in the in-person visit and 74% of patients in the virtual visit arm were able to complete their assigned visit type. There were no differences in the secondary outcomes or need for additional clinic or emergency department (ED) visits or patient satisfaction.[4] In another randomized Canadian trial of 65 women undergoing breast reconstruction, the intervention group was assigned to receive postoperative care via mobile app versus usual standard of care, which consisted of in-person postoperative visits at week 1 and week 4. Through the app, the patients were instructed to submit photographs of the surgical site, respond to an analog visual pain scale, and fill out a quality of recovery survey with daily asynchronous monitoring for the first 2 weeks and then weekly monitoring for the subsequent 2 weeks. The mobile app group reported a decreased need for in-person visits and no difference in rates of postoperative complications, which were surgical site infection and seroma.[5]

In a virtual care home recovery study, 30 patients were randomized after minimally invasive colectomy to standard of care enhanced recovery after surgery (ERAS) protocol or ERAS protocol with preplanned accelerated discharge on postoperative day 1 with home recovery monitoring using a tablet computer with a planned postoperative video televisit on postoperative day 2 and instant messaging with the care team as needed. Most of the patients in the accelerated discharge arm were able to safely recover at home, with 4 patients returning to the ED for abdominal pain, *Clostridium difficile* colitis, anastomotic leak, and port site hernia. None of these complications were attributed to accelerated discharge, and use of the app did not result in a delay in needed care.[6]

Further examples of randomized clinical trials involving telemedicine interventions in various surgical specialties are highlighted in **Table 2**.

PATIENT SAFETY OPPORTUNITIES IN THE OUTPATIENT SETTING

These studies demonstrate that in carefully selected patients, telemedicine interventions to replace and augment routine postoperative care are safe, are feasible, and may improve patient satisfaction when compared with routine in-person postoperative care. The low risk of complications in these studies also calls into question whether routine follow-up with a surgeon is necessary in most low-risk patients undergoing low-risk surgery. Very few studies show the ability of these interventions to enhance clinical outcomes or decrease complications. Lee and colleagues'[10] study was one of the few studies that demonstrated an improvement in 90-day readmissions in a liver transplant population using a tablet computer coupled with vital sign monitoring and on-demand instant messaging, phone calls, and video encounters with the care team (28% vs 58%; $P = .004$). The value of telemedicine interventions in improving patient safety may be better demonstrated in higher-risk surgeries and higher-risk populations where there is greater variance in outcomes.

Many telehealth interventions for the postoperative phase of care were initially focused on substitution of care for follow-up. However, as pressure for value-based payment grows, more recent studies have focused on new telehealth strategies to improve length of stay while maintaining or improving patient safety during the recovery phase and preventing readmissions. Although telehealth interventions have demonstrated potential savings to patients in terms of time and travel costs in the outpatient setting, few studies have examined the return on investment from the institutional or surgeon perspective. The few economic studies of telemedicine in postoperative care have focused on reallocation of provider time or improved clinic access.[17,18]

Another area of potential study is whether telehealth platforms can predict impending complications. In a prospective cohort study, Panda and colleagues[19] captured smartphone accelerometer data from 1 week before surgery to 6 months after surgery in patients with cancer. Accelerometer data were used as a proxy measure of physical

Table 2
Randomized controlled trials in the evaluation of telemedicine applications in the outpatient setting

Surgical Discipline	Procedure Types	Intervention	Outcomes	References
General surgery	Inguinal hernia, laparoscopic cholecystectomy, laparoscopic appendectomy	Video follow-up visit vs in-person visit	Feasibility of completing scheduled visit type. No difference in 30-d complications, 30-d ED visits, or patient satisfaction	Cremades et al,[4] 2020
	Stoma creation	Stoma nurse follow-up by teleconsultation video visit with patient presenting to district medical center vs in-person visit at university hospital	No differences in quality of life as measured by EQ-5D index, number of 30-d hospital appointments or readmissions; communication rated as poorer in the teleconsultation group	Augestad et al,[7] 2020
Surgical oncology	Colectomy	Accelerated discharge after ERAS protocol with computer tablet remote monitoring vs standard ERAS protocol	Lower length of stay in accelerated discharge group without increase in severe adverse events	Bednarski et al,[6] 2019
Plastic surgery	Breast reconstruction	Smartphone app with 1-way pain reporting and incision photograph submission in lieu of in-person visit	No difference in 30-d in-person visits composite (PCP, ED, surgeon), 30-d complications, or patient satisfaction scores	Armstrong et al,[5] 2017
Thoracic surgery	Thoracotomy	Automated telephone calls to the patient for symptom monitoring with e-mail alert to care team for severity triggers vs monitoring without e-mail to clinicians	Reduction in number of reports of severe symptoms	Cleeland et al,[8] 2011
Transplant surgery	Kidney transplant	Smartphone app integrated with wireless blood pressure monitor and medication box	Improved medication adherence and systolic blood pressure measurement at months 1 and 3	McGillicuddy et al,[9] 2013

	Liver transplant	Tablet computer with vital sign transmission, on demand instant messaging and video visit vs standard of care	Lower 90-d readmission rate	Lee et al,[10] 2019
Urology	Prostatectomy	Video visit in lieu of in-person visit	Equivalent visit efficiency, patient satisfaction; decreased patient cost	Viers et al,[11] 2015
Orthopedic surgery	Rotator cuff repair	Video visit in lieu of in-person visit	Detection of surgical site drainage in 3 patients in telehealth group, 4 in control group; 1 patient in telemedicine group with postoperative myocardial infarction; similar pain scores and patient satisfaction	Kane et al,[12] 2020
	Total knee replacement	Smartphone app with daily instruction via push notification vs smartphone app with twice a week instruction (information provided across 2 groups are the same)	Lower pain scores, higher quality of life, activities of daily living, and patient satisfaction in the daily instruction group	Timmers et al,[13] 2019
Vascular	Lower-extremity revascularization via groin incision	Telehealth electronic monitoring system including tablet computer for image capture, weight scale, blood pressure cuff, thermometer, and pulse oximeter reviewed by care manager vs usual standard of care with no remote monitoring	No difference in 30-d readmissions or surgical site infection; increased patient satisfaction in intervention group	Mousa et al,[14] 2019
Gynecology	Pelvic floor surgery	Telephone interviews vs in-person visit for postoperative care	No difference in adverse events, ED visits, or PCP visits	Thompson et al,[15] 2019
Pediatric surgery	Nonoperative and operative hospitalization	Video visit vs in-person follow-up	No missed clinical findings in video visit group; travel time, days off from school/work lower in the telemedicine group	Goedeke et al,[16] 2019

Data from Refs.[4–16]

activity. Twenty-seven percent of patients had at least 1 postoperative event, which included readmission, ED visit, wound complication, reoperation, respiratory complication, sepsis, and death. Before surgery, physical activity levels as measured through accelerometer data were similar between groups with and without postoperative events. However, postoperative accelerometer data demonstrated a decreased level of activity in the group with a postoperative event.

Although telemedicine has been used on a limited basis for preoperative triage, no randomized trials have been performed to date to evaluate the safety of telemedicine consultation in the preoperative setting. Before the COVID-19 pandemic, many US states prohibited the use of telemedicine for initial consultation. Since then, state regulations have rapidly evolved to accommodate new patient visits. Studies carried out over the next 2 years will likely determine which patients and procedures can be safely brought to the operating room without an in-person physical examination at the time of initial consultation.

FUTURE DIRECTIONS IN OUTPATIENT TELEHEALTH

Although 80% of Americans use smartphones or tablets, it is important to recognize that new technologies may exacerbate existing disparities.[20] Initial pilots of new programs may only be designed for English speakers and rely on patients to have access to self-purchased home-monitoring equipment or mHealth devices. This need may disadvantage minority, immigrant, nontechnologically adept, and low-income patients.[5,21] Furthermore, results from such trials may not be generalizable to wider populations and may fail to show safety equivalence or improved outcomes when more broadly implemented.

Design of future telemedicine interventions must take into account patient preferences and limitations. For example, the effect of smartphone applications on medication compliance after transplant surgery has been studied in multiple studies with varying results.[22,23] Some studies report low levels of engagement with the application limiting the effectiveness of potential interventions, whereas others show sustained improvements not only in medication adherence but also in clinical outcomes. In Timmers and colleagues,[13] the same patient volume and content of educational material were given to total knee replacement patients in both arms of the study through a smartphone application with the only difference being the format and frequency of instruction. This study suggests that the timing, volume, and delivery format of the information make a difference in patient-reported outcomes.

TELE-INTENSIVE CARE UNITS

Intensive care units (ICUs) across the country are under substantial strain because of the relative shortage of intensivist physicians and increasing US elderly population requiring complex levels of care.[24] Most ICUs in the United States are unable to be staffed by intensivists, despite evidence from multiple studies that intensivist-staffed ICUs have both lower length of stays and mortalities.[25,26] In addition to the shortage of intensivists, burnout plays a significant role in intensivist productivity and longevity. Guntupalli and Fromm[27] studied emotional exhaustion, depersonalization, and personal accomplishment using the Maslach Burnout Inventory, in which one-third of intensivists scored in the high range. In order to "battle intensivist burnout," research has focused on workload management through tele-ICU implementation and improved workflows rather than merely relying on resilience training.[28]

Tele-ICUs leverage an intensivist's care across multiple ICUs, significantly decreasing workload. A remote intensivist is able to care for distant patients in multiple

ICUs via an audiovisual interface, document findings within an EMR, and administer treatments via computerized physician order entry tools. Initial technology used tele-conferencing video and spacelabs bedside data to provide remote intensivist access to patients.[29] Today, advances in technology continue to expand tele-ICU technologies while driving down costs, making tele-ICU more scalable. In addition, tele-ICU can be categorized into continuous, episodic, and response care models that are tailored to the hospitals' needs.[30] Although technology plays an integral role in tele-ICU, successful implementation is also contingent on patient and staff acceptance, as well as organizational management.

Tele-ICU uses audio-video technology, telemetry, and EMRs to allow a centralized intensivist to care for multiple distant ICUs.[31] Early attempts at tele-ICU were curtailed by a lack of technology and high costs. Rosenfeld and colleagues[29] were one of the first groups to trial tele-ICU on a large scale in 1997, evaluating the feasibility of 24-hour telemedicine coverage in a 10-bed surgical ICU. They performed an observational time series triple cohort study over 16 weeks and found that 24-hour telemedicine coverage decreased length of stay, costs, complications, and mortality. The Rosenfeld and colleagues study served as a proof-of-concept model, confirming that tele-ICU is feasible and improves overall quality of care for the patients.

Lilly and colleagues[32] performed a single-academic center prospective study of 6290 adults across 7 ICUs comparing preintervention traditional ICUs and postintervention tele-ICUs. The postintervention tele-ICUs were associated with increased adherence to best practice guidelines, lower rates of preventable complications, shorter lengths of stay, and decreased mortality. However, a multi-institutional observational pre-post study by Nassar and colleagues[33] in 2012 found no significant decreases in mortality or length of stay. Nassar and colleagues and Lilly and colleagues highlight the complexity of tele-ICU implementation across complex health care systems. Tele-ICU implementation requires reengineering of the ICU to integrate technology, standards of care, and cultural change within individual health care organizations.

Three metaanalyses have been performed on tele-ICU interventions examining mortality and length of stay. In 2011, Young and colleagues[34] identified 13 studies from 35 ICUs revealing a decrease in ICU and hospital mortality, and ICU length of stay. Hospital length of stay was not significantly decreased following tele-ICU intervention. Chen and colleagues[35] revealed similar results in 2018, showing a reduction in ICU mortality, hospital mortality, and ICU length of stay, but no significant reduction in hospital length of stay (confidence interval -1.14 to -0.59 days) following tele-ICU implementation. Wilcox and Adhikari[36] included 11 observational studies showing tele-ICU was associated with lower overall hospital and ICU mortalities, and lower ICU lengths of stay. However, these results must be taken with caution, as nonrandomized trials can overestimate significant results. Hospitals must also be careful to tailor tele-ICUs technology and workflow to their organization, as there is no one-size-fits-all tele-ICU model.

PATIENT SAFETY OPPORTUNITIES IN TELE-INTENSIVE CARE UNITS

The recent advent of tele-ICU has led to the development of a unique set of patient safety advancements and concerns. Outside of mortality and length of stay outcomes, tele-ICU has improved patient safety through adherence to standard of care. Pre-post tele-ICU interventional studies have shown improved adherence for deep vein thrombosis prophylaxis (odds ratio [OR] 15.4), stress ulcer prophylaxis (OR 4.57), cardiovascular protection (OR 30.7), and ventilator-associated pneumonia (OR 2.2).[32] The overall tele-ICU decrease in patient mortality and length may be attributed to both the adherence to standard of care best practices and the tele-ICU technologies.

In addition, tele-ICU can improve patient care through the use of team-based systems. Patient monitoring technology has significantly increased ICU staff alerts with a single 10-bed ICU study showing as many as 100,000 alarms per year. Tele-ICU systems can include centralized command centers staffed with nurses and physicians who are able to better monitor and readily respond to critical patient alerts. Traditional ICUs respond to a threshold 90% of critical alarms within 3 minutes 45% of the time, compared with tele-ICUs that respond to 71% (P<.001).[37] Importantly, studies show that ICUs with response times less than 3 minutes have shorter lengths of stay for ICU patients.[38] Comparing traditional ICU care with supplemental tele-ICU, studies show a noninferiority or improved patient care in favor of supplemental tele-ICU care.

Tele-ICU medicine moves away from the traditional doctor-patient relationship, and research regarding its effect on patient satisfaction is lacking. Patient and family satisfaction has been shown to be dependent on the understanding that both care teams, on-site and remote, are present to care for the patient.[39] No standardized tools have been developed to properly assess satisfaction in the tele-ICU (**Box 1**).

FUTURE DIRECTIONS IN TELE-INTENSIVE CARE UNITS

Future tele-ICU studies are focused on technology integration, data analysis, and systems implementation. Current tele-ICU technology relies on multiple platforms to integrate patient information regarding radiology, documentation, and order entry.[40] Integration will help standardize best practices and nomenclature across institutions, allowing for improved analysis of tele-ICU effectiveness.

The COVID-19 pandemic has also created an opportunity to study not only patient safety but also health care worker safety in the context of tele-ICU. Tele-ICU may minimize some of the need for physical interaction between the patient and the caregiver, save personal protective equipment, and prevent the spread of nosocomial infection between patients. Tele-ICU can also enable family members to visit with ventilated, isolated patients without exposing the bedside nurse. Furthermore, tele-ICU can be used to reallocate intensivists to areas of greater need during surge events.

Intensivists have the daunting task of analyzing vast amounts of patient information produced by tele-ICU technologies on multiple platforms to help guide patient care. Machine learning (ML) software is being developed to help establish connections between the vast heterogenous information to guide patient care. Current ML software uses classical models that can detect sepsis early, identify light versus deep sedation in mechanically ventilated patients, and predict the risk of hospital-acquired pressure ulcers.[41] Newer ML models use deep neural networks centered on novel algorithms that better integrate large and heterogenous data.[42]

Last, with improvements in technology integration and data analysis must come system implementation strategies. Differences between mortality and length of stay

---

Box 1
General applications of tele-intensive care units

Extension of limited local workforce

Remote consultation/supervision

Family visits in patients under isolation precautions (such as COVID-19)

in Lilly and colleagues[32] and Nassar and colleagues[33] emphasize that tele-ICU success depends on proper implementation. Implementation requires successful change in behavior, acceptance from all staff, and an extensive information support system. Future studies are needed on managerial organization, clearly defined tele-ICU implementation steps, and examination of individual steps that are improving patient care.[42]

SUMMARY

Pilot studies and small clinical trials have demonstrated the feasibility and safety of telehealth interventions in both the inpatient and the outpatient setting. The next iteration of outpatient telehealth evaluation should focus on expanding telehealth studies to more diverse populations, evaluating the cost-effectiveness of these interventions, and seeking to demonstrate improved outcomes rather than equivalence. For inpatient telehealth, tele-ICU shows promise to improve adherence to best practices and enables better outcomes by sorting and prioritizing information for intensivists. Future design of telehealth interventions must also address interoperability standards, user preferences and needs, and data privacy and ownership issues.

CLINICS CARE POINTS

- Telemedicine visits may be safe in lieu of in-person visits for low-risk surgeries in low-risk patients and is well accepted by patients.
- Tele-ICUs may improve efficiency of allocation of scarce intensivist resources and shows promise to improve adherence to evidence-based practices.
- Design of telehealth platforms in the inpatient and outpatient setting must take into account institutional resources and culture, staff acceptance and training, user interface, and adult learning principles.

DISCLOSURE

The authors have nothing to disclose.

REFERENCES

1. Hebert M. Telehealth success: evaluation framework development. Stud Health Technol Inform 2001;84(Pt 2):1145–9.
2. Hwa K, Wren SM. Telehealth follow-up in lieu of postoperative clinic visit for ambulatory surgery: results of a pilot program. JAMA Surg 2013;148(9):823–7.
3. Eisenberg D, Hwa K, Wren SM. Telephone follow-up by a midlevel provider after laparoscopic inguinal hernia repair instead of face-to-face clinic visit. JSLS 2015; 19(1). e2014.00205.
4. Cremades M, Ferret G, Pares D, et al. Telemedicine to follow patients in a general surgery department. A randomized controlled trial. Am J Surg 2020;219(6): 882–7.
5. Armstrong KA, Coyte PC, Brown M, et al. Effect of home monitoring via mobile app on the number of in-person visits following ambulatory surgery: a randomized clinical trial. JAMA Surg 2017;152(7):622–7.
6. Bednarski BK, Nickerson TP, You YN, et al. Randomized clinical trial of accelerated enhanced recovery after minimally invasive colorectal cancer surgery (RecoverMI trial). Br J Surg 2019;106(10):1311–8.
7. Augestad KM, Sneve AM, Lindsetmo RO. Telemedicine in postoperative follow-up of STOMa PAtients: a randomized clinical trial (the STOMPA trial). Br J Surg 2020;107(5):509–18.

8. Cleeland CS, Wang XS, Shi Q, et al. Automated symptom alerts reduce postoperative symptom severity after cancer surgery: a randomized controlled clinical trial. J Clin Oncol 2011;29(8):994–1000.

9. McGillicuddy JW, Gregoski MJ, Weiland AK, et al. Mobile health medication adherence and blood pressure control in renal transplant recipients: a proof-of-concept randomized controlled trial. JMIR Res Protoc 2013;2(2):e32.

10. Lee TC, Kaiser TE, Alloway R, et al. Telemedicine based remote home monitoring after liver transplantation: results of a randomized prospective trial. Ann Surg 2019;270(3):564–72.

11. Viers BR, Lightner DJ, Rivera ME, et al. Efficiency, satisfaction, and costs for remote video visits following radical prostatectomy: a randomized controlled trial. Eur Urol 2015;68(4):729–35.

12. Kane LT, Thakar O, Jamgochian G, et al. The role of telehealth as a platform for postoperative visits following rotator cuff repair: a prospective, randomized controlled trial. J Shoulder Elbow Surg 2020;29(4):775–83.

13. Timmers T, Janssen L, van der Weegen W, et al. The effect of an app for day-to-day postoperative care education on patients with total knee replacement: randomized controlled trial. JMIR MHealth UHealth 2019;7(10):e15323.

14. Mousa AY, Broce M, Monnett S, et al. Results of telehealth electronic monitoring for post discharge complications and surgical site infections following arterial revascularization with groin incision. Ann Vasc Surg 2019;57:160–9.

15. Thompson JC, Cichowski SB, Rogers RG, et al. Outpatient visits versus telephone interviews for postoperative care: a randomized controlled trial. Int Urogynecol J 2019;30(10):1639–46.

16. Goedeke J, Ertl A, Zoller D, et al. Telemedicine for pediatric surgical outpatient follow-up: a prospective, randomized single-center trial. J Pediatr Surg 2019; 54(1):200–7.

17. Zheng F, Park KW, Thi WJ, et al. Financial implications of telemedicine visits in an academic endocrine surgery program. Surgery 2019;165(3):617–21.

18. Nikolian VC, Williams AM, Jacobs BN, et al. Pilot study to evaluate the safety, feasibility, and financial implications of a postoperative telemedicine program. Ann Surg 2018;268(4):700–7.

19. Panda N, Solsky I, Huang EJ, et al. Using smartphones to capture novel recovery metrics after cancer surgery. JAMA Surg 2019;155(2):123–9.

20. Smartphones in the U.S. - Statistics & Facts. Available at: https://nam03.safelinks. protection.outlook.com/.

21. Gunter RL, Chouinard S, Fernandes-Taylor S, et al. Current use of telemedicine for post-discharge surgical care: a systematic review. J Am Coll Surg 2016; 222(5):915–27.

22. Gomis-Pastor M, Roig E, Mirabet S, et al. A mobile app (mHeart) to detect medication nonadherence in the heart transplant population: validation study. JMIR MHealth UHealth 2020;8(2):e15957.

23. Han A, Min SI, Ahn S, et al. Mobile medication manager application to improve adherence with immunosuppressive therapy in renal transplant recipients: a randomized controlled trial. PLoS One 2019;14(11):e0224595.

24. Lois M. The shortage of critical care physicians: is there a solution? J Crit Care 2014;29(6):1121–2.

25. Angus DC, Kelley MA, Schmitz RJ, et al, Committee on manpower for pulmonary and critical care societies (COMPACCS). Caring for the critically ill patient. Current and projected workforce requirements for care of the critically ill and patients

with pulmonary disease: can we meet the requirements of an aging population? JAMA 2000;284(21):2762–70.

26. Pronovost PJ, Angus DC, Dorman T, et al. Physician staffing patterns and clinical outcomes in critically ill patients: a systematic review. JAMA 2002;288(17): 2151–62.

27. Guntupalli KK, Fromm RE. Burnout in the internist–intensivist. Intensive Care Med 1996;22(7):625–30.

28. Lilly CM, Cucchi E, Marshall N, et al. Battling intensivist burnout: a role for workload management. Chest 2019;156(5):1001–7.

29. Rosenfeld BA, Dorman T, Breslow MJ, et al. Intensive care unit telemedicine: alternate paradigm for providing continuous intensivist care. Crit Care Med 2000;28(12):3925–31.

30. Herasevich V, Subramanian S. Tele-ICU technologies. Crit Care Clin 2019;35(3): 427–38.

31. Kumar G, Falk DM, Bonello RS, et al. The costs of critical care telemedicine programs: a systematic review and analysis. Chest 2013;143(1):19–29.

32. Lilly CM, Cody S, Zhao H, et al. Hospital mortality, length of stay, and preventable complications among critically ill patients before and after tele-ICU reengineering of critical care processes. JAMA 2011;305(21):2175–83.

33. Nassar BS, Vaughan-Sarrazin MS, Jiang L, et al. Impact of an intensive care unit telemedicine program on patient outcomes in an integrated health care system. JAMA Intern Med 2014;174(7):1160–7.

34. Young LB, Chan PS, Lu X, et al. Impact of telemedicine intensive care unit coverage on patient outcomes: a systematic review and meta-analysis. Arch Intern Med 2011;171(6):498–506.

35. Chen J, Sun D, Yang W, et al. Clinical and economic outcomes of telemedicine programs in the intensive care unit: a systematic review and meta-analysis. J Intensive Care Med 2018;33(7):383–93.

36. Wilcox ME, Adhikari NKJ. The effect of telemedicine in critically ill patients: systematic review and meta-analysis. Crit Care 2012;16(4):R127.

37. Lilly CM, Fisher KA, Ries M, et al. A national ICU telemedicine survey: validation and results. Chest 2012;142(1):40–7.

38. Fuhrman SA, Lilly CM. ICU telemedicine solutions. Clin Chest Med 2015;36(3): 401–7.

39. Golembeski S, Willmitch B, Kim SS. Perceptions of the care experience in critical care units enhanced by a tele-ICU. AACN Adv Crit Care 2012;23(3):323–9.

40. Sapirstein A, Lone N, Latif A, et al. Tele ICU: paradox or panacea? Best Pract Res Clin Anaesthesiol 2009;23(1):115–26.

41. Kindle RD, Badawi O, Celi LA, et al. Intensive care unit telemedicine in the era of big data, artificial intelligence, and computer clinical decision support systems. Crit Care Clin 2019;35(3):483–95.

42. Lilly CM, Zubrow MT, Kempner KM, et al. Critical care telemedicine: evolution and state of the art. Crit Care Med 2014;42(11):2429–36.